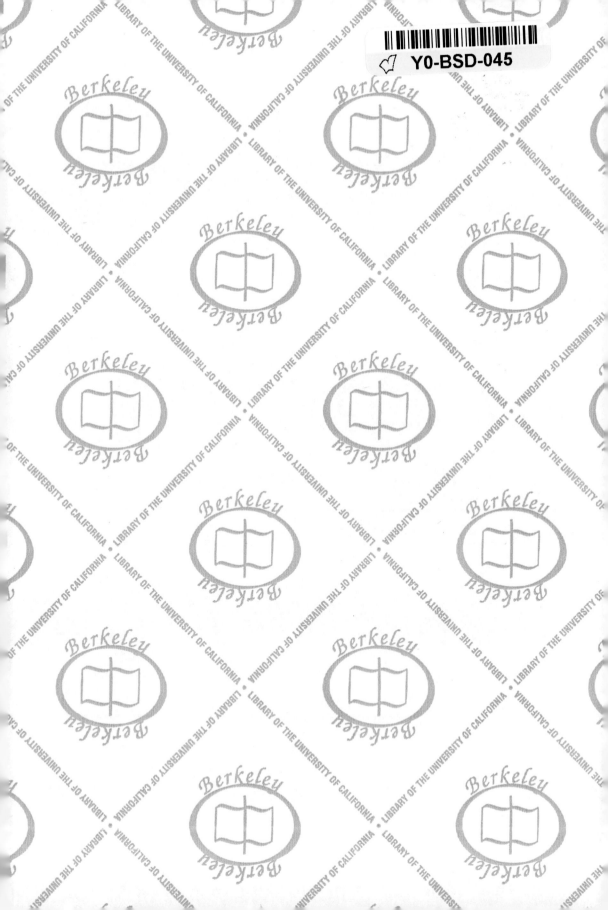

Ecology of Pathogenic Bacteria

Royal Netherlands Academy of Arts and Sciences
P.O. Box 19121, 1000 GC Amsterdam, the Netherlands

Proceedings of the colloquium
'Ecology of Pathogenic Bacteria;
Molecular and Evolutionary Aspects'
Amsterdam, 1–3 February 1995

ISBN 0-444-85802-4

Koninklijke Nederlandse Akademie van Wetenschappen
Verhandelingen, Afd. Natuurkunde, Tweede Reeks, deel 96

Ecology of Pathogenic Bacteria

Molecular and Evolutionary Aspects

Edited by B.A.M. van der Zeijst, W.P.M. Hoekstra, J.D.A. van Embden and
A.J.W. van Alphen

North-Holland, Amsterdam/Oxford/New York/Tokyo, 1997

Index

Introduction

Bacteria have been present on earth for some 3.4 billion years, but the study of the evolution of bacteria is only decades old. Not that microbiologists lacked fascination for the evolution and phylogeny of bacteria. They shared the widely present human urge to classify living creatures. Early classification of plants and animals was based on comparative anatomy. Later on classification became phylogenetic, i.e. followed the lineages of the evolution. Bacteriologists have tried to apply the principles used in zoology to develop a phylogenetic system for bacteria. This was a failure (Van Niel, 1955) since the morphologic variation of bacteria is very limited: a sphere, a rod or a spiral. The only other criterion is the cell wall: either gram-negative or gram-positive.

A solution was indicated in 1965 by Zuckerkandl and Pauling in their paper 'Molecules as documents of evolutionary history' in which they argued that nucleic acid would be the master molecule, providing the basis for a molecular phylogeny. At that time it was still impossible to determine DNA and RNA sequences. When RNA sequencing became operational, Woese argued that the 16S ribosomal RNA (rRNA) subunit is well suited to measure phylogenetic relationships among bacteria. The pioneering work of Woese and coworkers demonstrated that 16S rRNA sequences are a proper basis for the phylogeny and evolution in bacteria (Woese *et al.*, 1983, Woese *et al.*, 1990). Indeed 16S rRNA sequences of bacteria have now become the basis of a phylogenetic classification system. Results presented in two chapters of this volume demonstrate that fluorescent probes to 16S rRNA can be used to enumerate the various phylogenetic groups of intestinal bacteria *in situ*.

Bacterial evolution and genetic exchange

To discriminate between closely related species, and certainly to follow subtle changes in the genome within a species, the sequence of other genes than those encoding rRNA have to be analyzed and compared. The first section of this volume focusses on the molecular mechanisms promoting and limiting the generation of genetic variation and gives a number of important, well-researched, examples of the effects of genomic changes in pathogenic bacteria.

The emphasis on pathogenic bacteria in this book, and the meeting on which it is based, is deliberate in view of the many selective pressures to which these bacteria are exposed. These pressures shorten the time frame of evolution; often widespread changes are detected in bacteria isolated from the population within a few years after selection. In the analysis of the evolution of pathogenic bacteria one has to realize that, in the long era before these bacteria became pathogenic, they followed the 'normal' course of evolution. After that period, starting at the beginning of plant and animal life, a superimposed, more recent evolution took place. Selective factors that directed this evolution have been adaptation to symbiosis with the host and the immune selection of the host. Only very recently in this time scale more profound selective pressures, originating from human activities/civilization, came in force. Relevant factors are crowding of man and his domestic animals, changes in the environment, the use of antibiotics, vaccination. Some bacteria probably only became pathogenic after close contact with man (e.g. Vibrio).

Population genetics and clonal spread

Crowding would favor bacteria with virulence factors contributing to spread by diarrhea and coughing. Vaccination or natural immunity select for antigenic variants. Antibiotic resistance has been the sad consequence of improper use of these drugs. This volume gives several examples of genetic changes fitting in the above scenario. Gene transfer between bacteria appears to play an important role in acquiring and changing virulence factors and in the development of penicillin-resistant bacteria.

Throughout the years this ongoing evolution resulted in some bacterial clones that became so well-adapted to their hosts that they had an advantage over other clones of the same species. When such an adaptation coincides with pathogenicity it results in a rapid epidemic expansion of the clone followed by only a few additional mutations. Later on the population becomes heterogeneous (panmictic) again by horizontal gene exchange between bacteria. Some pathogens are not clonal. The third section of this book illuminates and explains the situation in this field.

Host-parasite interactions

Another major insight that is discussed is the interplay between pathogenic bacteria and their host cells. The middle part of this volume is devoted to this topic. One example is the very stable interaction between some insects and bacteria. Other reports focus on the dynamic interaction between bacteria and host cells. It is now clear that bacteria are continually monitoring their environment and answer the signals they receive by increasing or decreasing the transcription of genes. The activity of some genes is needed for survival and multiplication in the host. Five chapters demonstrate the powerful methods available to study host-parasite interactions. One approach for the systematic identification of host-regulated bacterial genes is promoter-cloning followed by selection of differentially regulated promoters. Another is to use transposon mutagenesis. A very powerful modification of the latter method was reported at the meeting (Hensel et al., 1995).

Future developments

Looking back over the unexpected scientific developments in the field of bacterial evolution during the last 10 years makes one cautious to predict too far ahead. But certain developments are already visible. First, new and reemerging infectious diseases will require attention. New outbreaks can lead to a better understanding of the evolution of virulence and the effects of human activity on this evolution. A new journal 'Emerging Infectious Diseases' focusses on these topics.

Second, it is now clear that the complete genomic DNA sequence of the most important pathogenic bacteria and a number of apathogenic bacteria will be available within 10 years. This will have an enormous impact on both the understanding of host-parasite interactions and the evolution of bacteria. Regions present in pathogenic bacteria which are absent in their apathogenic counterparts will be identified. Also the role and spread of 'pathogenicity islands', discrete segments of DNA that encode virulence traits (Hacker et al., 1990), can be evaluated.

Bacterial evolution went on for more than 10^9 years before man arrived on the scene, and, about 10^4 years ago, started to affect the course of this evolution. The challenge will be to use our understanding of bacterial evolution and ecology in controlling infectious diseases.

References

Hacker, J., L. Bender, M. Ott, J. Wingender, B. Lund, R. Marre and W. Goebel, 1990 - Deletions of chromosomal regions coding for fimbriae and hemolysins occur *in vitro* and *in vivo* in various extraintestinal *Escherichia coli* isolates, *Microb. Pathogen.* **8**, 213–225.

Hensel, M., J.E. Shea, C. Gleeson, M.D. Jones, E. Dalton and D.W. Holden, 1995 - Simultaneous identification of bacterial virulence genes by negative selection, *Science* **269**, 400–403.

Van Niel, C.B., 1955 - Classification and taxonomy of the bacteria and bluegreen algae, in: *A century of progress in the natural sciences 1853–1953*, California Acadamy of Sciences, San Francisco, 89–114.

Woese, C.R., R. Gutell, R. Gupta and H.F. Noller, 1983 - Detailed analysis of the higher-order structure of 16S-like ribosomal ribonucleic acids, *Microbiol. Rev.* **47**, 621–669.

Woese, C.R., O. Kandler and M.L. Wheelis, 1990 - Towards a natural system of organisms: proposal for the domains Archaea, Bacteria & Eucarya, *Proc. Nat. Acad. Sci. USA* **87**, 4576–4579.

Zuckerkandl, E. and L. Pauling, 1965 - Molecules as documents of evolutionary history, *J. Theor. Biol.* **8**, 357–366.

Bacterial evolution and genetic exchange

Werner Arber

Genetic Bases for Evolutionary Development of Microorganisms [1]

Abstract

A synoptic view is given here to molecular mechanisms promoting and limiting the generation of genetic variation. These mechanisms include (a) the production of conventional spontaneous mutations resulting from DNA replication infidelity and from the action of environmental mutagens, (b) enzymatically mediated repair processes acting on DNA mismatches caused by those processes of mutagenesis listed under (a), (c) various types of DNA rearrangements such as transposition and site-specific recombination at secondary crossing over sites, (d) DNA acquisition upon transformation, conjugation and phage-mediated transduction, and (e) processes modulating the efficiency of DNA acquisition such as effects of restriction-modification systems. Many of these processes are mediated by specific gene products and these often act as generators of genetic variations, hence in a not strictly reproducible way with regard to their site of action on DNA. It is proposed that at least part of the enzymes and organelles involved in these processes function primarily for the evolutionary development of microorganisms and had also been selected for this property.

Introduction

Biological evolution ensures a steady development, long-term maintenance and diversification of life on earth. In this contribution I discuss evidence for the view that the evolutionary process does not only rely on illegitimate chance events, but is importantly influenced by genetically determined biological functions with evolutionary implications. A number of arguments taken from microbial genetics will give support to the following *thesis*:

Specific genes carried in the genome (and on accessory genetic elements) encode products that fulfil evolutionary functions
1. by generating genetic variation or
2. by limiting genetic plasticity to tolerable, but evolutionarily useful levels.
In spite of this genetic determination, biological evolution is not directed.

[1] This is a modified and extended version of a contribution to the UNESCO-COGENE Symposium 'Uniqueness and Universality in a Biological World' to be published in 'Biology International' by the International Union of Biological Sciences' (IUBS)

Prokaryotes as objects of studies on mechanisms of biological evolution

Evolutionary processes are known to rely on mutation, selection and isolation. They can ideally be studied with haploid microorganisms which rapidly manifest phenotypic alterations due to mutation events. Bacteria and their viruses have extremely short generation times and are ideally suited for population genetic investigations, e.g. for studies on competition between mixtures of parental and mutant types submitted to various selection pressures. In addition, molecular genetic approaches can reveal the molecular nature of individual mutations, such as nucleotide substitution, small deletions and insertions, and larger DNA rearrangements. For simplicity, spontaneous mutation will here be defined as any alteration occurring to DNA sequences without an intended intervention by an investigator. More often such mutations will be detrimental, sometimes even lethal, than beneficial to the organisms. Therefore, tolerable mutation rates should be smaller than one mutation per genome and per generation. However, we should be aware that generation time is difficult to define for resting bacteria in their stationary phase. In cultures of exponentially growing *E. coli* bacteria the rate of mutagenesis is in the order of 10^{-2} new genetic alterations per cell and per generation. This results in a relatively high degree of genetic polymorphism in colonies grown from a single cell. Natural, spontaneous mutagenesis thus seriously limits the size of clones formed by genetically fully identical individuals upon propagation of bacteria. By mutations occurring in phases of rest, members of pure clones undergo further genetic diversification.

Sources of genetic variation

Many mechanistically different processes contribute in parallel to the generation of mutations. For this discussion, we group these processes into four categories (Arber, 1991 and 1993):

a. reproductive infidelity
b. effects of environmental and internal mutagens
c. DNA rearrangements
d. DNA acquisition

The action of these processes on individuals in large populations generates new genetic diversity (Fig. 1). However, overall genetic diversity is kept in balance by natural selection and, after all, the size of the biosphere, which can hold in the order of 10^{30} living cells. In addition, the efficiency of processes of the first two categories, reproductive infidelity and effects of environmental mutagens, is considerably attenuated by the activity of various enzymatic repair processes, while DNA acquisition (category d) encounters a number of natural limits to DNA transfer.

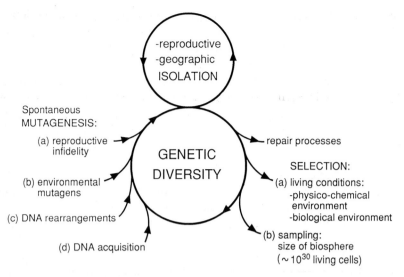

Fig. 1. Genetic diversity is steadily increased by various mutagenesis processes generating genetic variation, while natural selection acting on mixed populations of organisms limits the degree of diversity. Repair processes reduce the probability for some primary alterations on DNA to become fixed as mutations. Geographic and reproductive isolation can modulate genetic diversity. From Arber et al. (1994).

It is generally thought that a major source of nucleotide substitution is the occurrence of short-living tautomeric forms of the nucleotides, that are structural variants of the normal forms presenting different specificity of base pairing. A mispairing which results when an incorporated tautomeric base reassumes its normal form should thus not be qualified as a mistake in the incorporation, it is rather the consequence of a statistically occurring structural variation of a biochemical compound. Many, but not all of such cases of primary infidelity are efficiently repaired before such mutations become fixed.

DNA rearrangements

The following discussion on DNA rearrangements will be limited to bacterial systems. In these haploid organisms, homologous recombination cannot be attributed the same role in the generation of genomic diversity as is done for higher, sexually reproducing organisms with diploid genomes, although bacterial conjugation may sometimes substitute for the lacking recombinational reassociation of alleles from different sets of chromosomes. General recombination can also bring about major alterations in the genome structure and content by unequal crossing over at homologous sequences located at different sites in the genome.

In bacteria, enzymatic systems of site-specific recombination and of transposition are widespread. These and still other processes, often referred to as illegitimate recombination, widely contribute to genomic plasticity. Most of these processes are catalyzed by specific enzymes and thus result from the action of genetic determinants. Some of the DNA rearrangements mediated by these systems have been studied to great mechanistic details and are thus well understood. This is e.g. the case for site-specific DNA inversion (Glasgow et al., 1989) and transposition of IS elements (Galas and Chandler, 1989).

DNA inversion

Site-specific DNA inversion is a source both of gene fusion and operon fusion. In the well-studied genetic flip-flop systems, one of two - or in some cases more - possible, alternative genomic arrangements is periodically assumed. This process can rapidly result in mixed populations of individuals with different phenotypic properties, if different genomic structures influence gene expression differently. Examples are the connection or disconnection of a promoter with an open reading frame (Silverman et al., 1981) or the fusion of a variable part with a constant part of a gene (Giphart-Gassler et al., 1982; Iida, 1984). The sites of crossing over in this enzymatically mediated process are consensus DNA sequences. Deviations from the consensus can still serve in DNA inversion, although with different efficiencies (Iida and Hiestand-Nauer, 1986 and 1987).

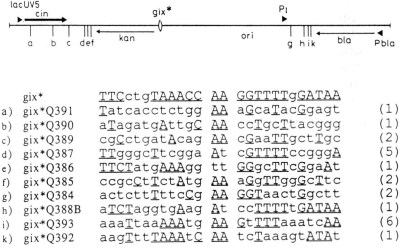

Fig. 2. Nucleotide sequences used as secondary crossing over sites in Cin-mediated site-specific DNA inversion. On plasmid pSHI383 rare DNA inversion between the natural crossing over site *gix** and a secondary crossing over site brought the expression of the kanamycin resistance gene *kan* under the control of either promoter lacUV5 (sites a to f) or promoter PI (sites g and h). The plasmid also underwent unequal cointegration using *gix** and either site i or k and resulting in the fusion of *kan* with the operon under control of promoter P*bla*. Nucleotides corresponding to the *dix* consensus sequence of efficient crossing over sites are shown as underlined capital letters. Numbers in parenthesis refer to the number of independent isolates having used the crossing over site in question. The data were pooled from Iida and Hiestand-Nauer (1987).

Interestingly, the reaction can still take place with very low probability on DNA sequences widely diverting from the consensus (Fig. 2). It is possible that short-term structural variations of the interacting partners, recombinase and its substrate DNA, thereby play a critical role. Many different DNA sequences can thus occasionally serve for DNA inversion. This rare use of secondary crossing over sites is thought to represent an important natural source of novel gene fusions and novel operon fusions with evolutionary relevance (Arber, 1990).

Transposition

Another source of genomic rearrangements is the transpositional activity of mobile genetic elements. A number of different such 'inserted sequence' elements, IS elements, reside each in a number of copies in bacterial genomes. Once in a while they undergo enzymatically mediated DNA rearrangements, which include simple transposition, the formation of an adjacent deletion and DNA inversion, as well as the cointegration of plasmids or of a plasmid with the chromosome.

Interestingly, transposition also occurs in resting bacteria. E.g., bacterial sub-clones kept alive for decades in a stab culture accumulate genetic polymorphism due to transposition, and the resulting diversity increases linearly with the time of storage of the bacteria (Naas et al., 1994 and 1995). The degree of genetic diversity thus obtained largely depends on the target selection criteria of the participating IS elements. Depending on the IS element these criteria show different levels of sequence specificities.

A relatively strong target specificity is e.g. exerted by IS30, although other target sequences than the preferred ones are also used occasionally (Caspers et al., 1984; Stalder and Arber, 1989). The 1221-bp IS30 element is a resident of *E. coli* K12. A constitutively expressed open reading frame covers practically the entire length of the element and encodes the transposase (Dalrymple et al., 1984). This is a bifunctional DNA recombinase and it efficiently mediates site-specific recombination and less efficiently transpositional DNA rearrangements (Olasz et al., 1993). The level of these activities are controlled by a leaky transcription terminator located within the reading frame of the transposase (Dalrymple and Arber, 1986), a constitutively expressed anti-sense RNA complementary to the middle part of the transposase gene (A. Arini, M. Keller and W. Arber, to be published) and possibly by an autorepression exerted by the transposase itself (Stalder et al., 1990).

Evidence has been obtained that IS30 transposition goes through a structural intermediate, (IS30)$_2$ formed by two directly repeated IS30 elements separated by normally a 2-bp spacer (Olasz et al., 1993). This intermediate structure originates from the action of the site-specific recombinase, and its resolution is usually also brought about by site-specific deletion formation, which occurs upon standard growth conditions with a frequency in the order of 10^{-1} per cell and per generation. However, (IS30)$_2$ also gives rise to different kinds of transpositional DNA rearrangements such as intramolecular DNA inversion and deletion formation, as well as intermolecular inverse transposition (Fig. 3). In the presence of efficient target sequences for IS30 transposition, these DNA rearrangements occur with frequencies in the range of 10^{-3} per cell and per generation. For these reasons, IS30, which is in principle remarkably stable, can occasionally give rise to a burst of transposition, once an intermediate form has been produced. In such a burst different subclones with various DNA rearrangements can arise with high frequency, thereby providing a population of bacteria with different genetic variants (Naas et al., 1994).

That a large fraction of lethal mutations is also caused by transposition of IS elements had been demonstrated by a study of bacteriophage P1 mutations affecting the vegetative reproduction of the phage but not its maintenance as prophage in the lysogenic condition (Arber et al., 1981; Sengstag and Arber, 1983). In these studies about 95% of the detected lethal mutations were caused by the insertion of an IS element originating from the bacterial chromosome. A study of the integration sites of these IS elements on the P1 prophage showed that most IS elements did not randomly select their target sites. Rather, some elements such as IS30 highly preferred a particular site as already mentioned,

IS30-mediated DNA rearrangements

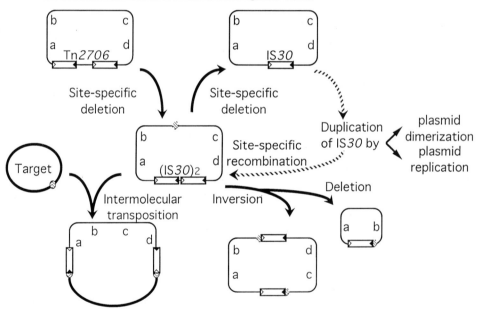

Fig. 3. Pathways of IS30-mediated DNA rearrangements. The recombinogenic (IS30)$_2$ structure shown in the center results from site-specific recombination involving the two IS30 ends. The (IS30)$_2$ structure can resolve by site-specific deletion, but it also gives rise to transpositional DNA rearrangements shown in the lower part of the figure. Drawn after Olasz et al. (1993) and reproduced from Arber et al. (1994).

Genetic bases for evolutionary development of microorganisms while IS2, the element most active under the experimental conditions used, preferred particular regions of the phage genome for its insertion, but within these regions, many different target sequences were used (Fig. 4). This illustrates how some genome regions can more often be affected by spontaneous mutation than others and how recombination processes can occur at a large number of possible crossing over sites, each of which may have its characteristic probability to serve for transposition. We thus count transposable genetic elements to genetically determined variation generators.

Composite transposons are defined as two identical IS elements flanking one or several genes unrelated to the transposition process. Composite transposons can originate when two copies of the same IS element subsequently insert into different sites of a DNA segment (Iida et al., 1981). Although the two participating IS elements can still transpose alone, they sometimes transpose together as a unit with the DNA segment carried between them. This can happen intramolecularly as well as intermolecularly, e.g. to a natural gene vector such as a conjugative plasmid or a phage genome. This then opens the possibility of horizontal transfer not only of the IS element involved, but also of the gene(s) carried between the two IS elements.

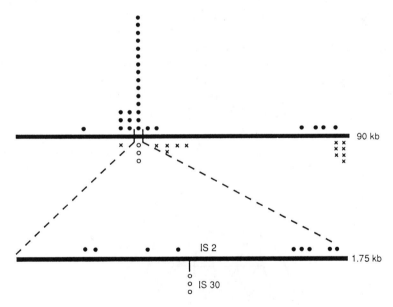

Fig. 4. Location of independent IS insertions into the genome of bacteriophage P1 and resulting in mutants affected in the vegetative reproduction of the phage. The circular 90-kb genome of P1 is shown linearized in the upper part. Dots shown above the genome identify independent IS2 insertions, crosses shown below the genome refer to insertions of IS1, IS3, IS5, Tn1000 and circles to IS30 insertions. As shown in the lower part, each of nine sequenced IS2 insertions into the hot region for IS2 transposition had occurred into a different sequence, while the 3 independent IS30 insertions had occurred between the same base pairs and both orientations had been used. After Sengstag and Arber (1983).

Gene acquisition

The process of horizontal gene transfer has been widely documented, e.g. by the horizontal spreading of genetic determinants for antibiotic resistances. This latter example also nicely illustrates the important role played by selection for genetically altered derivatives in dependence of changes in the environmental conditions.

The acquisition of genetic information from a donor by a receptor strain is at the basis of classical microbial genetics, i.e. (1) transformation of a receptor strain by the uptake of free DNA originating from a donor strain, (2) conjugation, in which donor and receptor bacteria enter in close contact and in which a conjugative plasmid serves as vector for the transfer of donor genes to recipient bacteria, and (3) phage-mediated transduction, in which a viral genome serves as gene vector. In all of these processes gene transfer is followed by the establishment of the acquired genes in the receptor cell. This can be brought about by a recombination process or else by the establishment of the transferred vector together with its passenger DNA as an autonomous replicon.

As was already mentioned, various limitations reduce the efficiency of gene acquisition. These limits include (a) the requirement of surface compatibilities for the DNA uptake in transformation, for interaction between donor and receptor cells in conjugation and for phage infection in transduction, (b) the action of restriction-modification systems on penetrating DNA molecules, (c) the requirements for the already described establishment step, and finally (d) the responses given by the receptor cell to the expression of the acquired functions, which may risk to perturb the functional harmony of the host cell. This latter limitation is less severe for the acquisition of only small portions of genetic information, a condition strongly favored by the action of restriction endonucleases.

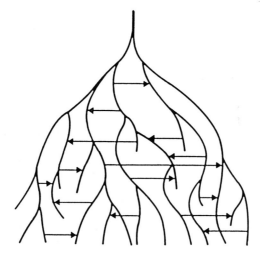

Fig. 5.   The tree of microbial evolution drawn with horizontal connectors to symbolize the occasional occurrence of horizontal gene transfer between different branches of the tree.

These enzymes cleave large DNA molecules into small fragments, the free ends of which are recombinogenic. DNA acquisition thus follows a strategy of acquisition in small steps.

In view of the multitude of processes contributing not only to vertical biological evolution by alterations occurring within the genome of an organism, but also to horizontal biological evolution by the occasional acquisition of small portions of foreign genetic information, the evolutionary tree should schematically be drawn with horizontal connections allowing for a gene flux between different branches (Fig. 5).

Conclusions

It should be emphasised that the mechanistically different processes providing genetic diversity can only partially substitute for each other. Rather, they often fulfil different evolutionary functions. This can be seen in a comparison of the processes of (1) nucleotide substitution resulting from infidelity upon DNA replication, (2) intragenomic DNA rearrangements and (3) DNA acquisition. The first of these processes serves in the strategy to stepwise develop new biological functions and to improve and adjust available biological functions. The second process, DNA rearrangement by any of the described enzyme-mediated recombinations, can lead to an improvement of available capacities, particularly by the fusion of different functional domains and by the fusion of expression control signals with coding sequences thereby leading to different expression controls. Finally, the acquisition of sequence domains and motifs, of functional genes, and of clusters of genes offers the receptor cell a chance to profit of a successful development made by others.

The attribution of primarily evolutionary biological functions to DNA recombination systems acting as generators of genetic variations, to systems providing means for horizontal gene transfer, and also to natural limiters of genetic plasticity, such as mismatch repair systems or restriction-modification systems, is largely a matter of attitude of an investigator towards the object of his investigations, nature and life. Is it reasonable to assume that genetically encoded biological functions serve only to meet the needs of individual lives, by providing housekeeping and accessory functions required during the life span of the organisms? Alternatively, one can consider the process of a steady biological evolution as sufficiently important to justify the presence of genetic determinants specified and mainly responsible for both the past and the future development of a multitude of life forms able to adapt to changing living conditions and to withstand some of the contra-selective forces such as those found under extreme life conditions.

What has been described here for bacteria with a few selected examples might well have a more general validity. Analogous genetic variation generators act also in the development of variations in the immune response of higher animals. I am aware that a very strict subdivision of biological functions into (1) those serving to maintain intact the cellular physiology, (2) those others serving for developmental purposes of multicellular organisms and (3) still others serving for the biological evolution of populations would not correspond to reality. Indeed, some genetically determined products serve for more than one of these purposes. But some specific gene products may very well primarily be used for the needs of biological evolution and they may also have been in the long term selected for this purpose. Since the selection of genetic variation generators is made mostly on variations concerning gene products which are not determined by the evolutionary genes in question, this kind of group selection - or selection between bacterial clones - must be exerted at the population level and must depend on the presence of enough appropriate variants to fulfil the selective needs. This can help to explain why in spite of the genetic determination of the evolutionary process, the direction of evolution remains undetermined and is a matter of interplay between the aleatoric occurrence of particular mutations and the action of natural selection exerted on the sustained mixed populations of organisms.

Affiliation of author

Department of Microbiology
Biozentrum, University of Basel
Klingelbertstr. 70
CH-4056 Basel, Switzerland
phone 061 267 2130
Fax 061 267 2118

References

Arber, W., 1990 - Mechanisms in microbial evolution. *J. Struct. Biol.* **104**, 107–111.

Arber, W., 1991 - Elements in microbial evolution. *J. Mol. Evol.* **33**, 4–12.

Arber, W., 1993 - Evolution of prokaryotic genomes. *Gene* **135**, 49–56.

Arber, W., Hümbelin, M., Caspers, P., Reif, H.J., Iida, S. and Meyer, J., 1981 - Spontaneous mutations in the *Escherichia coli* prophage P1 and IS-mediated processes. *Cold Spring Harbor Symp. Quant. Biol.* **45**, 38–40.

Arber, W., Naas, T. and Blot, M., 1994 - Generation of genetic diversity by DNA rearrangements in resting bacteria. *FEMS Microbiol. Ecol.* **15**, 5–14.

Caspers, P., Dalrymple, B., Iida, S. and Arber, W., 1984 - IS*30*, a new insertion sequence of *Escherichia coli* K12. *Mol. Gen. Genet.* **196**, 68–73.

Dalrymple, B. and Arber, W., 1986 - The characterization of terminators of RNA transcription on IS*30* and an analysis of their role in IS element-mediated polarity. *Gene* **44**, 1–10.

Dalrymple, B., Caspers, P. and Arber, W., 1984 - Nucleotide sequence of the prokaryotic mobile genetic element IS*30*. *EMBO J.* **3**, 2145–2149.

Galas, D.J. and Chandler, M., 1989 - Bacterial insertion sequences. In: Mobile DNA, Berg, D.E. and Howe, M.M. (Eds.), *Am. Soc. Microbiol.*, Washington, DC, pp. 109–162.

Giphart-Gassler, M., Plasterk, R.H.A. and van de Putte, P., 1982 - G inversion in bacteriophage Mu: a novel way of gene splicing. *Nature* **297**, 339–342.

Glasgow, A.C., Hughes, K.T. and Simon, M.I., 1989 - Bacterial DNA inversion systems. In: Mobile DNA, Berg, D.E. and Howe, M.M. (Eds.), *Am. Soc. Microbiol.*, Washington, DC, pp. 637–659.

Iida, S. and Hiestand-Nauer, R., 1986 - Localized conversion at the crossover sequences in the site-specific DNA inversion system of bacteriophage P1. *Cell* **45**, 71–79.

Iida, S. and Hiestand-Nauer, R., 1987 - Role of the central dinucleotide at the crossover sites for the selection of quasi sites in DNA inversion mediated by the site-specific Cin recombinase of phage P1. *Mol. Gen. Genet.* **208**, 464–468.

Iida, S., 1984 - Bacteriophage P1 carries two related sets of genes determining its host range in the invertible C segment of its genome. *Virology* **134**, 421–434.

Iida, S., Meyer, J. and Arber, W., 1981 - Genesis and natural history of IS-mediated transposons. *Cold Spring Harbor Symp. Quant. Biol.* **45**, 27–37.

Naas, T., Blot, M., Fitch, W. and Arber, W., 1995 - Dynamics of IS-related genetic rearrangements in resting *Escherichia coli* K12. *Mol. Biol. Evol.* **12**, 198–207.

Naas, T., Blot, M., Fitch, W.M. and Arber, W., 1994 - Insertion sequence-related genetic variation in resting *Escherichia coli* K-12. *Genetics* **136**, 721–730.

Olasz, F., Stalder, R. and Arber, W., 1993 - Formation of the tandem repeat (IS*30*)$_2$ and its role in IS*30*-mediated transpositional DNA rearrangements. *Mol. Gen. Genet.* **239**, 177–187.

Sengstag, C. and Arber, W., 1983 - IS*2* insertion is a major cause of spontaneous mutagenesis of the bacteriophage P1: non-random distribution of target sites. *EMBO J.* **2**, 67–71.

Silverman, M., Zieg, J., Mandel, G. and Simon, M., 1981 - Analysis of the functional components of the phase variation system. *Cold Spring Harbor Symp. Quant. Biol.* **45**, 17–26.

Stalder, R. and Arber, W., 1989 - Characterization of *in vitro* constructed IS*30*-flanked transposons, *Gene* **76**, 187–193.

Stalder, R., Caspers, P., Olasz, F. and Arber, W., 1990 - The N-terminal domain of the insertion sequence *30* transposase interacts specifically with the terminal inverted repeats of the element. *J. Biol. Chem.* **265**, 3757–3762.

Martin C.J. Maiden, Janet Suker and Ian M. Feavers

Horizontal Genetical Exchange in the Evolution of *Neisseria meningitidis* outer Membrane Proteins

Abstract

Antigenic variability contributes significantly to the ability of many pathogens to evade host immune responses. Understanding the genetical mechanisms underlying the evolution of such variation enhances our ability to design and evaluate novel vaccines rationally. Horizontal genetical exchange has played a major role in the evolution of the porin proteins of *Neisseria meningitidis* and the implications of this have to be considered when novel meningococcal vaccines based on these, or other antigens, are being assessed.

Antigenic variation, evolution, and vaccination

A major selective pressure on microorganisms that live in close association with humans is their need to prevent or evade the lethal effects of their host's immune response. There are a number of possible strategies for achieving this including: hiding from the immune response (e.g. intracellular growth); preventing or interfering with the immune response (immune modulation); and evading the immune response (e.g. antigenic variation, or the production of poorly immunogenic surface components). The adoption of these strategies, particularly antigenic variation, has resulted in an 'arms race' between the immune system of the host and the invading or colonising microbes. This has, in turn, lead to the co-evolution of microbe survival strategies and host immune responses (Brunham *et al.* 1993). Many of the complex interactions that have arisen in this way remain poorly understood and it is possible that some of the 'antigenic variation' observed in pathogenic microorganisms is the result of selective pressures other than immune selection (Virji *et al.* 1993).

Since Jenner's experiments into Smallpox vaccination almost 200 years ago, vaccines have become increasingly important for the prevention and control of infectious disease. Priming the immune system by means of vaccination aims to alter the balance between host and parasite in favour of the vaccinated individual; however; mass vaccination can also alter the selective pressures experienced by the target organism. If the vaccine is effective and administered to sufficient members of the host population, the extinction of the parasite may ensue, the eradication of Smallpox providing a spectacular example (Fenner *et al.* 1988). However, Smallpox remains the sole example of the eradication of a major human pathogen by vaccination, despite a number of international vaccination programs and much research into new vaccines. Of course, it may not always be desirable to eradicate a microbial colonist that rarely causes disease, lest a more aggressive organism should fill the vacated niche. It is therefore desirable to understand the population biology as well as the pathology of disease causing microorganisms.

A further spur to research is the number of disease-causing organisms for which there are no satisfactory vaccines. Antigenic variability is often a major reason for vaccine failure, and also presents difficulties for vaccine design. Bacteria that normally have a commensal relationship with their host, but which can cause disease, present particular problems in vaccine design and assessment. The continual exposure of these bacteria to host immune responses during colonisation has led to the evolution of sophisticated genetical mechanisms for the generation of antigenic variants (Seifert & So, 1988). Populations of such bacteria may contain strains that express diverse surface antigens in almost limitless combinations. This presumably promotes carriage in the host by enabling the bacterium to avoid immune responses induced by its presence. Although progress has been made in defining genetical mechanisms for intra-strain variation for a number of antigens in several microbial species (Robertson & Meyer, 1992), the population genetics of inter-strain variation is less well understood. The increasing demand for novel, defined, vaccines necessitates an understanding of the population genetics of antigenic variation which is essential for rational vaccine design and assessment. It is particularly important in anticipating selective effects of vaccine implementation on the population of the target organism. This article describes the contribution of horizontal genetical exchange to the generation of antigenic diversity of the major outer membrane proteins (OMPs) of *Neisseria meningitidis*.

Vertical and horizontal genetical exchange

In asexual organisms, such as the bacteria which divide by binary fission, cell division normally gives rise to two daughter cells which are clones of their mother cell. In this case genetic information is transferred 'vertically' from single parent to offspring, and the result is a clonal population. The first studies on the population genetics of bacteria identified clonal population structures, characterised by linkage disequilibrium of alleles, and this was considered to be the model for all bacterial populations (Selander & Levin, 1980; Selander *et al.* 1986; Selander *et al.* 1987). However, there is increasing evidence that sexual processes such as transformation, transduction, and conjugation, can play an important part in the evolution of bacterial species (Lorenz & Wackernagel, 1994) and can disrupt such clonal structures (Maynard Smith *et al.* 1993). 'Horizontal genetical exchange' normally involves the movement of relatively small parts of the chromosome between strains and has been referred to as 'localised sex' (Maynard Smith et al. 1991; Maynard Smith, 1995). It requires both a mechanism for DNA transfer and an opportunity for exchange, in other words there must be a sufficient level of association among genetically diverse strains. The balance between horizontal and vertical genetical exchange is different between different species of bacteria and even differs within some species, resulting in different degrees of clonality (Maynard Smith et al. 1993; Spratt et al. 1995)

The most compelling evidence for horizontal genetical exchange is the observation that bacterial genes are mosaics. A mosaic gene is one in which different segments of the gene have different evolutionary histories; such structures become apparent when genes from many natural isolates are compared (DuBose et al. 1988; Coughter & Stewart, 1989; Halter et al. 1989; Milkman & Bridges, 1990; Feavers et al. 1992a; Spratt et al. 1989; Milkman & McKane, 1995). A number of antigen genes from various species have been shown to comprise mosaics, implying involvement of horizontal genetical exchange in their evolution, including: flagella genes in *Salmonella enteritica* (Li et al. 1994); *Streptococcus pneumoniae emm*-like genes (Whatmore & Kehoe, 1994); the capsulation genes of *Haemophilus influenzae* (Kroll & Moxon, 1990); IgA protease and pilin genes of *Neisseria gonorrhoeae* (Halter et al. 1989; Haas et al. 1992); and a number of antigens of *N. meningitidis*, including the porin and *opa* genes (Maiden, 1993; Hobbs et al. 1994).

Neisseria meningitidis and horizontal genetical exchange

N. meningitidis is a major cause of childhood disease world wide and is an example of a normally commensal organism that occasionally causes a life-threatening infection. The *Neisseria* are a group of genetically closely related species only two of which, *N. meningitidis* and *N. gonorrhoeae*, commonly cause disease. The meningococcus normally colonises the nasopharynx asymptomatically and carriage rates in a country such as the UK can be high, in some cases exceeding 10% of the population (Cartwright et al. 1987). A very small proportion of colonisations, usually fewer than 1 per thousand (Peltola, 1983; Schwartz et al. 1989), result in the organism invading the host, crossing the mucus membrane into blood stream. This invasion can develop rapidly into a highly dangerous meningitis and/or septicaemia. If the fulminant stage of the infection is reached prognosis is poor, even with aggressive antibiotic treatment and intensive supportive therapy. Although the serious nature of meningococcal infection has provided much of the impetus for research of this organism, the meningococcus also rewards investigation with the elegance of its mechanisms of antigenic variation and as a model for the interrelationships between epidemiology and population genetics. For example, there are at least four different epidemiologies of meningococcal infection and these are associated with distinct population structures (Maiden & Feavers, 1995).

In common with a number of other bacteria that colonise the upper respiratory tract, *N. meningitidis* has the property of autolysis and is naturally competent for DNA uptake. High carriage rates, autolysis and natural competence combine to provide both the mechanism and opportunity for horizontal genetical exchange mediated by transformation and homologous recombination. Recently, evidence of the major influence of horizontal genetical exchange on the population genetics and epidemiology of the meningococcus has accumulated (Maiden, 1993; Maiden & Feavers, 1995). Nucleotide sequence and other analyses have demonstrated mosaic DNA structures in numerous meningococcal genes including those encoding: 'housekeeping' genes (Zhou & Spratt, 1992); penicillin binding proteins (Spratt *et al.* 1989; Spratt *et al.* 1992); IgA protease (Morelli *et al.* 1994); Opa proteins (Hobbs *et al.* 1994); sulphonamide resistance (Radstrom *et al.* 1992); and outer membrane proteins (OMPs) (Feavers *et al.* 1992a). In addition to evidence inferred by comparison of nucleotide sequence data, there have been a number of *in vitro* demonstrations of horizontal genetical exchange: (i) exchange of putative virulence determinants on co-cultivation of distinct *N. meningitidis* strains (Frosch & Meyer, 1992); (ii) the transfer of *penA* genes, important in penicillin resistance, from *Neisseria flavescens* to *N. meningitidis* (Bowler *et al.* 1994); and (iii) the use of transformation to construct multivalent meningococcal vaccine strains (van der Ley *et al.* 1993).

The outer membrane proteins of the *Neisseria*

In common with other Gram negative organisms the *Neisseria* express porins, pore proteins, in their cell envelope (Nikaido, 1992). These are the most abundant OMPs and constitute a major part of the outer membrane. Most species of *Neisseria* express one porin, the meningococcus being unusual in expressing two simultaneously (Suker *et al.* 1993). On isolation most meningococcal strains express: (i) a class 1 outer membrane protein (OMP), encoded by the gene *porA*; and (ii) either a class 2 or a class 3 OMP, encoded by separate alleles of the *porB* locus (Hitchcock, 1989; Tsai *et al.* 1981). There are many antigenic variants of each of these porin classes (Mocca & Frasch, 1982; Maiden *et al.* 1991; Wolff & Stern, 1991; Feavers *et al.* 1992b; Mee *et al.* 1993).

The antigenically variable porins of both of the pathogenic *Neisseria*, the meningococcus and the gonococcus, have formed the basis of serological typing of isolates for a number of years (Frasch *et al.* 1985). They have also been proposed as vaccine components, particularly against the meningococcus (Saukkonen *et al.* 1989; Bjune *et al.* 1991; Frasch *et al.* 1991; Zollinger & Moran, 1991; van der Ley & Poolman, 1992). These considerations have stimulated work on the antigenic variation of the *Neisseria* porins. The availability of rapid nucleotide sequencing techniques, based on the polymerase chain reaction (PCR), has enabled the determination of the sequences of genes encoding many antigenic variants of these proteins (Barlow *et al.* 1989; McGuinness *et al.* 1990; Maiden *et al.* 1991; McGuinness *et al.* 1991; Feavers *et al.*

1992b; McGuinness *et al.* 1993; Zapata *et al.* 1992; Suker *et al.* 1994). Comparisons of the sequences obtained have demonstrated that all the *Neisseria* porins are related, forming a family (Ward *et al.* 1992; Suker *et al.* 1993). These relationships are illustrated by the phenogram in Fig. 1.

Evidence for horizontal genetical exchange between species can be inferred from these interrelationships, particularly when the meningococcal class 2 and 3 OMPs (Nme P2 and Nme P3 in Fig. 1) and the equivalent porins from *N. gonorrhoeae*, PIA and PIB (Ngo PIA and Ngo PIB in Fig. 1) are considered. The three meningococcal porins are located on different branches and, with the exception of the class 1 OMP which is distantly related to all of the other porins, they are more closely related to porins from other species than they are to each other. This implies that during evolution different species of the *Neisseria* have exchanged porins. The same is true for the gonococcal PIA and PIB porins, each of which is more closely related to porins in other species than they are to each other.

At the nucleotide sequence level, the meningococcal class 2 and 3 OMPs share around 70% nucleotide sequence identity, whereas the class 3 OMP gene is about 80% identical to the PIA protein of the gonococcus. On the other hand,

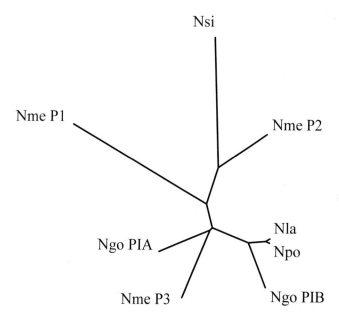

Fig. 1. Relationships among the *Neisseria* Porins. The (unrooted) tree was constructed from aligned amino acid sequences with the programs DRAWTREE and NEIGHBOR using a distance matrix constructed by the program PROTDIST. All these programs were from the PHYLIP (Phylogeny Inference) package written by J. Felsenstein, Department of Genetics, University of Washington, Seattle, WA, USA, down loaded by anonymous FTP from evolution.genetics.washington.edu (directory pub/phylip). The *Neisseria* porins included are: *N. meningitidis* class 1 OMP, NmeP1; *N. meningitidis* class 2 OMP, NmeP2; *N. meningitidis* class 3 OMP, NmeP3; *N. gonorrhoeae* PIA protein, NgoPIA; *N. gonorrhoeae* PIB protein, NgoPIB; *N. sicca* porin, Nsi; *N. lactamica* porin, Nla; *N. polysaccharae* porin, Npo.

the PIB protein from *N. gonorrhoeae* is nearly 90% identical to the porins from the commensal organisms *N. lactamica* and *N. polysaccharae*, although it shares less than 80% identity with the PIA protein. In all cases the precise figures for per cent sequence identity vary slightly, depending on the antigenic variants used in the comparison. It is also noteworthy that the meningococcal class 1 OMP (Nme P1) is the most distantly related *Neisseria* porin described to date, and only shares around 50% nucleotide sequence identity with each of the other porins (Maiden, 1993).

These patterns of sequence identity have important implications for horizontal genetical exchange between and within *Neisseria* species. Efficient homologous recombination is unlikely to occur in sequences that are less than 77% identical. Thus, whilst it is unlikely for a class 2 OMP gene from the meningococcus to recombine with a class 3 OMP gene to form a mosaic, it is much more likely for hybrid class 3 - PIA genes to occur or for the gonococcal PIB gene to recombine with the porin from *N. lactamica*, assuming that there is adequate mixing of the populations. Recombination may occur on either side of the porin genes, if regions of sufficient homology are present, and this is presumably the mechanism for the gene replacement from a class 2 OMP gene to class 3 OMP gene in the meningococcus or from a PIA to PIB gene in the gonococcus. One example of the transfer of a gonococcal PIB porin to a meningococcal strain has been reported (J. Vazquez and B. Spratt, personal communication), and such events may explain the occasional reports of isolates that appear to belong to both species.

Patterns of recombination in the PorA proteins

The class 1 OMP, or PorA, protein of the meningococcus has attracted more study than the other *Neisseria* porins to date, largely because of interest in its use as a major component of novel meningitis vaccines. Initial work on the protein was related to its use as the meningococcal serosubtyping antigen and studies using the monoclonal serosubtyping antibodies targeted against this protein suggested that a limited number of antigenic variants of the PorA proteins existed (Abdillahi & Poolman, 1987; Abdillahi & Poolman, 1988; Poolman & Abdillahi, 1988). This has subsequently proved not to be the case: nucleotide sequence analysis has shown that PorA is antigenically more variable than suggested by the data obtained with monoclonal serosubtyping reagents. The structure of the PorA protein and the genetic basis of variation of the *porA* gene also make it an excellent model for the study of the evolution of antigenic variation by horizontal genetical exchange.

Molecular analyses and sequence comparisons have identified the structural basis for the antigenic variation of the PorA protein (Maiden *et al.* 1991; van der Ley *et al.* 1991). A model for the structure of the porin is shown in Fig. 2A. In common with other porins it is assumed to have a ß-barrel structure, with the C- and N-termini of the polypeptide located on the periplasmic side of the outer

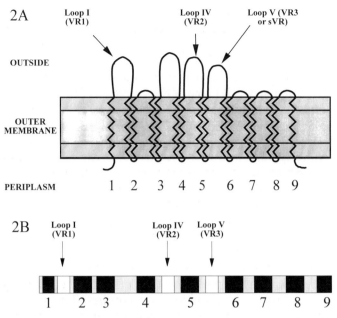

Fig. 2. Molecular basis of the antigenic variation of the class 1 OMP. A: Structural model of the PorA protein adapted from Maiden *et al.* (1991) and van der Ley *et al.* (1991). Antigenic variability resides in the surface exposed loops particularly, in PorA, loops I, IV and, to a lesser extent, loop V. Conserved regions of the protein are indicated by arabic numerals. B: Sequence features of the *porA* gene reflect the protein structure. The regions encoding the structural regions are conserved in different strains (CRs 1–9; dark shading and indicated by arabic numerals) while the regions encoding the surface loops, particularly loops I, IV, and V are variable in different strains (VRs 1, 2 and 3, light shading).

membrane (Nikaido, 1992). The ß-barrel structure comprises eight anti-parallel ß-strands, seven of which are formed by contiguous peptide sequences folding back on themselves by means of a turn located on the periplasmic side of the membrane. The eighth ß-strand is formed from the C- and N-terminal segments of the protein which form an anti-parallel structure with each other. This has the effect, in three dimensions, of forming the barrel which enables the protein to fulfill its function as an aqueous pore in the outer membrane. Between these ß-strands, on the outside of the cell surface, are eight loops of variable length that project away for the cell surface. It is in these loops that antigenic variability of these proteins reside. In the PorA protein most variation occurs in loops I (VR1) and IV (VR2) with minor variation in loop V (VR3 or sVR). In other *Neisseria* porins different surface loops are significant in antigenic variation (Ward *et al.* 1992; Feavers *et al.* 1992b; Suker *et al.* 1993), with the exception of loop III, which by analogy with the crystal structure of the *E. coli* porins, is probably folded into the pore and not surface exposed (Cowan *et al.* 1992).

As a result of the constraints imposed by the protein's structure, there are nine conserved regions (CRs 1–9) in all of the porin genes (illustrated by dark shading and arabic numerals in Fig. 2B) where little variation between different porin classes or the porin genes of different species. The nucleotide sequence changes observed in these regions are normally synonymous or biochemically conservative. In the meningococcal *porA* genes there are three variable regions (illustrated by the open boxes in Fig. 2B) encoding loops I, IV and V. There are a range of very diverse sequences which encode distinct epitopes for each of these locations, particularly VR1 and VR2. Some sequence diversity also occurs in regions of the gene encoding other loops, these are illustrated in Fig. 2B with light shading. The structure of a conserved gene with a number of variable segments is ideal for the detection of mosaics as it is relatively simple to detect the diverse variable regions and therefore to investigate the reassortment of the variable regions without needing to sequence the entire gene. In addition, although there are relatively few mutations in the conserved regions, it is possible to identify fingerprints of mutations within the CRs. These mutations enable the evolutionary lineage of the entire sequence to be determined and the location of recombination events outside the VRs to be identified.

The epitopes present in loops I and IV of different meningococcal isolates are highly diverse. The relationships of some of the amino acid sequences described to date are illustrated in Fig. 3. The variation of epitope-containing sequences is not continuous and they can be divided into families. The families are named using an extension of the serosubtype designations originally adopted for typing with monoclonal antibodies. Each of the epitope-containing sequences is

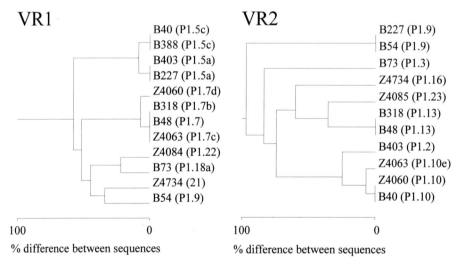

Fig. 3. Variable region families. There are a number distinct amino acid sequence families in the loop I and loop IV regions, originally defined by their reaction with monoclonal antibodies. Within each sequence family there are minor variants. The peptide sequence variants of VR1 and VR1 found in the serogroup A are shown on the dendrograms, with the variant name (P1.5 etc.) and the strain name given for each branch. The dendrograms are based on the similarity of the aligned peptide sequences calculated by the program DISTANCES from the GCG software package (Devereux *et al.* 1984). Note that the two dendrograms are not congruent, indicating that there has been reassortment of the DNA encoding loops I and IV of the PorA protein during the evolution of these genes.

assigned a number which is placed after the notation 'P1.' to indicate a class 1 OMP (P1.1, P1.2 etc.) Unfortunately, because the original designation was adopted before the molecular basis of the antigenic variation was established the numbers are arbitary and do not indicate the location of the epitope-containing sequence in loop I (VR1) or loop IV (VR2). This is addressed by placing the epitopes in the order VR1 VR2 separated by a comma, e.g. P1.7,16 (P1.7 is a VR1 epitope whereas P1.16 is a VR2 epitope). The original monoclonal antibodies did not identify minor variants within these families, which are now distinguished with lower case letters e.g. P1.7, P1.7a, P1.7b etc. So far a total of 24 distinct families have been described, 9 in VR1 and 15 in VR2 and many of these families have several minor variants (Maiden and Feavers, unpublished observations).

Many complete *porA* genes have now been sequenced and there is nucleotide sequence data for the VRs of many more (Barlow *et al.* 1989; McGuinness *et al.* 1990; Maiden *et al.* 1991; McGuinness *et al.* 1991; McGuinness *et al.* 1993; Rosenqvist *et al.* 1993; Suker *et al.* 1994). There are a number of general conclusions from this data set which will be discussed briefly before a more detailed discussion of the evolution of *porA* genes in different epidemiological situations. First, there is a global gene pool of *porA* genes; second this gene pool contains numerous mosaics as determined by reassortment of VRs; third, the rates of change and mechanisms of change of *porA* genes differ in meningococci associated with distinct epidemiologies of meningococcal disease.

Horizontal genetical exchange of *porA* genes in different epidemiological situations

Four epidemiologies of meningococcal disease have been described: epidemic/pandemic; localised epidemic; hyperendemic; and endemic (Schwartz *et al.* 1989). Comparison of data on the electrotypes (ETs) of meningococcal isolates, obtained by multilocus enzyme electrophoresis, with epidemiological data has shown that genetically distinct meningococci are associated with different meningococcal populations (Maiden & Feavers, 1995). As well as being genetically different, these groups of meningococci also exhibit diverse population structures, as defined by Maynard Smith *et al.* (1993). The epidemic/pandemic meningococci (largely serogroup A) are clonal, the localised epidemic and hyperendemic meningococci are 'epidemic' clonal (the result of the rapid spread of a recently arising clone), and the endemic meningococci are non-clonal or panmictic. The population structures of the *Neisseria* and the inter-relationships of population genetics and epidemiology are discussed in more detail in Spratt *et al.* (1995) and Maiden & Feavers (1995).

As the PorA protein is likely to be under immunological selection, it is a sensitive measure of the opportunity for horizontal genetical exchange to occur among different groups of meningococci, as novel products of recombination are likely to be positively selected and recovered during strain isolation. If the disruption of clonality is due to widespread recombination, as envisaged by Maynard Smith *et al.*, there would be relatively little recombination in the *porA* genes of the clonal organisms, whereas extensive recombination would be found in the panmictic meningococci. A different pattern of recombination might be expected in the 'epidemic clonal' meningococci. The data is at present incomplete for some of these groups and is almost certainly biased by epidemiological sampling (Maiden & Feavers, 1995). However, the available sequence data from *porA* genes confirms these predictions. The most complete data are available for serogroup A meningococci and these will be discussed first.

Pandemic meningococci

Meningococci belonging to serogroup A are responsible for the most epidemiologically serious form of meningococcal disease: large scale epidemics and pandemics, spreading across several continents causing a high incidence of disease in third world countries (Achtman, 1990; Moore, 1992). Extensive genetical analyses have demonstrated that each of the pandemics that have occurred this century have been caused by one of the genetically related subgroups of serogroup A (Olyhoek *et al.* 1987; Wang *et al.* 1992; Achtman, 1994). These subgroups represent clones which are genetically homogenous. In a survey of the *porA* genes in serogroup A subgroups, 55 strains chosen to be genetically, geographically and temporally representative were examined either by nucleotide sequence analysis or 'T-track' analysis (comparing multiple samples by running only one of the nucleotide sequence termination reactions) of the entire gene (Suker *et al.* 1994).

These analyses gave detailed information of the evolution of the genes which allowed the following conclusions to be drawn: (i) there was a limited number of *porA* gene types (4) in the serogroup A meningococci; (ii) these were stable over the sample period (up to 50 years) and during intercontinental spread; (iii) the gene types had originally arisen by recombination, and ultimately derived from a global pool of *porA* genes shared by all meningococci; (iv) with very rare exceptions all members of the same subgroup had the same *porA* gene, probably reflecting the acquisition of a novel *porA* gene type on subgroup divergence; (v) therefore, the *porA* gene types present in serogroup A meningococci were probably older than the subgroups in which they occurred; (vi) the few recombination events that had occurred in these meningococci over the time period sampled had not spread; (vii) two of the gene types had been spread around the world by successive waves of pandemic disease. The association of *porA* gene types with subgroup are illustrated in Fig. 4.

Thus the *porA* genes of serogroup A behave as predicted by the clonal population structure of these meningococci and show little evidence of recent recombination events. There were a number of possible reasons for the limited amount recombination observed in these bacteria. One is that during the rapid epidemic spread of these organisms they simply do not meet other meningococci, and the opportunity of exchange is thereby reduced. It is also possible that serogroup A

Genetic Distance   *porA* Gene Type

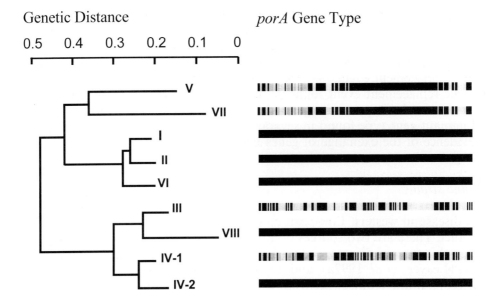

Fig. 4.   Distribution of *porA* gene types in the subgroups (clones) of serogroup A meningococci. There are only four main gene types found in the serogroup A meningococci and these are stable within clonal subgroups. The genetic relationships of each of the subgroups is shown, together with a graphical representation of the sequence relationships between the each of the *porA* genes. Similar patterns of shading indicate where two genes are similar, diverse patterns show where the genes differ.

meningococci are less competent for DNA uptake than other meningococci. It should also be noted that antibodies against the serogroup A capsule, in contrast to antibodies against serogroup C and B capsules prevent both disease and carriage and this may have a substantial effect on the selective pressures experienced by the subcapsular antigens, including the porins. The stability of the serogroup A subgroups and their fate between pandemics are yet to be fully explained.

Localized epidemic and hyperendemic meningococci

Meningococci associated with localized epidemic and hyperendemic disease are thought to exhibit the 'epidemic' clonal population structure. There is rather less comprehensive evidence for the evolution of the *porA* gene in these meningococci but two distinct complexes of related meningococci have been studied in sufficient detail for some conclusions to be drawn: the ET-37 complex, which has been responsible for numerous localised epidemics throughout the world over the last 50 years or so (Wang *et al.* 1993); and the ET-5 complex which spread causing hyper-endemic disease in a number of countries in the late 1970s and 1980s (Caugant *et al.* 1986; Caugant *et al.* 1987).

   Meningococci belonging to the ET-37 complex generally only express one type of *porA* gene which encodes the P1.5,2 epitopes or close relatives which have probably arisen by accumulation of mutations in the gene. A few gene replacements were observed (Wang *et al.* 1993). The ET-5 meningococci are antigenically much less stable and there are a number of class 1 OMPs which have been associated with this complex, most of which appear to been imported by gene replacement events, although there is one mosaic reported. Interestingly one gene replacement event found in a ET-5 strain isolated in Worcester, England, was the import of a gene identical at every base position to the predominant gene type found in several serogroup A subgroups, perhaps providing evidence of the exchange of genes between serogroup A and ET-5 meningococci.

Endemic strains

Most disease in western European countries is endemic, sporadic, and difficult to predict. There are two sources of information on *porA* genes for meningococci causing this type of disease: the nucleotide sequence of serological reference strains (Feavers *et al.* 1992a); and a study of VRs 1 and 2 in 250 strains, chosen to be representative of isolates from England and Wales during the period 1989-1991 (Maiden, Fox, and Feavers, unpublished observations). Unlike the genetically related collections of Ets discussed above, the serological reference strains were chosen because of their antigenic diversity, rather than their genetical relatedness. Comparative analysis of a set of 15 strains revealed mosaic gene structures which had been generated by at least five separate recombinational events. In addition, analysis of the chromosome structure of the isolates by pulsed field gel electrophoresis fingerprinting, demonstrated that in some cases similar or identical *porA* genes occurred in genetically distinct meningococci and, in other cases, genetically similar strains had diverse *porA* genes.

More extensive data on the reassortment of VRs comes from the study of 250 isolates by a combination of DNA-dot blot analysis and nucleotide sequence analysis. In this study the epitopes present in both VR1 and VR2 were identified for 240 of the 250 isolates examined: the results are summarised in Fig. 5. There were representatives of seven VR1 families and 13 VR2 families in this strain collection. In one strain the region of the *porA* gene encoding VR2 had been deleted. Some VR families, e.g. the P1.13 VR2 family, were associated with a number of VR1 family sequences. Others, for example the P1.4 and P1.10 VR2 families, occur with a limited range of VR1 sequence families.

These data show that whilst recombination can lead to reassortment of VR1 and VR2 within *porA* genes, strain collections of endemic meningococci do not comprise a completely random assortment of VR1 and VR2 associations. There are three possible explanations for this: (i) sampling; (ii) presence of predominant clones in the meningococcal population; and (iii) structural constraints. As most meningococci derive from case isolates the strain collections may be biased by sampling and some epitope combinations, e.g. P1.5,10, may be prevalent in strains with a higher pathogenic potential. On the other hand, at any one time it is possible that certain clones which happen to have a particular epitope

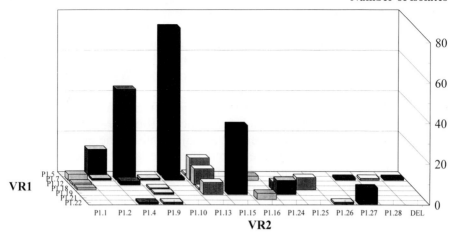

Fig. 5. Non-random association of variable region families in meningococci. The association of VR1 with VR2 epitope families in a set of 250 meningococci is illustrated. Note that while some VR2 epitope families, e.g. P1.13, occur with a number of VR1 epitope families others, e.g. P1.10 are much more limited in the range of VR1 with which they are associated.

combination predominate in the population. Finally, all meningococcal porins have to be able to fold correctly in the outer membrane and to perform their biochemical function. While the structural versatility of the ß-barrel is indicated by the diverse sequences that occur in VR1 and VR2, it is possible that certain epitope combinations lead to unstable or dysfunctional porin. These explanations are not mutually exclusive and it is possible that a combination of more than one of these explanations accounts for the results observed.

Conclusions

Nucleotide sequence comparisons provide extensive evidence of horizontal genetic exchange in the genes encoding the porin proteins of *N. meningitidis*. The differences in the clonal and epidemiological behaviour of different meningococci enable the effect of horizontal genetical exchange in different time-frames to be observed in one species. In serogroup A, where clones persist over decades and during global spread, evidence for 'ancient' exchange events, with a subsequent accumulation of point mutation can be seen. This is similar to the types of mosaics observed in clonal species such as *Escherichia coli* (Hartl *et al.* 1986; DuBose *et al.* 1988; Milkman & Bridges, 1990; Milkman & McKane, 1995). The antigenic diversity of the serogroup A subgroups, or clones, is limited and reassortment of the lineages suggests that the mosaics are in this case older than the clonal subgroups in which they occur.

In other meningococci there is evidence for much more recent exchange, resulting in either the reassortment of PorA epitopes within the *porA* gene or gene replacement of the complete *porA* gene. Gene replacement has enabled the ET-5 meningococci, for example, to express a number of antigenically different porin genes during its spread around the world. It is interesting to note, however, that there is little evidence for exchange playing a major role in antigenic variation of ET-37 meningococci, although isolates from around the world over a protracted time-scale have been collected. When isolates representing endemic meningococci are examined, there appears to be much recombination of relatively small fragments of the genome resulting not in gene replacement, but reassortment of PorA epitope families within *porA* genes. Thus horizontal genetical exchange has played a major role in the evolution of novel antigenic variants of the porin proteins but this role, and the balance of exchange events to other mutational events, varies in genetically and epidemiologically distinct meningococci.

Acknowledgements

The serogroup A studies were carried out in collaboration with Dr. M. Achtman, Max-Planck-Institut für molekulare Genetik, Berlin, Germany. We would like to thank Dr. D.M. Jones and Dr. A. Fox of the Meningococcal Reference Unit, Withington Hospital, Manchester, UK, for the provision of strains, and Professor B.G. Spratt and Dr. N.H. Smith of the University of Sussex, for discussion of data prior to publication.

The authors are at the Division of Bacteriology, National Institute for Biological Standards and Control, South Mimms, Potters Bar, Herts, EN6 3QG.

References

Abdillahi, H. and J.T. Poolman, 1987 - Whole-cell ELISA for typing *Neisseria meningitidis* with monoclonal antibodies, *FEMS Microbiol. Lett.* **48**, 367–371.

Abdillahi, H. and J.T. Poolman, 1988 - *Neisseria meningitidis* group B serosubtyping using monoclonal antibodies in whole-cell ELISA, *Microb. Pathog.* **4**, 27–32.

Achtman, M., 1990 - Molecular epidemiology of epidemic bacterial meningitis, *Rev. Med. Microbiol.* **1**, 29–38.

Achtman, M., 1994 - Clonal spread of serogroup A meningococci. A paradigm for the analysis of microevolution in bacteria, *Mol. Microbiol.* **11**, 15–22.

Barlow, A.K., J.E. Heckels and I.N. Clarke, 1989 - The class 1 outer membrane protein of *Neisseria meningitidis*: gene sequence and structural and immunological similarities to gonococcal porins, *Mol. Microbiol.* **3**, 131–139.

Bjune, G., E.A. Hoiby, J.K. Gronnesby, O. Arnesen, J.H. Fredriksen, A. Halstensen, E. Holten, A.K. Lindbak, H. Nokleby, E. Rosenqvist *et al.*, 1991 - Effect of outer membrane vesicle vaccine against group B meningococcal disease in Norway, *Lancet* **338**, 1093–1096.

Bowler, L.D., Q.Y. Zhang, J.Y. Riou and B.G. Spratt, 1994 - Interspecies recombination between the *penA* genes of *Neisseria menningitidis* and commensal *Neisseria* species during the emergence of penicillin resistance in *N. meningitidis*: natural events and laboratory simulation, *J. of Bacteriol.* **176**, 333–337.

Brunham, R.C., F.A. Plumer and R.S. Stephens, 1993 - Bacterial antigenic variation, host immune response, and pathogen-host coevolution, *Infect. Immun.* **61**, 2273–2276.

Cartwright, K.A.V., J.M. Stuart, D.M. Jones and N.D. Noah, 1987 - The Stonehouse survey: nasopharyngeal carriage of meningococci and *Neisseria lactamica*, *Epidemiol. Infect.* **99**, 591–601.

Caugant, D.A., L.O. Froholm, K. Bovre, E. Holten, C.E. Frasch, L.F. Mocca, W.D. Zollinger and R.K. Selander, R.K. 1986 - Intercontinental spread of a genetically distinctive complex of clones of *Neisseria meningitidis* causing epidemic disease, *Proc. Nat. Acad. Sci. USA* **83**, 4927–4931.

Caugant, D.A., L.O. Froholm, K. Bovre, E. Holten, C.E. Frasch, L.F. Mocca, W.D. Zollinger and R.K. Selander, 1987 - Intercontinental spread of *Neisseria meningitidis* clones of the ET-5 complex, *Antonie van Leeuwenhoek* **53**, 389–394.

Coughter, J.P. and G.J. Stewart, 1989 - Genetic exchange in the environment, *Antonie van Leeuwenhoek* **55**, 15-22.

Cowan, S.W., T. Schirmer, G. Rummel, M. Steiert, R. Ghosh, R.A. Paupit, J.N. Jansonius and J.P. Rosenbusch, 1992 - Crystal structures explain functional properties of two *E. coli* porins, *Nature* **358**, 727–733.

Devereux, J.P., P. Haeberli and O. Smithies, 1984 - A comprehensive set of sequence analysis programs for the VAX, *Nucleic Acids Res.* **12**, 387–395.

DuBose, R.F., D.E. Dykhuizen and D.L. Hartl, 1988 - Genetic exchange among natural isolates of bacteria: recombination within the *phoA* gene of *Escherichia coli*, *Proc. Nat. Acad. Sci. USA* **85**, 7036–7040.

Feavers, I.M., A.B. Heath, J.A. Bygraves and M.C. Maiden, 1992a - Role of horizontal genetic exchange in the antigenic variation of the class 1 outer membrane protein of *Neisseria meningitidis*, *Mol. Microbiol.* **6**, 489–495.

Feavers, I.M., J. Suker, A.J. McKenna, A.B. Heath and M.C.J. Maiden, 1992b - Molecular analysis of the serotyping antigens of *Neisseria meningitidis*, *Infect. Immun.* **60**, 3620–3629.

Fenner, F., D.A. Henderson, I. Arita, Z. Jezek and I.D. Ladnyi, 1988 - Smallpox and its eradication, Geneva: World Health Organization.

Frasch, C.E., W.D. Zollinger and J.T. Poolman, 1985 - Serotype antigens of *Neisseria meningitidis* and a proposed scheme for designation of serotypes, *Rev. Infect. Dis.* **7**, 504–510.

Frasch, C.E., C.T. Sacchi, M.C. Brandiolone, V.S. Vieiera and L.C. Leite, 1991 - Development of a second generation group B meningococcal vaccine. *NIPH. Ann.* **14**, 225–230.

Frosch, M. and T.F. Meyer, 1992 - Transformation-mediated exchange of virulence determinants by co-cultivation of pathogenic Neisseriae, *FEMS Microbiol. Lett.* **100**, 345–349.

Haas, R., S. Veit and T.F. Meyer, 1992 - Silent pilin genes of *Neisseria gonorrhoeae* MS11 and the occurrence of related hypervariant sequences among other gonococcal isolates, *Mol. Microbiol.* **6**, 197–208.

Halter, R., J. Pohlner and T.F. Meyer, 1989 - Mosaic-like organization of IgA protease genes in *Neisseria gonorrhoeae* generated by horizontal genetic exchange *in vivo*, *EMBO J.* **8**, 2737–2744.

Hartl, D.L., M. Medhora, L. Green, D.E. Dykhuizen, M. Medhora and L. Green, 1986 - The evolution of DNA sequences in *Escherichia coli, Philos. Trans. R. Soc. Lond. [Biol]* **312**, 191–204.

Hitchcock, P.J., 1989 - Unified nomenclature for pathogenic *Neisseria* species, *Clin. Microbiol. Rev.* **2**, S64–S65.

Hobbs, M.M., A. Seiler, M. Achtman and J.G. Cannon, 1994 - Microevolution within a clonal population of pathogenic bacteria: recombination, gene duplication and horizontal genetic exchange in the *opa* gene family of *Neisseria meningitidis. Mol. Microbiol.* **12**, 171–180.

Kroll, J.S. and E.R. Moxon, 1990 - Capsulation in distantly related strains of *Haemophilus influenzae* type b: genetic drift and gene transfer at the capsulation locus, *J. Bacteriol.* **172**, 1374–1379.

Li, J., K. Nelson, A.C. McWhorter, T.S. Whittam and R.K. Selander, 1994 - Recombinational basis of serovar diversity in *Salmonella enterica, Proc. Nat. Acad. Sci. USA* **91**, 2552–2556.

Lorenz, M.G. and W. Wackernagel, 1994 - Bacterial Gene Transfer by Natural Genetic Transformation in the Environment, *Microbiol. Rev.* **58**, 563–602.

Maiden, M.C.J., J. Suker, A.J. McKenna, J.A. Bygraves and I.M. Feavers, 1991 - Comparison of the class 1 outer membrane proteins of eight serological reference strains of *Neisseria meningitidis, Mol. Microbiol.* **5**, 727–736.

Maiden, M.C.J., 1993 - Population genetics of a transformable bacterium: the influence of horizontal genetical exchange on the biology of *Neisseria meningitidis, FEMS Microbiol. Lett.* **112**, 243–250.

Maiden, M.C.J. and I.M. Feavers, 1995 - Population genetics and global epidemiology of the human pathogen *Neisseria meningitidis*, in, Baumberg, S., J.P.W. Young, J.R. Saunders and E.M.H. Wellington (eds), *Population genetics of bacteria*, Cambridge, Cambridge University Press, pp. 269–293.

Maynard Smith, J., C.G. Dowson and B.G. Spratt, 1991 - Localized sex in bacteria, *Nature* **349**, 29–31.

Maynard Smith, J., N.H. Smith, M. O'Rourke and B.G. Spratt, 1993 - How clonal are bacteria?, *Proc. Nat. Acad. Sci. USA* **90**, 4384–4388.

Maynard Smith, J., 1995 - Do bacteria have population genetics?, in, Baumberg, S., J.P.W. Young, E.M.H. Wellington and J.R. Saunders (eds), *Population genetics of bacteria*, Cambridge, Cambridge University Press, pp. 1–12.

McGuinness, B.T., A.K. Barlow, I.N. Clarke, J.E. Farley, A. Anilionis, J.T. Poolman and J.E. Heckels, 1990 - Deduced amino acid sequences of class 1 protein *PorA* from three strains of *Neisseria meningitidis*, *J. Exp. Med.* **171**, 1871–1882.

McGuinness, B.T., I.N. Clarke, P.R. Lambden, A.K. Barlow, J.T. Poolman, D.M. Jones and J.E. Heckels, 1991 - Point mutation in meningococcal *porA* gene associated with increased endemic disease, *Lancet* **337**, 514–517.

McGuinness, B.T., P.R. Lambden and J.E. Heckels, 1993 - Class 1 outer membrane protein of *Neisseria meningitidis*: epitope analysis of the antigenic diversity between strains, implications for subtype definition and molecular epidemiology, *Mol. Microbiol.* **7**, 505–514.

Mee, B.J., H. Thomas, S.J. Cooke, P.R. Lambden and J.E. Heckels, 1993 - Structural Comparison and Epitope Analysis of Outer Membrane Protein PIA from Strains of *Neisseria gonorrhoeae* with Differing Serovar Specificities, *J. Genet. Microbiol.* **139**, 2613–2620.

Milkman, R. and M.M. Bridges, 1990 - Molecular evolution of the *Escherichia coli* chromosome. III. Clonal frames, *Genetics* **126**, 505–517.

Milkman, R. and M. McKane, 1995 - Variation and recombination in *E. coli*, in, Baumberg, S., J.P.W. Young, E.M.H. Wellington and J.R. Saunders (eds), *Population genetics of bacteria*, Cambridge, Cambridge University Press, pp. 127–142.

Mocca, L.F. and C.F. Frasch, 1982 - Sodium dodecyl sulfate polyacrylamide-gel typing system for characterisation of *Neisseria meningitidis* isolates, *J. Clin. Microbiol.* **16**, 240–244.

Moore, P.S., 1992 - Menigococcal meningitis in Sub-Saharan Africa: A model for the epidemic process, *Clin. Infect. Dis.* **14**, 515–525.

Morelli, G., J. del Valle, C.J. Lammel, J. Pohlner, K. Müller, M.S. Blake, G.F. Brooks, T.F. Meyer, B. Koumarg, N. Brieske and M. Achtman, 1994 - Immunogenicity and evolutionary variability of epitopes within IgA1 proteases from serogroup A *Neisseria meningitidis*, *Mol. Microbiol.* **11**, 175–187.

Nikaido, H., 1992 - Porins and specific channels of bacterial outer membranes, *Mol. Microbiol.* **6**, 435–442.

Olyhoek, T., B.A. Crowe and M. Achtman, 1987 - Clonal Population Structure of *Neisseria meningitidis* Serogroup A Isolated from Epidemics and pandemics Between 1915 and 1983, *Rev. Infect. Dis.* **9**, 665–682.

Peltola, H., 1983 - Meningococcal disease: still with us. *Rev. Infect. Dis.* **5**, 71–91.

Poolman, J.T. and H. Abdillahi, 1988 - Outer Membrane Protein Serotyping of *Neisseria meningitidis*, *Eur. J. Clin. Microbiol. Infect. Dis.* **7**, 291–292.

Radstrom, P., C. Fermer, B.E. Kristiansen, A. Jenkins, O. Skold and G. Swedberg, 1992 - Transformational Exchanges in the Dihydropterate Synthase Gene of *Neisseria meningitidis*: a novel mechanism for the Acquisition of Sulfonamide Resistance, *J. Bacteriol.* **174**, 5961–5968.

Robertson, B.D. and T.F. Meyer, 1992 - Antigenic variation in bacterial pathogens, in, Hormaeche, C.E., C.W. Penn and C.J. Smyth (eds), *Molecular Biology of Bacterial Infection: Society for General Microbiology, Symposium* **49**, Cambridge, Cambridge University Press, pp. 61–74.

Rosenqvist, E., E.A. Hoiby, E. Wedege, D.A. Caugant, L.O. Froholm, B.T. McGuinness, J. Brooks and P.R. Lambden, 1993 - A new variant of serosubtype P1.16 in *Neisseria meningitidis* from Norway associated with increased resistance to bactericidal antibodies induced by a serogroup B outer membrane protein vaccine, *Microb. Pathogen.* **15**, 197–205.

Saukkonen, K., M. Leinonen, H. Abdillahi and J.T. Poolman, 1989 - Comparative evaluation of potential components for group B meningococcal vaccine by passive protection in the infant rat and *in vitro* bactericidal assay, *Vaccine* **7**, 325–328.

Schwartz, B., P.S. Moore and C.V. Broome, 1989 - Global epidemiology of meningococcal disease, *Clin. Microbiol. Rev.* **2**, s118–s124.

Seifert, H.S. and M. So, 1988 - Genetic mechanisms of bacterial antigenic variation, *Microbiol. Rev.* **52**, 327–336.

Selander, R.K., D.A. Caugant, H. Ochman, J.M. Musser, M.N. Gilmour and T.S. Whittam, 1986 - Methods of multilocus enzyme electrophoresis for bacterial population genetics and systematics, *Appl. Environ. Microbiol.* **51**, 837–884.

Selander, R.K., J.M. Musser, D.A. Caugant, M.N. Gilmour and T.S. Whittam, 1987 - Population genetics of pathogenic bacteria, *Microb. Pathogen.* **3**, 1–7.

Selander, R.K. and B.R. Levin, 1980 - Genetic diversity and structure in *Escherichia coli* populations, *Science* **210**, 545–547.

Spratt, B.G., Q.-Y. Zhang, D.M. Jones, A. Hutchison, J.A. Brannigan and C.G. Dowson, 1989 - Recruitment of a penicillin-binding protien gene from *Neisseria flavescens* during the emergence of penicillin resistance in *Neisseria meningitidis*, *Proc. Nat. Acad. Sci. USA* **86**, 8988–8992.

Spratt, B.G., L.D. Bowler, Q.Y. Zhang, J. Zhou and J.M. Smith, 1992 - Role of interspecies transfer of chromosomal genes in the evolution of penicillin resistance in pathogenic and commensal Neisseria species, *J. Mol. Evol.* **34**, 115–125.

Spratt, B.G., N.H. Smith, J. Zhou, M. O'Rourke and E. Feil, 1995 - The population genetics of the pathogenic *Neisseria*, in, Baumberg, S., J.P.W. Young,

E.M.H. Wellington and J.R. Saunders (eds), *Population genetics of bacteria*, Cambridge, Cambridge University Press, pp. 143–160.

Suker, J., I.M. Feavers and M.C.J. Maiden, 1993 - Structural analysis of the variation in the major outer membrane proteins of *Neisseria meningitidis* and related species, *Biochem. Soc. Trans.* **21**, 304–306.

Suker, J., I.M. Feavers, M. Achtman, G. Morelli, J.-F. Wang and M.C.J. Maiden, 1994 - The *porA* gene in serogroup A meningococci: evolutionary stability and mechanism of genetic variation, *Mol. Microbiol.* **12**, 253–265.

Tsai, C.-M., C.E. Frasch and L.F. Mocca, 1981 - Five structural classes of major outer membrane proteins in *Neisseria meningitidis*, *J. Bacteriol.* **146**, 69–78.

van der Ley, P., J.E. Heckels, M. Virji, P. Hoogerhout and J.T. Poolman, 1991 - Topology of outer membrane proteins in pathogenic *Neisseria* species, *Infect. Immun.* **59**, 2963–2971.

van der Ley, P., J. van der Biezen, P. Hohenstein, C. Peeters and J.T. Poolman, 1993 - Use of transformation to construct antigenic hybrids of the class 1 outer membrane protein in *Neisseria meningitidis*, *Infect. Immun.* **61**, 4217–4224.

van der Ley, P. and J.T. Poolman, 1992 - Construction of a multivalent meningococcal vaccine strain based on the class 1 outer membrane protein, *Infect. Immun.* **60**, 3156–3161.

Virji, M., J.R. Saunders, G. Sims, K. Makepeace, D. Maskell and D.J.P. Ferguson, 1993 - Pilus-faciltitated adherence of *Neisseria meningitidis* to human epithelial and endothelial cells: modulation of adherence phenotype occurs concurrently with changes in primary amino acid sequence and the glycosylation status of pilin, *Mol. Microbiol.* **10**, 1013–1028.

Wang, J.-F., D.A. Caugant, X. Li, X. Hu, J.T. Poolman, B.A. Crowe and M. Achtman, 1992 - Clonal and antigenic analysis of serogroup A *Neisseria meningitidis* with particular reference to epidemiological features of epidemic meningitis in China, *Infect. Immun.* **60**, 5267–5282.

Wang, J.-F., D.A. Caugant, G. Morelli, B. Koumaré and M. Achtman, 1993 - Antigenic and epidemiological properties of the ET-37 complex of *Neisseria meningitidis*, *J. Infect. Dis.* **167**, 1320–1329.

Ward, M.J., P.R. Lambden and J.E. Heckels, 1992 - Sequence analysis and relationships between meningococcal class 3 serotype proteins and other porins of pathogenic and non-pathogenic *Neisseria* species, *FEMS Microbiol. Lett.* **94**, 283–290.

Whatmore, A.M. and M.A. Kehoe, 1994 - Horizontal gene transfer in the evolution of group A streptococcal emm-like genes: gene mosaics and variation in Vir regulons, *Mol. Microbiol.* **11**, 363–374.

Wolff, K. and A. Stern, A. 1991 - The class 3 outer membrane protein (PorB) of *Neisseria meningitidis*: gene sequence and homology to the gonococcal porin PIA, *FEMS Microbiol. Lett.* **83**, 179–185.

Zapata, G.A., W.F. Vann, Y. Rubinstein and C.E. Frasch, 1992 - Identification of Variable Region Differences in *Neisseria meningitidis* Class 3 Protein Sequences Among Five Group B Serotypes, *Mol. Microbiol.* **6**, 3493–3499.

Zhou, J. and B.G. Spratt, 1992 - Sequence diversity within the *argF*, *fbp* and *recA* genes of natural isolates of *Neisseria meningitidis*: interspecies recombination within the *argF* gene, *Mol. Microbiol.* **6**, 2135–2146.

Zollinger, W.D. and E. Moran, 1991 - Meningococcal vaccines - present and future, *Trans. R. Soc. Trop. Med. Hyg.* **85** Suppl. 1, 37–43.

Thomas F. Meyer

Ecology and Infection Mechanisms of Pathogenic *Neisseria* Species

Abstract

Pathogenic and commensal *Neisseria* species form a large 'collective' linked by a constant horizontal flow of genetic information via natural transformation. Two basic processes, i.e. horizontal exchange and mutational events, govern the neisserial population structure which is described here as a 'clonal network'. Environmental factors such as spatial separation and selective advantage of certain traits determine the shape of the network allowing individual clones and seemingly autonomous species to emerge. The thus sustainable long-term flexibility of *Neisseria* species is supplemented by rapid DNA rearrangements in the neisserial genome which facilitate both short-term adaptive and escape processes.

Both pathogenic *Neisseria* spp. colonize human mucosal surfaces but rarely cause systemic infections. Despite their different disease spectrum, both pathogens use similar infection strategies. Crucial steps of the infection process include (i) the pilus-mediated attachment to epithelial cells, (ii) the *opacity* (Opa/Opc) protein-mediated entry into these cells and (iii) the interaction with, and intracellular accommodation within, professional phagocytes. In recent years, molecular biological approaches taken have provided astounding insights into the structure and function of factors which play a part in the interactions between the pathogens and their cellular targets. Current investigations with the *Neisseria* model aim towards an improved understanding of the phenomenon of bacterial pathogenesis.

Introduction

The pathogenic *Neisseria* species, discovered in 1879 and 1887 by Albert Neisser (gonococci) and Anton Weichselbaum (meningococci), respectively, are the causative agents of gonorrhoea and meningitis. The *Neisseria*e are gram-negative organisms usually with a diplococcal shape. They include a wide variety of commensal species and two pathogenic species. Meningococci and gonococci as well as some of their commensal relatives infect man who is their sole natural host. They represent typical mucosal colonizers. While localized infections with *N. meningitidis* (e.g. of the nasopharynx) of normal human individuals occur frequently and are usually asymptomatic, therefore reminiscent of infections with

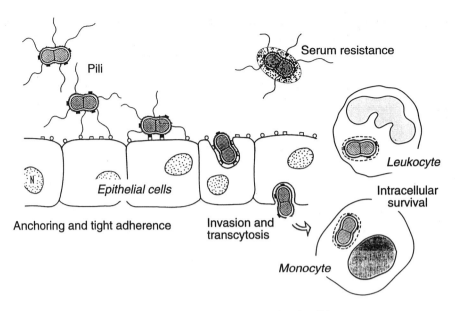

Fig. 1. Model of the neisserial infection process (see text for details).

commensal *Neisseria* species. Under rare, still undefined, conditions pathogenic *Neisseria* disseminate to cause life-threatening or other severe diseases including meningitis, bacteremia, pelvic inflamatory disease and septic arthritis.

Localized neisserial infections involve a series of receptor-mediated interactions between the bacteria and the primary target cells. The formation of pili is a prerequisite for the neisserial attachment to the epithelial cell surface. Often the surface-attached bacteria penetrate the epithelial cells and - while contained in a vacuole - may transcytose towards subepithelial tissues. The pathogenic *Neisseriae* strongly interact with phagocytic cells, such as neutrophils and macrophages, which seem to provide them with an intracellular habitat (Fig. 1).

Neisserial pathogenesis is characterized by the strong inflamatory response to the infection rather than by the action of distinct bacterial toxins. The neisserial infection is the result of a multifactorial process. With regard to their putative virulence attributes meningococci and gonococci are similarly equipped, with perhaps one major difference which is the lack of a polysaccharide capsule in gonococci. Therefore, most of the topics discussed here are relevant to both species, despite the different disease spectra caused by the two pathogens.

Evolution and microecology of the pathogenic *Neisseria* spp.

Horizontal exchange

Several recent studies emphasize the significance of horizontal genetic exchange in the evolution and ecology of *Neisseria* species. It appears that a continuous horizontal flow of genetic material affects the chromosomal composition not only of the pathogenic *Neisseria* species, but also of many commensal species. In fact, there exists ample circumstantial evidence for horizontal exchange of genes between commensal and pathogenic *Neisseria* species, between meningococci and gonococci, and within distinct *Neisseria* species, generating mosaic genes (Halter 1989; Feavers 1992; Spratt 1992). It is difficult to give precise estimates of the frequencies with which such horizontal exchanges occur in nature, however, in a few cases it is plausible that events may have happened in recent years (Achtman 1994). Conceivably, horizontal genetic exchange can be envisioned as a long-term adaptive mechanism suitable for responding to gross environmental changes and for securing the genetic flexibility of *Neisseria* species as a collective group of seemingly independent but truly inter-connected traits. Consistent with the fact that the *Neisseria* species evolved from, and still rely on, a common pool of genes, these organisms can be regarded as a 'collective' rather than entirely distinct species.

Clonal networks

How does this concept of a 'species collective' fit with the clonality of *Neisseria* species as is particularly evident in the case of *N. meningitidis* (Wang 1992; Achtman 1994)? This issue was recently addressed by Maynard Smith and collegues (1993) who proposed a significant difference in the clonal structures of *N. meningitidis* versus other clonal species, such as *Salmonella* and *Escherichia coli*, based on gene linkage disequilibrium measurements. The authors define several types of population structures, an entirely clonal structure, the epidemic structure and, at the other extreme, the panmictic structure with no evidence of linkage disequilibrium. These population structures are the direct consequence of two competing genetic processes, i.e. the genetic drift (mutagenesis) occurring within the scope of a species, and horizontal exchange (recombination) affecting this species extrinsically. *Salmonella* is little influenced by horizontal exchange and thus appears as a clonal population. Contrastingly, *N. gonorrhoeae* constitutes a panmictic population where horizontal exchange is overwhelming (O'Rourke 1994). *N. meningitidis* occupies an intermediate position where occasional clonal outgrowths occur within an otherwise panmictic context.

The latter population structure could also be termed a 'clonal network' comprising both sexual and clonal elements. Interestingly, such a clonal network structure is evident at several levels of the genus *Neisseria* as a whole. Likewise the species of *N. gonorrhoeae* can be regarded as a 'large epidemic clone' of the genus *Neisseria*, still connected with the remainder of the network by horizontal exchange (Hobbs 1994). Conversely, on a short scale, following up the infection route of individual *N. gonorrhoeae* strains among sexual contacts, a similar clonal network structure is generated under the influence of genetic variation (a rapid and specialized form of mutagenesis discussed below) and horizontal exchange, for example, in individuals infected with multiple strains. Thus, a clonal network is evident at several levels, i.e. strains, epidemic clones, and species. The fine-structure of a clonal network is influenced by several parameters, (i) the sexual activity between species, epidemic clones and strains, (ii) their spatial relationship and (iii) the selective advantage of novel recombinants. According to this theory, *N. gonorrhoeae*, despite being part of the *Neisseria* network, developed and functioned as an 'independent' *Neisseria* species because it was unaffected by dramatic sexual exchange with the rest of the genus, owing to its ecological isolation (Vázquez 1993). The theory of context dependent selective advantage also explains why, despite active horizontal exchange among the *Neisseria* species, some genotypes, including that for the polysaccharide capsule and IgA protease, are restricted to distinct *Neisseria* species (Facius 1993; Frosch 1989) while the distribution of many other putative virulence determinants is not species-restricted, not even to the pathogenic *Neisseriae* (Aho 1987).

Natural competence for transformation

The ability of *N. gonorrhoeae* to undergo DNA transformation under natural conditions was recognized more than 30 years ago (Catlin 1961). Till today no natural process other than transformation that might account for the horizontal exchange of chromosomal genes has been reported for *Neisseria*. Bacteriophages and transducing phages in particular have not been identified and, although many conjugative plasmids exist, conjugative (Hfr-like) mobilization of chromosomal determinants is not known to occur under natural conditions. Thus, the only known mechanism that could account for the observed horizontal exchange among *Neisseria* is transformation.

Horizontal exchange of chromosomal markers via transformation is readily observed by co-cultivation of different *Neisseria* strains *in vitro* (Frosch 1992; Zhang 1992). In a typical experiment the efficiency of transfer between two gonococcal strains after one hour of co-cultivation was in the order of 10^{-5} per cell and genetic locus. The process is completely inhibited in the presence of DNase in the culture medium indicating that, despite of the apparent viability of the cultured cells, there is a substantial release of DNase-accessible DNA into the medium. How the DNA is released into the medium has not been studied in detail, however, the spontaneous autolysis observed for the gonococcus is one explanation (Hebeler 1975).

Natural transformation competence differs markedly from artificial transformation used for the cloning of genes e.g. in *E. coli*. For, in *Neisseria* the transforming DNA is taken up as a linear molecule and requires the RecA function and homologous sequences in the resident DNA of the recipient cell in order to allow re-circularization of a plasmid or incorporation of the DNA into the chromosome (Biswas 1986; Koomey 1987). The DNA homology requirement is probably the most effective mechanism of protection against bacterial transformation with unrelated DNA. Whether there is any role of the DNA restriction and methylation systems (Sullivan 1989; Gunn 1992) which are highly abundant among the *Neisseria* species on the transformation-mediated exchange is currently not well understood. Above these restrictions, the *Neisseria* species recognize a specific DNA sequence, 8 bp in length, that serves as a signal for the efficient uptake of DNA (Goodman 1988). Usually, the uptake signal is part of a transcriptional terminator where it constitutes the palindromic stem region; thus a typical neisserial terminator consists of two inverted uptake signals. Whether the uptake signal only serves for the DNA recognition or whether it also represents a site for the DNA linearization and/or a signal for the direction of the DNA transport is currently not known.

A panel of chemical mutants have been generated which led to the dissection of the gonococcal transformation into (i) uptake and conversion of the transforming DNA into a DNase-resistant state and (ii) the subsequent processes (Biswas 1989). One such DNA uptake deficient mutant (*dud1*) has been further characterized biochemically (Dorward 1989). Early studies suggested a role of gonococcal pili (which belong to the type 4 or N-methyl-Phe class of pili) in transformation competence (Sparling 1966). This interesting observation has recently been specified in that pilin (PilE), the major pilus subunit, rather than intact pili are required for DNA uptake (Gibbs 1989; Rudel 1995a). This not only results in an absolute transformation defect but also implicates the definite loss of ability to produce pili representing essential determinants in the infection process.

In addition to PilE, the minor pilus-associated protein, PilC (Jonsson 1991), is required for DNA uptake (Rudel 1995a). The involvement of pilus-associated factors in neisserial transformation competence is not unexpected since DNA import (for example in *Bacillus*) and type 4 pilus assembly obviously share common structural elements (Hobbs 1993). That competence gene products are often involved in other essential cellular processes may explain why respective defects are often pleiotropic. Such pleiotropic effects are evident for two peptidoglycan-associated factors (ComL and Tpc) which have recently been implicated in gonococcal competence (Fussenegger 1996). An example of a nonessential competence determinant is *comA* also identified in *N. gonorrhoeae* and other competent *Neisseria* species. ComA appears to be a typical inner membrane protein and is involved in a transformation step subsequent to the initial DNA uptake (Facius 1993). Its distribution among neisserial species suggest that the transformation mechanism is similar in different *Neisseria* species. Future studies on the natural transformation will hopefully shed more light on the significance of this interesting process for the genetic evolution and the pathogenic properties of the *Neisseria* species.

Rapid microenvironmental adaptation strategies

Genetic variation versus gene regulation

Microbial populations not only need to adapt to gross environmental changes encountered during evolution but, in addition, encounter frequent microenvironmental usually recurrent changes, for example, during the course of an infection. In order to respond to such recurrent changes, microorganisms maintain retrievable genetic programs. There are two principle types of adaptive programs used by microorganisms: (i) Genetic variation concerns spontaneous changes in the DNA which are inherited by the progeny and are often reversible. These changes, although temporarely random, take place at spatially distinct loci and ultimately lead to the synthesis of altered gene products. As a consequence, genetic variation generates heterogeneous populations of a distinct microbial strain, such that a fraction of this population is likely to show an improved micro-environmental adaptation. (ii) By contrast, the second microbial adaptation strategy, gene regulation, influences the bacterial population as a whole. In response to a certain environmental stimulus, such as temperature, osmolarity, or specific substances, the bacteria coordinatedly alter the expression of responsive genes.

Obviously both strategies bear specific advantages for microorganisms: While genetic variation better protects (minor parts of the population) against a large variety of unpredictable changes, gene regulation effects a well-determined adaptive process to the benefit of the whole population. However, genetic variation and gene regulation are not exclusive and often are interconnected: Likewise, the frequency or the direction of a switch may be influenced by environmental effectors, and conversely, a phase-variable regulator protein may control the expression of genes (Robertson 1992).

Although *Neisseria* represents a paradigm of genetic variability, gene regulation processes seem to play equally important roles in these bacteria. Likewise, stress-responsive systems sensitive to heat shock and/or other stress conditions, such as nutrient starvation and iron limitation, have been identified. The genetics of some of these systems, including the regulation of pilin synthesis are being studied (Taha 1992). Furthermore, recent investigations suggest the possibility of global regulatory changes, such as DNA superhelicity, in the regulation of certain gonococcal genes and the modulation of their virulence properties (Riemann, submitted).

Gene families and mechanisms of genetic variation in Neisseria

An interesting feature of some (but not all) variable surface proteins in *Neisseria* is that they are represented in the genome by gene families rather than individual genes. This applies for at least three variable surface proteins which have essential functions in the infection process, i.e., the PilE, PilC and Opa proteins (Robertson 1992), while other variable factors, such as the meningococcal Opc (Olyhoek 1991) and class I (PorA) porins (Barlow 1989), are encoded by single copy genes. Two principle mechanisms by which these proteins vary their structures can be distinguished based upon whether or not the variation process requires a functional RecA protein (Koomey 1987; Robertson 1992).

The best known example of RecA-dependent variation represents the major pilus subunit, PilE or pilin, which operates by intragenic recombination: In the bacterial genome multiple gene copies exist most of which are unexpressed, incomplete (silent/cryptic) gene copies (*pilS*) and one or two of which represent the expressed gene copies (*pilE*). The *pilS* copies constitute the variant sequence repertoire which is used for the recombination with *pilE* and thus in the generation of variant pilin molecules. In *N. gonorrhoeae* MS11 this repertoire is large enough to potentially produce $\sim 10^7$ variant pilin proteins (Swanson 1987; Haas 1992). Owing to this remarkable variability the bacterial pili can effectively escape the human immune response, as the variability of antibodies and T-cell receptors of the immune system, which uses a similar variation mechanism, is within the same order of magnitude. Recent studies have provided evidence that the recombination of *pil* genes can occur by at least three pathways, i.e., reciprocal, non-reciprocal (gene conversion-like) and transformation-mediated recombination (see Robertson 1992).

In contrast to the *pilE* genes, the genes encoding Opa and PilC proteins represent complete, rather than incomplete, variant genes (Stern 1986; Jonsson 1991) which undergo frequent phase transitions (ON/OFF switches) but rarely recombine with each other. These switches occur via a RecA-independent DNA slippage mechanism involving homo- or heteropolymeric repeated nucleotide sequences within the coding sequences of the genes (Robertson 1992); variation of the number of the repeating units alters the reading frame and consequently affects the translation into functional gene products. In case of the *opa* genes, the repeating unit is a pentameric (CTCTT) sequence whereas the *pilC* genes are controlled by a run of C residues; both 'coding repeats' (CR) are located in the secretory signal peptide-encoding part of the genes. Another method to control the expression of a gene via a repetitive sequence is realized in the meningococcal *opc* gene where a variable homopolymer of C residues is positioned between the -10 and -35 boxes of the *opc* promoter, thus giving rise to altered transcriptional activities. Recently, homopolymeric G runs have been identified in association with neisserial LPS genes suggesting that LPS variation is modulated by the same RecA-independent mechanism (Gotschlich 1994).

Functional significance of genetic variation

Neisserial type 4 pili

The type 4 pili, fine, hair-like organelles protruding from the bacterial cell surface, probably represent the most variable structures produced by the pathogenic *Neisseria* spp. They are absolutely required for the initiation of an infection (Kellogg 1968) in that they confer attachment of the bacteria to epithelial cells (McGee 1981). The binding of pili appears to be specific for human cells and the pili therefore represent major determinants of the neisserial species tropism. Owing to their exposed location, they are also strong targets of an antibody response that could interfere with receptor recognition. However, efforts in generating a pilus-based vaccine have thus far failed due to the enormous variability of the pili, and in particular of the pilin (Johnson 1991). It is therefore a prime question how the pili deceive the immune system in spite of fulfilling their function as adhesins. This problem clearly bears important practical and theoretical implications not necessarily restricted to the *Neisseria* model.

What components of pili are involved in receptor recognition? Early studies suggested a direct role of pilin (PilE), the major subunit, in adherence to various cellular substrates (Virji 1984; Rothbard 1985). At least three distinct adherence specificities, one for epithelial cells, one for erythrocytes and one allowing inter-gonococcal adherence, can be distinguished either genetically or otherwise (Rudel 1992). This does not exclude the association of pili with yet other adherence properties, e.g. for endothelial, phagocytic and sperm cells. Even more, *N. meningitidis* can produce two different classes of major subunits (class I and class II pilins) which may influence the adherence properties (Virji 1989). Interestingly, adherence to epithelial cells and interbacterial interaction are influenced by the pilin variation while the pilus-dependent haemagglutination is not (Lambden 1980; Rudel 1992; Nassif 1993). Pilin can be modified by phosphorylation and/or glycosylation (Robertson 1977; Schoolnik 1984; Virji 1993b) and variant-specific glycosylation of gonococcal pilin has been suggested to influence receptor recognition (Virji 1993b). However, the observed effect of pilin variation on adherence might be indirect and does not preclude a role of potential minor subunits in adherence.

Recent studies, in fact, suggest an association of minor protein components with the gonococcal pilus (Muir 1988; Parge 1990). One of these components, the PilC proteins, has been characterized genetically and implicated in the biogenesis of pili (Jonsson 1991) and transformation competence (Rudel 1995a). Nonetheless, pili can be assembled in the absence of both PilC1 and PilC2 proteins (Rudel 1992 and 1995bc), probably by utilizing an alternative PilC-like assembly factor. Such pili still haemagglutinate but lack the potential to adhere to epithelial cells indicating a role of PilC in epithelial cell adherence. We recently succeeded in purifying a gonococcal PilC protein to homogeneity from a PilE-negative strain, and in raising specific antibodies (Rudel 1995b). Experiments done with these reagents firmly indicate that PilC proteins represent epithelial cell-specific pilus-associated adhesins. Furthermore, the purified PilC protein effectively competes with the binding to epithelial cells of both gonococci and meningococci producing a variety of different PilC and PilE proteins. This, and additional recent results (Rudel 1995c; Ryll submitted; Scheuerpflug submitted), led us to the intriguing conclusion that the pili of pathogenic *Neisseria* species, irrespective of their structural variability, recognize the same, or a group of closely related receptors.

Cell tropisms conferred by the opacity *(Opa) proteins*

The Opa proteins (previously referred to as class 5 proteins of the meningococcus and P.II proteins of the gonococcus) are major constituents of the outer membranes mainly of the pathogenic *Neisseria* spp. Computer predictions suggest a β-pleated sheat structure of Opa proteins, typical of many outer membrane proteins, whereby three variable loop regions and a fourth conserved loop are oriented towards the bacterial surface (Meyer 1986; Bhat 1991). The number of variant *opa* genes present in gonococci (~ 11) is considerably higher than that in meningococci (3–4) and *N. lactamica* (~ 2). Interestingly, independent *N. gonorrhoeae* isolates rarely possess *opa* genes of identical sequence, indicating that the repertoire of variant *opa* genes within the gonococcal population is substantially larger than that of a single strain.

The role of Opa proteins in various adherence functions such as interbacterial adhesion and interaction with human epithelial and phagocytic cells has long been recognized. Recent work suggests that Opa proteins not only cause bacterial adherence but also trigger important cellular functions. Invasion of *N. gonorrhoeae* MS11 into human epithelial cells was shown to depend on the production of one distinct variant Opa protein produced by this strain (Makino 1991). Using a reverse genetics approach, the remainder Opa proteins of the same strain were subsequently shown to confer binding to human polymorphonuclear cells (PMNs) but not to epithelial cells (Kupsch 1993). Consistently, chemoluminescense of PMNs could only be induced with certain Opa proteins (Belland 1992). Yet, a different set of Opa proteins, including the one that reacts with epithelial cells, triggers uptake and chemoluminescense in human peripheral blood monocytes (PBMs). Interestingly, for all Opa proteins of strain MS11 at least one binding specificity is observed, indicating that each variant gene encodes a functional protein. The specific properties of Opa proteins are maintained if the genes are cloned and expressed in a different neisserial host (Kupsch 1993). A similar pattern of functional variation is seen for other *N. gonorrhoeae* strains some of which have also been assessed with regard to the interaction with endothelial cells. In the much smaller Opa protein repertoire of meningococci, Opa proteins required for epithelial cell invasion and PMN stimulation have been identified. This species often carries a copy of the phase variable *opc* gene whose product, although structurally unrelated, has a function similar to the epithelial cell-specific Opa proteins (Virji 1992b). It is thus evident, that the variable Opa and Opc adhesins represent important cell tropism determinants of *N. gonorrhoeae* and *N. meningitidis* and that the variability of these proteins allows multiple cellular interactions.

Immune escape versus structural adaptation

It is useful to distinguish between two principal functions of genetic variation, i.e. an escape function and an adaptive function, examples of which seem to be given by the *pil* and the *opa* systems, respectively. A typical escape mechanism is antigenic variation: This term describes the competition between two variable systems operating with similar mechanisms, i.e. the host immune system and a bacterial population. In this case, it is the pivotal interest on the bacterial side to *avoid* molecular interaction, e.g., with an antibody. The opposite applies for the adaptive variation model: Here any structural change must lead to a productive molecular fit; an error and trial mechanism would, instead, cause unnecessary bacterial extinction. We will briefly discuss to which extent the genetic systems underlying pili and Opa variation conform this model.

The extreme variability of the major pili subunit (PilE) classifies it as an escape factor. The mechanism used for its variation, i.e. more or less random intragenic recombination, provides little chance that novel recombinants attain, rather than lack, a specific molecular fit. Thus interaction with, e.g., antibody could be efficiently avoided. The question, however, arises how functional integrity is maintained? At least two conserved functions of the pili must be postulated, i.e., one for pili polymerization and - as our recent results suggest - one for the interaction with a conserved receptor (Rudel 1995b). The polymerization function is non-problematic because it involves the conserved hydrophobic regions of PilE which are neither surface-exposed nor immuno-susceptible. The dilemma, however, is how to accomodate a conserved receptor binding function in the highly variable context of the pili? To solve the problem the bacteria make use of a minor, pilus-associated adhesin, PilC, which is far less variable. In conclusion, therefore, PilE variation primarily serves to protect pili from interacting with immunoglobulins but is probably inadequate to modulate the receptor specificity.

For adaptive variation, the underlying genetic mechanisms ought to avoid mutation and recombination which could lead to non-productive phenotypes, and rather to utilize a selected set of preexisting genes. This situation is found in the *opa* gene system which exhibits limited phenotypic variability: Recombination, bearing the risk of generating non-productive hybrids, is a rare event among the *opa* genes (Stern 1986; Connell 1988) and all native *opa* genes encode functional Opa proteins capable of recognizing distinct cellular targets (Kupsch 1993). In contrast, *in vitro* engineered hybrid *opa* genes often encode non-functional Opas. It is hence evident that the mechanism of Opa variation favours productive interaction with target cells but its overall variability is probably too small in order to support an efficient immune escape reaction. If this applies, why is it so essential for the pili rather than for the Opa proteins to vary antigenically? Why is it that many other surface proteins of *Neisseria*, such as the major outer membrane porin proteins, are able to withstand host immunity without undergoing any intrastrain variation at all?

This question leads us to variation system of the neisserial lipopolysacharide (LPS). In contrast to the highly exposed pili, the neisserial membrane-associated proteins seem to be efficiently protected against host immunity through a variable carbohydrate coat produced by the bacteria. The *Neisseria* species produce a short type of lipopolysaccharide (LPS or LOS) which lacks any repetitive O-side chains but, instead, reveal multiple size classes indicating a structural heterogeneity of the neisserial LPS (Schneider 1988). A major difference among the variant LPS molecules is the presence of additional terminal galactose residues in the longer LPS forms which can be externally modified by a membrane-associated bacterial sialyltransferase using host-derived or endogenous CMP-NANA as sialyl donor (Smith 1991; Mandrell 1993; van Putten 1993). Given the presence of CMP-NANA, LPS variation thus determines whether or not the LPS is sialylated.

The functional relevance of the LPS phase transitions has recently been elucidated (van Putten, 1993) and appears to lie in the expression of variable amounts of sialic acid incorporated in the different forms of LPS. A low sialylation phenotype, as found early in the infection (Schneider 1991), enables entry of the bacteria into mucosal cells, but makes them susceptible to bactericidal activity. In contrast, highly sialylated bacteria are incapable of entering epithelial cells but are resistant to phagocytosis and killing by antibodies and complement, allowing persistence of infection. Thus, depending on the degree of sialylation the bacteria either adapt to the extracellular environment capable of resisting humoral immune mechanisms, or they become sensitive to bacteriocidal activities but then readily enter the intracellular milieu via Opa-mediated cellular interactions.

The function of highly sialylated LPS has many similarities with that of polysialic capsules produced by *N. meningitidis* and many commensal *Neisseria* species (Frosch 1989), in that they protect extracellular bacteria against both specific and non-specific host responses. Capsule expression appears to be influenced by genetic rearrangements (M. Frosch, pers. communication) as well as environmental factors. Loss of capsule expression favours Opa and Opc-mediated interactions of *N. meningitidis* with target cells and probably is a pre-requisite for cellular invasion (Virji 1993a). Therefore recent advances made in the analysis of capsular (cps) gene organisation and function (Edwards 1994) are important for our understanding of the conditions favouring invasive meningococcal infections.

Molecular cross-talk between pathogenic *Neisseria*e and target cells

Mucosal cell receptors

Despite extensive investigations, the exact nature of the pilus receptor(s) on host cell surfaces has not yet been identified. Since pilus-dependent adherence of neisserial strains seems to be restricted to human cells and some closely related avian species, this receptor resembles a crucial species-specific determinant. It is hoped that the recent identification of PilC as a pilus adhesin (Rudel *et al.*, 1995b) will facilitate the search for the corresponding structure(s). In many *in vitro* cell culture systems, pili are not required for bacterial adherence, but adherence can be conferred by members of the Opa protein family (Lambden 1979, Makino 1991; Virji 1992a). Recently, a host cell binding site for members of the Opa protein family was identified (van Putten 1995). This receptor resolved as a syndecan-like proteoglycan which is present on many epithelial cell lines. It appears that the heparan sulfate side chains specifically recognize the gonococcal Opa protein associated with tight adherence and cellular entry, and its meningococcal homologue Opc, but hardly binds other members of the Opa protein family. Purified receptor and receptor analogues, but not other basic proteins, totally block Opa/Opc protein mediated bacterial adherence to eukaryotic cells *in vitro*, and cell lines defective in receptor expression are only sparsely colonized with bacteria, suggesting that the missing structure is an essential component in the adherence process.

Entry of Neisseria *into mucosal cells*

The initial attachment phase is followed by the entry of *Neisseria* into mucosal cells, providing the organisms express the appropriate phenotype. Morphologically the entry process involves an elongation of the microvilli, and, in order to encompass the bacteria, the formation of zones of intimate contact between the bacterial and the host cell membranes, along with the engulfment of the bacteria via a zipper-like mechanism (Watt 1980; Weel 1991a; Stephens, 1989). As for most other pathogens, the molecular basis of these events is a current topic in *Neisseria* research. Experiments using inhibitors of different endocytic pathways and confocal microscopy of stained actin filaments and actin-binding proteins suggest that the Opa/Opc protein-associated internalization event involves an actin-filament process without a function for receptor-mediated endocytosis (Shaw 1988; Makino 1991; Grassmé submitted). The factor initiating the bacteria-directed endocytosis is unclear. Expression of the appropriate Opa protein in *E. coli* results in a very low level of internalization compared to native gonococcci (maximal 2 versus 30–50 bacteria per cell, respectively) (Simon 1992; Kupsch 1993), suggesting that additional, possibly newly synthesised factors are required to create the invasive phenotype (Chen 1991; Kupsch 1993; Kahrs 1994). It has been speculated that the insertion of the major neisserial ion channel PorB (known as the gonococcal P.I and the meningococcal class 2/3 proteins) into target cell membranes (Lynch 1984; Young 1983; Layh-Schmitt 1989) is a critical determinant for entry (Blake, 1985; Weel 1991b). PorB interferes with cell signalling, induces a transient membrane hyperpolarization and inhibits phosphatidylcholine phospholipase C activity (Haines 1988 and 1991; Lorenzen submitted). Complete internalization of the bacteria requires phosphorylation of host proteins at tyrosine residues (Grassmé submitted), but whether Opa protein, PorB and/or other bacterial factors trigger this event is still unclear.

Accomodation within professional phagocytes

Neisserial colonization of the human mucosa is characteristically associated with an inflammatory response involving recruitment and activation of professional phagocytes. Morphological data suggest that in the natural infection, the pathogenic *Neisseria* may reside inside phagocytes (Ward 1972; DeVoe 1973; Swanson 1974). Interaction of *Neisseria* with professional phagocytes is independently conferred by the pili and the variant Opa proteins. A striking difference is that the Opa- but not the pilus-mediated interaction causes a respiratory burst (Knepper submitted). Inhibition of the respiratory burst is due to the translocation of the neisserial PorB into the target cell membrane (Haines 1988; Lorenzen submitted). A function of PorB within phagocytes is the prevention of degranulation and phagosome acidification, which correlates with the intracellular survival of the bacteria (Weel 1991b). Thus, PorB is considered a key factor for cell infection, the accommodation of the pathogens within cells and the overall process of host infection (Brunham 1985; Cannon 1983; Sandström 1984). Contrasting with the situation of *Salmonella* or *Shigella* species which use the intracellular environment for rapid multiplication, intracellular accomodation of the pathogenic *Neisseriae* is considered a means for the long-term survival and escape from the humoral immune response rather than as a mechanism for bacterial multiplication, despite of the fact that prolonged intracellular survival has been difficult to establish *in vitro* (Swanson 1975; for review see Shafer 1989).

PorB shows interesting structural and functional similarities to mitochondrial porins suggesting that intraphagosomal accommodation of *Neisseriae* is to some extent related to mitochondrial endosymbiosis (Rudel submitted). For example, like eukaryotic porins PorB binds and is regulated by ATP/GTP. Patch clamp studies indicate that the PorB channel activity is decreased after insertion into human cells, however, it also opens at short intervals. It is speculated that PorB channel activity is regulated by additional cellular factors and thus prevents phagolysosome fusion by an as yet unknown mechanism. Interestingly, ATP/GTP binds to the gonococcal cell surface via PorB. However, ATP binding is lethal to most gonococcal strains, probably due to interference with PorB function. Revertible phase variants resistant to ATP can be isolated which exhibit an altered outer membrane profile. The ATP-resistant phenotype might be biologically significant, e.g. with respect to a possible cytosolic location of gonococci. In fact, cytosolic locations have been occasionally observed in the case of gonococcci and meningococci (e.g. Shaw 1988), indisputable evidence, however, is missing.

Conclusions and outlook

In addition to providing the fundament for the development of vaccines and novel drugs in order to prevent disease, bacterial pathogenesis models serve as a platform to study the complexity of interactions between microbial populations and higher organisms. The strength, and to the same extent a weakness, of the *Neisseria* model is the narrow host range of the species included. This minimizes the number of interactions a microbe can possibly encounter and therefore may help us specify the evolutionary forces governing microbial behaviour. Thus far the biological meaning of many genetic processes remains obscure, an example being the irreversible loss of essential infection determinants, such as *pilE* (Segal 1985) and similar examples in other systems, which seems to drive the bacteria into a dead end. Understanding the evolutionary basis is crucial if we are to explain the pathogenesis which presently is best described as an accidental case (Falkow 1990). In this field, the genus *Neisseria* offers a wide scenario for the comparison on multiple levels of pathogenic and non-pathogenic species inter-connected by the flow of genetic material.

Apart from evolutionary considerations, the *Neisseria* model represents a paradigm of escape and adaptive functions and contributes significantly to the current adventure of unravelling the biochemical processes of cellular cross-talk. Despite the experimental obstactle of genetic variability and the lack of an animal model, neisserial adhesins playing critical roles in target cell interaction have been sucessfully defined and other signalling factors have been identified, such as the PorB channel which inserts into target cell membranes and the Iga polyproteins which are capable of entering the nuclei of human cells. As in other systems, cytoscelletal reorganisation and phosphorylation of host cell proteins upon neisserial entry into epithelial cells can be demonstrated and the intracellular processing of bacteria contained in professional phagocytes is being studied. Research along these lines will not only extend our knowledge in terms of isolated pathogen host cell interactions but undoubtedly lead to a better understanding of the interplay between *Neisseria* and the immune system: Key questions relate to the modulation of antigen presentation and cytokine production, and finally to the mechanism of the inflamatory response associated with neisserial infections.

Acknowledgements

I am particular grateful to my past and present coworkers for their respective contributions to our understanding of the molecular basis of neisserial infections.

References

Achtman, M., (1994) - Clonal spread of serogroup A meningococci. A paradigm for the analysis of microevolution in bacteria. *Mol. Microbiol.* **11**, 15–22.

Aho, E.L., G.L. Murphy and J.G. Cannon, 1987 - Distribution of specific DNA sequences among pathogenic and commensal *Neisseria* species. *Infect. Immun.* **55**, 1009–1013.

Barlow, A.K., J.E. Heckels and I.N. Clarke, 1989 - The class 1 outer membrane protein of *Neisseria meningitidis*: cloning and structure of the gene. *Gene* **105**, 125–128.

Belland, R.J., T. Chen, J. Swanson and S.H. Fischer, 1992 - Human neutrophil response to recombinant neisserial Opa proteins. *Mol. Microbiol.* **6**, 1729–1737.

Bhat, K.S., C.P. Gibbs, O. Barrera, S.G. Morrison, F. Jähnig, A. Stern, E.M. Kupsch, T.F. Meyer and J. Swanson, 1991 - The repertoire of opacity proteins displayed by *Neisseria gonorrhoeae* MS11 outer surface are encoded by a family of 11 complete genes. *Mol. Microbiol.* **5**, 1889–1901; Corrigendum (1992) **6**, 1073–1076.

Biswas, G.D., K.L. Burnstein and P.F. Sparling, 1986 - Linearization of donor DNA during plasmid transformation in *Neisseria gonorrhoeae*. *J. Bacteriol.* **168**, 756–761.

Biswas, G.D., S.A. Lacks and P.F. Sparling, 1989 - Transformation-deficient mutants of piliated *Neisseria gonorrhoeae*. *J. Bacteriol.* **171**, 657–664.

Blake, M.S., 1985 - Functions of outer membrane proteins of *Neisseria gonorrhoeae*. In: G.G. Jackson, H. Thomas (eds.). The pathogenesis of bacterial infections. Springer-Verlag KG, Berlin, pp. 51–66.

Brunham, R.C., F. Plummer, L. Slaney and F. de Witt, 1985 - Correlation of auxotype and protein I type with expression of disease due to *Neisseria gonorrhoeae*. *J. Infect. Dis.* **152**, 339–343.

Cannon, J.G., T.M. Buchanan and P.F. Sparling, 1983 - Confirmation of association of protein I serotype of *Neisseria gonorrhoeae* with ability to cause disseminated infection. *Infect. Immun.* **40**, 816–819.

Catlin, B.W. and L.S. Cunningham, 1961 - Transforming activities and base contents of desoxyribonucleate preparations from various *Neisseriae*. *J. Gen. Microbiol.* **26**, 303–312.

Chen, J.C.R., P. Bavoil and V.L. Clark, 1991 - Enhancement of the invasive ability of *Neisseria gonorrhoeae* by contact with Hec1B, an adenocarcinoma endometrial cell line. *Mol. Microbiol.* **5**, 1531–1538.

Connell, T.D., W.J. Black, T.H. Kawula, D.S. Barritt, J.A. Dempsey, K. Kverneland, A. Stephenson, B.S. Schepart, G.L. Murphy and J.G. Cannon, 1988 - Recombination among 11 genes of *Neisseria gonorrhoeae* generates new coding sequences and increases structural variability in the protein I family. *Mol. Microbiol.* **2**, 227–236.

DeVoe, I.W., J.E. Gilchrist and D.W. Storm, 1973 - Ultrastructural studies on the fate of group B meningococci in human peripheral blood leukocytes. *Can. J. Microbiol.* **19**, 1355–1359.

Dorward, D.W. and C.F. Garon, 1989 - DNA-binding proteins in cells and membrane blebs of *Neisseria gonorrhoeae*. *J. Bacteriol.* **171**, 4196–4201.

Edwards, U., A. Müller, S. Hammerschmidt, R. Gerardy-Schahn and M. Frosch, 1994 - Molecular analysis of the biosynthesis pathway of the alpha-2,8 polysialic acid capsule by *Neisseria meningitidis* serogroup B. *Mol. Microbiol.* **14**, 141–149.

Facius, D. and T.F. Meyer, 1993 - A novel determinant (*comA*) essential for natural transformation competence in *Neisseria gonorrhoeae* and the effect of a *comA* defect on pilin variation. *Mol. Microbiol.* **10**, 699–712.

Falkow, S., 1990 - The 'Zen' of bacterial pathogenicity. In: Iglewski B.H., Clark V.L. (eds.). Molecular basis of bacterial pathogenesis. Academic Press, New York, pp. 3–9.

Feavers, I.M., A.B. Heath, J.A. Bygraves and M.C.J. Maiden, 1992 - Role of horizontal genetic exchange in the antigenic variation of the class 1 outer membrane protein of *Neisseria meningitidis*. *Mol. Microbiol.* **6**, 489–495.

Frosch, M., C. Weiseberger and T.F. Meyer, 1989 - Molecular characterization and expression in *Escherichia coli* of the gene complex encoding the polysccharide capsule of *Neisseria meningitidis* group B. *Proc. Natl. Acad. Sci. USA* **86**, 1669–1673.

Frosch, M. and T.F. Meyer, 1992 - Transformation-mediated exchange of virulence determinants by co-cultivation of pathogenic Neisseriae. *FEMS Microbiol. Lett.* **100**, 3435–3439.

Fussenegger, M., 1996 - A novel peptidiglycan-linked lipoprotein (ComL) that functions in natural transformation competence of Neisseria gonorrhoeae, unpublished.

Gibbs, C.P., B.-Y. Reimann, E. Schultz, A. Kaufmann, R. Haas and T.F. Meyer, 1989 - Reassortment of pilin genes in *Neisseria gonorrhoeae* occurs by two distinct mechanisms. *Nature* **338**, 651–652.

Goodman, S.D. and J.J. Scocca, 1988 - Identifcation and arrangement of the DNA sequence recognized in specific transformation of *Neisseria gonorrhoeae*. *Proc. Natl. Acad. Sci. USA* **85**, 6982–6896.

Gotschlich, E.C., 1994 - Genetic locus for the biosynthesis of the variable portion of *Neisseria gonorrhoeae* lipooligosaccharide. *J. Exp. Med.* **180**, 2181–2190.

Gunn, J.S., A. Piekarowicz, R. Chien and D.C. Stein, 1992 - Cloning and linkage analysis of *Neisseria gonorrhoeae* DNA methyltransferases. *J. Bacteriol.* **174**, 5654–5660.

Haas, R., S. Veit and T.F. Meyer, 1992 - Silent pilin genes of *Neisseria gonorrhoeae* MS11 and the occurrence of related hypervariant sequences among gonococcal isolates. *Mol. Microbiol.* **6**, 197–208.

Haines, K.A., L. Yeh, M.S. Blake, P. Cristello, H. Korchak and G. Weissmann, 1988 - Protein 1, a translocatable ion channel from *Neisseria gonorrhoeae*, selectively inhibits exocytosis from human neutrophils without inhibiting O_2^- generation. *J. Biol. Chem.* **263**, 945–951.

Haines, K.A., J. Reibman, X.Y. Tang, M. Blake and G. Weissmann, 1991 - Effects of protein 1 of *Neisseria gonorrhoeae* on neutrophil activation - Generation of diacylglycerol from phosphatidylcholine via a specific phospholipase C is associated with exocytosis. *J. Cell Biol.* **114**, 433–442.

Halter, R., J. Pohlner and T.F. Meyer, 1989 - Mosaic-like organisation of IgA protease genes in *Neisseria gonorrhoeae* generated by horizontal genetic exchange in vivo. *EMBO J.* **8**, 2737–2744.

Hebeler, B.H. and F.E. Young, 1975 - Autolysis of *Neisseria gonorrhoeae*. *J. Bacteriol.* **122**, 385–391.

Hobbs, M. and J.S. Mattick, 1993 - Common components in the assembly of type-4 fimbriae, DNA transfer systems, filamentous phage and protein secretion apparatus. *Mol. Microbiol.* **10**, 233–243.

Hobbs, M.M., A. Seiler, M. Achtman and J.G. Cannon, 1994 - Microevolution within a clonal population of pathogenic bacteria: recombination, gene duplication and horizontal genetic exhange in the *opa* gene family of *Neisseria meningitidis*. *Mol. Microbiol.* **12**, 171–180.

Johnson, S.C., R.C.Y. Chung, C.D. Deal, J.W. Boslego, J.C. Sadoff, S.W. Wood, Jr. C.C. Brinton and E.D. Tramont, 1991 - Human immunization with Pgh 3–2 gonococcal pilus results in cross-reactive antibody to the cyanogen bromide fragment-2 of pilin. *J. Infect. Dis.* **163**, 128–134.

Jonsson, A.-B., G. Nyberg and S. Normark, 1991 - Phase variation of gonococcal pili by frame shift mutation in pilC, a novel gene for pilus assembly. *EMBO J.* **10**, 477–488.

Kahrs, A.F., A. Bihlmaier, D. Facius and T.F. Meyer, 1994 - Generalized transposon shuttle mutagenesis in *Neisseria gonorrhoeae*: a method for isolating epithelial cell invasion-defective mutants. *Mol. Microbiol.* **12**, 819–831.

Kellogg, Jr. D.S., I.R. Cohen, L.C. Norins, A.L. Schroeter and G. Reising, 1968 - *Neisseria gonorrhoeae*. II. colonial variation and pathogenicity during 35 months *in vitro. J. Bacteriol.* **96**, 596–605.

Koomey, J.M., E.C. Gotschlich, K. Robbins, S. Bergström and J. Swanson, 1987 - Effects of *recA* mutations on pilus antigenic variation and phase transitions in *Neisseria gonorrhoeae. Genetics* **117**, 391-398.

Kupsch, E.-M., B. Knepper, T. Kuroki, I. Heuer and T.F. Meyer, 1993 - Variable opacity (Opa) outer membrane proteins account for the cell tropisms displayed by *Neisseria gonorrhoeae* for human leukocytes and epithelial cells. *EMBO J.* **12**, 641–650.

Lambden, P.R., J.E. Heckels, L.T. James and P.J. Watt, 1979 - Variations in surface protein composition associated with virulence properties in opacity types of *Neisseria gonorrhoeae. J. Gen. Microbiol.* **114**, 305–312.

Lambden, P.R., J.N. Robertson and P.J. Watt, 1980 - Biological properties of two distinct pilus types produced by isogenic variants of *Neisseria gonorrhoeae* P9. *J. Bacteriol.* **141**, 393–396.

Layh-Schmitt, G., S. Schmitt and T.M. Buchanan, 1989 - Interaction of non-piliated *Neisseria gonorrhoeae* strain 7122 and protein IA with an epithelial cell monolayer. *Zbl. Bakteriol. Inf. J. Med. Microbiol.* **271**, 158–170.

Lorenzen, D., J. Pandit, T. Rudel, M. Ernst and T.F. Meyer, 1996 - Inhibition of Myeloperoxidase (MPO)-dependent oxidative metabolism in human phagocytes by the neisserial pore protein P. I. In preparation.

Lynch, E.C., M.S. Blake, E.C. Gotschlich and A. Mauro, 1984 - Studies on porins: Spontaneously transferred from whole cells and from proteins of *Neisseria gonorrhoeae* and *Neisseria meningitidis. Biophys. J.* **45**, 104–107.

Makino, S., J.P.M. van Putten and T.F. Meyer, 1991 - Phase variation of the opacity outer membrane protein controls the invasion of *Neisseria gonorrhoeae* into human epithelial cells. *EMBO J.* **10**, 1307–1315.

Mandrell, R.E. and M.A. Apicella, 1993 - Lipo-oligosaccharides (LOS) of mucosal pathogens: Molecular mimicry and host-modification of LOS. *Immunobiol.* **187**, 382–402.

Maynard Smith, J., N.H. Smith, M. O'Rourke and B.G. Spratt, 1993 - How clonal are bacteria? *Proc. Natl. Acad. Sci. USA* **90**, 4384–4388.

McGee, Z.A., A.P. Johnson and D. Taylor-Robinson, 1981 - Pathogenic mechanisms of *Neisseria gonorrhoeae*: observations on damage to human fallopian tubes in organ culture by gonococci of colony type 1 or type 4. *J. Infect. Dis.* **143**, 413–422.

Meyer, T. F., R. Haas, A. Stern, M. Frosch, F. Jähnig, K. Muraldharan and S. Veit, 1986 - Variable and conserved proteins on the surface of pathogenic Neisseria. In: Bacterial Vaccines and Local Immunity, *Annali Sclavo, Siena* **1-2**, 407–414.

Muir, L.L., R.A. Strugnell and J.K. Davies, 1988 - Proteins that appear to be associated with pili in *Neisseria gonorrhoeae. Infect. Immun.* **56**, 1743–1747.

Nassif, X, J. Lowy, P. Stenberg, P. O'Gaora, A. Ganji and M. So, 1993 - Antigenic variation of pilin regulates adhesion of *Neisseria meningitidis* to human epithelial cells. *Mol. Microbiol.* **8**, 719–725.

Olyhoek, A.J.M., J. Sarkari, M. Bopp, G. Morelli and M. Achtman, 1991 - Cloning and expression in *Escherichia coli* of *opc*, the gene for an unusual class 5 outer membrane protein from *Neisseria meningitidis* (meningococci/surface antigen). *Microb. Pathog.* **11**, 249–257.

O'Rourke, M. and E. Stevens, 1993 - Genetic structures of *Neisseria gonorrhoeae* populations: a non-clonal pathogen. *J. Gen. Microbiol.* **139**, 2603–11.

Parge, H.E., S.L. Bernstein, C.D. Deal, D.E. McRee, D. Christensen, M.A. Capozza, B.W. Kays, T.M. Fieser, D. Draper, M. So, E. Getzoff and J.A. Tainer, 1990 - Biochemical purification and crystallographic characterization of the fiber-forming protein pilin from *Neisseria gonorrhoeae. J. Biol. Chem.* **265**, 2278–2285.

Robertson, B.D. and T.F. Meyer, 1992 - Genetic variation in pathogenic bacteria. *Trends Genet.* **8**, 422–27.

Robertson, J.N., P. Vincent and M.E. Ward, 1977 - The preparation and properties of gonococcal pili. *J. Gen. Microbiol.* **102**, 169–177.

Rothbard, J.B., R. Fernandez, L. Wang, N.N.H. Teng and G.K. Schoolnik, 1985 - Antibodies to peptides corresponding to a conserved sequnec of gonococcal pilins block bacterial adhesion. *Proc. Natl. Acad. Sci. USA* **82**, 915–919.

Rudel, T., J.P.M. van Putten, C.P. Gibbs, R. Haas and T.F. Meyer, 1992 - Interaction of two variable proteins (pilE and pilC) required for pilus-mediated adherence of *Neisseria gonorrhoeae* to human epithelial cells. *Mol. Microbiol.* **6**, 3439–3450.

Rudel, T., D. Facius, R. Barten, I. Scheuerpflug, E. Nonnenmacher and T.F. Meyer, 1995a - Role of pili and the phase-variable PilC protein in natural competence for transformation of *Neisseria gonorrhoeae. Proc. Natl. Acad. Sci. USA.* **92**, 7986–7990.

Rudel, T., I. Scheuerpflug and T.F. Meyer, 1995b - PilC protein identified as a type IV pilus tip-located adhesin essential for the attachment of pathogenic *Neisseria* species to human epithelial cells. *Nature* **373**, 357–359.

Rudel, T., H.J. Boxberger and T.F. Meyer, 1995c - Pilus biogenesis and epithelial cell adherence of *Neisseria gonorrhoeae pilC* double knock-out mutants. *Mol. Microbiol.* **7**, 1057–1071.

Rudel, T., A. Schmid, R. Benz, H.A. Kolb, F. Lang and T.F. Meyer, 1996 - Modulation of Neisseria porin (PorB) by cytosolic ATP/GTP of target cells: parallels between pathogen accommodation and mitochondrial endosymbiosis. *Cell* **85**, 391–402.

Sandström, E.G., J.S. Knapp, L.B. Reller, S.E. Thompson, E.W. Hook III and K.K. Holmes, 1984 - Serogrouping of *Neisseria gonorrhoeae*: Correlation of serogroup with disseminated gonoccocal infection. *Sex. Transm. Dis.* **11**, 77–80.

Schneider, H., C.A. Hammack, M.A. Apicella and J.M. Griffis, 1998 - Instability of expression of lipooligosaccharides and their epitopes in *Neisseria gonorrhoeae. Infect. Immun.* **56**, 942–946.

Schneider, H., J.M. Griffis, J.W. Boslego, P.J. Hitchcock, K.M. Zahos and M.A. Apicella, 1991 - Expression of paragloboside-like lipooligosachharides may be a necessary component of gonococcal pathogenesis in men. *J. Exp. Med.* **174**, 1601–1606.

Schoolnik, G.K., R. Fernandez, J.Y. Tai, J. Rothbard and E.C. Gotschlich, 1984 - Gonococcal pili. Primary structure and receptor binding domain. *J. Exp. Med.* **159**, 1351–1370.

Segal, E., E. Billyard, M. So, S. Störzbach and T.F. Meyer TF, 1985 - Role of chromosomal rearrangement in *Neisseria gonorrhoeae* pilus phase variation. *Cell* **40**, 293–300.

Shafer, W.M. and R.F. Rest, 1989 - Interactions of gonococci with phagocytic cells. *Ann. Rev. Microbiol.* **43**, 121–145.

Shaw, J.H. and S. Falkow, 1988 - Model for invasion of human tissue culture cells by *Neisseria gonorrhoeae. Infect. Immun.* **56**, 1625–1632.

Simon, D. and R.F. Rest, 1992 - *Escherichia coli* expressing *Neisseria gonorrhoeae* opacity -associated outer membrane protein invade human cervical and endometrial epithelial cells. *Proc. Natl. Acad. Sci. USA* **89**, 5512–5516.

Smith, H., 1991 - The Leeuwenhoek lecture 1991. The influence of the host on microbes that cause disease. *Proc. R. Soc. Lond. B* **246**, 97–105.

Sparling, P.F., 1966 - Genetic transformation of *Neisseria gonorrhoeae* to streptomycin resistance. *J. Bacteriol.* **92**, 1364–1371.

Spratt, B.G., L.D. Bowler, Q.-Y. Zhang, J. Zhon and J.M. Smith, 1992 - Role of interspecies transfer of chromosomal genes in the evolution of penicillin resistance in pathogenic and commensal Neisseria species. *J. Mol. Evol.* **34**, 115–125.

Stephens, D.S., 1989 - Gonococcal and meningococcal pathogenesis as defined by human cell, cell culture, and organ culture assays. *Clin. Microbiol. Rev.* **2**, S104–111.

Stern, A., M. Brown, P. Nickel and T.F. Meyer, 1986 - Opacity genes in *Neisseria gonorrhoeae*: control of phase and antigenic variation. *Cell* **47**, 61–71.

Sullivan, K.M. and J.R. Saunders, 1989 - Nucleotide sequence and genomic organization of the *Ngo*PII restriction-modification system of *Neisseria gonorrhoeae. Mol. Gen. Genet.* **216**, 380–387.

Swanson, J., G. King and B. Zeligs, 1975 - Studies on gonococcus infection VII. *In vitro* killing of gonococci by human leukocytes. *Infect. Immun.* **11**, 65–68.

Swanson, J., K. Robbins, O. Barrera and J.M. Koomey, 1987 - Gene conversion variants generate structurally distinct pilin polypepetides in *Neisseria gonorrhoeae. J. Exp. Med.* **165**, 1016–1025.

Swanson, J. and B. Zeligs, 1974 - Studies on the gonococcus infection. VI. Electron microscopic study on *in vitro* phagocytosis by human leukocytes. *Infect. Immun.* **10**, 645–656.

Taha, M.-K., M. Larribe, B. Dupuy, D. Giorgini and C. Marchal, 1992 - Role of pilA, an essential regulatory gene of *Neisseria gonorrhoeae*, in the stress response. *J. Bacteriol.* **174**, 5978-5981.

van Putten, J.P.M., 1993 - Phase variation of lipopolysaccharide directs interconversion of invasive and immuno-resistant phenotypes of *Neisseria gonorrhoeae. EMBO J.* **12**, 4043–4051.

van Putten, J.P.M. and S.M. Paul, 1995 - Binding of a syndecan-like cell surface proteoglycan receptors is required for *Neisseria gonorrhoeae* entry into human mucosal cells. *EMBO J.* **14**, 2144–2154.

Vázquez, J.A., L. de la Fuente, S. Berron, M. O'Rourke, N.H. Smith, J. Zhou and B.G. Spratt, 1993 - Ecological separation and genetic isolation of *Neisseria gonorrhoeae* and *Neisseria meningitidis. Curr. Biol.* **3**, 567–572.

Virji, M., C. Alexandrescu, D.J.P. Ferguson, J. Saunders and E.R. Moxon, 1992a - Variations in the expression of pili: the effect on adherence of *Neisseria meningitidis* to human epithelial and endothelial cells. *Mol. Microbiol.* **6**, 1271–1279.

Virji, M. and J.E. Heckels, 1984 - The role of common and type-specific antigenic domains in adhesion and virulence of gonococci for human epithelial cells. *J. Gen. Microbiol.* **130**, 1089–1095.

Virji, M., J.E. Heckels, W.J. Potts, C.A. Hart and J.R. Saunders, 1989 - Identification of epitopes recognized by monoclonal antibodies SM1 and SM2 which react with all pili of *Neisseria gonorrhoeae* but which differentiate between two structural classes of pili expressed by Neisseria meningitidis and the distributions of their encoding sequence in the genomes of Neisseria spp. *J. Gen. Microbiol.* **135**, 3239–3251.

Virji, M., K. Makepeace, D.J.P. Ferguson, M. Achtman and E.R. Moxon, 1993a - Meningococcal Opa and Opc proteins: their role in colonization and invasion of human epithelial and endothelial cells. *Mol. Microbiol.* **10**, 499–510.

Virji, M., K. Makepeace, D.J.P. Ferguson, M. Achtman, J. Sarkari and E.R. Moxon, 1992b - Expression of the Opc protein correlates with invasion of epithelial and endothelial cells by *Neisseria meningitidis. Mol. Microbiol.* **6**, 2785–2795.

Virji, M., J.R. Saunders, G. Sims, K. Makepeace, D. Maskell and D.L.P. Feguson, 1993b - Pilus-facilitated adherence of *Neisseria meningitidis* to hman epithelial and endothelialcells: modulation of adherence phenotype occurs concurrently with changes in primary amino acid sequences and the glycosylation status of pilin. *Mol. Microbiol.* **10**, 1013–1028.

Ward, M.E., A.A. Glynn and P.J. Watt, 1972 - Fate of *Neisseria gonorrhoeae* in polymorphonuclear leukocytes: an electronmicroscopic study of the natural disease. *Br. J. Exp. Path* **53**, 289–294.

Watt, P.J. and M.E. Ward, 1980 - Adherence of *Neisseria gonorrhoeae* and other *Neisseria* species to mammalian cells. In: E.H. Beachey (ed.). Bacterial Adherence, Receptors and Recognition, Series b Vol 6. Chapman and Hall, New York, pp. 252–287.

Weel, J.F.L., C.T.P. Hopman and J.P.M. Van Putten, 1991a - In situ expression and localization of *Neisseria gonorrhoeae* opacity proteins in infected epithelial cells: Apparent role of Opa proteins in cellular invasion. *J. Exp. Med.* **173**, 1395–1405.

Weel, J.F.L., C.T.P. Hopman and J.P.M. van Putten, 1991b - Bacterial entry and intracellular processing of *Neisseria gonorrhoeae* in epithelial cells: immunomorphological evidence for alterations in the major outer membrane protein P.IB. *J. Exp. Med.* **174**, 705–715.

Young, J.D.E., M. Blake, A. Mauro and Z.A. Cohn, 1983 - Properties of the major outer membrane protein from *Neisseria gonorrhoeae* incorporated into model lipid membranes. *Proc. Nat. Acad. Sci.* **80**, 3831–3835.

Zhang, Q.Y., D. DeRyckere, P. Lauer and J.M. Koomey, 1992 - Gene conversion in *Neisseria gonorrhoeae*: evidence for its role in pilus antigenic variation. *Proc. Natl. Acad. Sci. USA* **89**, 5366–5370.

Frits R. Mooi, Elisabeth M. Bik and Annelies E. Bunschoten

Analysis of a Genetic Event Associated with the Birth of the Current Cholera Epidemic in Asia

Abstract

All three cholera pandemics since 1881 have been caused by *Vibrio cholerae* strains of serotype O1 and it was therefore assumed that only this serotype has epidemic potential. Thus it was unexpected that the recent cholera epidemic in Asia was caused by a non-O1 strain with the novel serotype O139. We provide evidence that the O139 strain arose by horizontal transfer of DNA, involved cell wall polysaccharide synthesis, from a *V. cholerae* non-O1 strain to an O1 El Tor strain. After transfer, homologous recombination occurred resulting in the replacement of a large part of O1 *rfb* genes by non-O1 DNA. The acquired DNA has changed the antigenic properties of the accepting strain, increasing its fitness in a region where cholera is endemic and natural immunity against *V. cholerae* O1 is high. This genetic event may have caused the present cholera epidemic in Asia.

Introduction

Vibrio cholerae strains are natural inhabitants of brackish water and estuarine systems (Colwell and Huq, 1994). More than 140 *V. cholerae* serotypes have been identified, only a few of which are known to cause disease in humans (Sanyal, 1992). Strains with the serotype O1 are the causative agents of all three cholera pandemics recorded since 1881 (Barua, 1992). Non-O1 serotypes have never been associated with cholera epidemics, although they may cause local outbreaks. On this basis it was assumed that only O1 strains were able to cause epidemic cholera. Therefore, it was totally unexpected that an epidemic of cholera, which started in Madras in 1992, was caused by a non-O1 strain with the novel serotype O139 (Albert *et al.*, 1993, Bhattacharya *et al.*, 1993, Ramamurthy *et al.*, 1993). Since its emergence, the O139 strain has affected hundreds of thousands of people and has replaced *V. cholerae* O1 strains as the predominant cause of cholera in South-East Asia. There is a large degree of natural immunity against O1 strains in this region, and the rapid spread of the O139 strain may have been facilitated by the fact that it is not affected by immunity to O1 strains (Albert *et al.*, 1994). O139 has already been isolated from travellers in California, Estonia, Germany, Singapore and Hong Kong, and it has been suggested that this strain may be the cause of the next cholera pandemic.

Two hypotheses were suggested for genesis of the O139 strain. The O139 strain could be a derivative of a non-O1 serotype that has acquired the potential to cause epidemic cholera, or the O139 strain could be a derivative of an O1 strain with an altered O-antigen. There is now abundant evidence for the latter hypothesis (Morris, 1994). The O1 serogroup can be further differentiated in two biotypes, designated classical and El Tor, and the O139 strain is most similar to the El Tor biotype. However, there are important differences between the O139 and O1 strains. In contrast to the O1 strains, the O139 strain expresses a capsule (Johnson *et al.*, 1994; Weintraub *et al.*, 1994). Further, the O1 and O139 strains express a different LPS: the O139 LPS has a shorter O-side chain and a different sugar composition (Manning *et al.*, 1994; Waldor *et al.*, 1995). Thus it seemed likely that the O139 strain arose from an El Tor strain by acquisition of DNA involved in O-antigen and capsule synthesis. The aim of our research was to characterize this DNA and the molecular events which led to the genesis of the O139 strain.

Results and Discussion

Characterization of a DNA region involved in synthesis of the O139 antigen

Since the O1 and O139 strains express distinct O-antigens, we investigated whether differences could be observed between these strains in their chromosomal regions coding for O-antigen synthesis (Bik *et al.*, 1995). Using probes derived from the O1 gene cluster (Stroeher *et al.*, 1992, Fig. 1) we

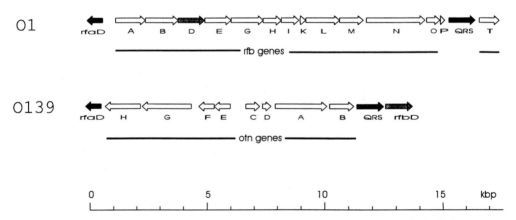

Fig. 1. Comparison of O1 and O139 DNA regions involved in cell wall polysaccharide synthesis. The representation of the O1 *rfb* region is based on Stroeher *et al.*, (1992). Homologous genes are indicated in black (>96% identity) or grey (68% identity). Abbreviation; kbp, kilo-base pairs.

Analysis of a genetic event

investigated whether genes, homologous to those involved in O1-antigen synthesis, could be detected in strain O139. Only *rfaD* and *rfbQRS* were detected in strain O139. This indicated that the genesis of O139 involved deletion of at least 15,000 base pairs (bp) of O1 chromosomal DNA. PCR analysis indicated that, like in the O1 strain, *rfaD* and *rfbQRS* were closely linked in the O139 chromosome, being separated by 12,000 bp of DNA. This DNA region was cloned and sequenced, and 11 open reading frames were found (Fig. 1). We have called this DNA region *otn*, for one-three-nine. As expected the *otn* DNA contained *rfaD* and *rfbQRS*. The O1 and O139 *rfaD* genes showed 2% sequence divergence, while *rfbQRS* genes showed 4% sequence divergence. Down stream of the *rfbQRS* genes, an open reading frame was observed which is homologous to the O1 *rfbD* gene, showing 32% sequence divergence with it. These observations suggest that the creation of strain O139 involved homologous recombination between the O1-antigen gene cluster and the *otn* DNA. One of the homologous regions involved in recombination could comprise *rfaD*, while the other region is probably located down stream of the *rfbQRS* genes.

It is also possible that the *rfbQRS* genes were involved in the genesis of strain O139. These genes comprise a putative insertion sequence element (Manning *et al.*, 1994), and a homologous element, designated the H-repeat, is found in *Escherichia coli* where it is involved in chromosomal rearrangements (Zhao *et al.*, 1993). More significantly, a homologous element is also found in *Salmonella enterica*, where it has been implicated in recombination between LPS gene clusters derived from different strains (Xiang *et al.*, 1994). It is an attractive hypothesis that the *rfbQRS* element has played a similar role in the creation of the O139 strain.

Homology searches indicated that the product of *otnA* showed significant similarity with an *E. coli* protein, KpsD, involved in transport of capsular precursors across the periplasmic space (Bronner *et al.*, 1993). The product of *otnB* showed significant similarity to a family of proteins found in *E. coli* and *S. enterica*, involved in regulation of O-antigen length (Batchelor *et al.*, 1992). This suggested that *otnA* and *otnB* are involved in O-antigen and/or capsule synthesis. To substantiate this assumption, we constructed an *otnA* mutant by allelic exchange, and analyzed this strain by means of the Ouchterlony double diffusion technique using sera raised against the O139 cell wall polysaccharides (not shown). The results indicated that the *otnA* mutant had lost the ability to synthesize cell wall polysaccharides which could be detected in the wild type strain by immune-precipitation.

The origin of the otn DNA

To determine the origin of the *otn* DNA, a probe consisting of *otnA* and *otnB* was used to screen more than 60 clinical and environmental *V. cholerae* isolates (Fig. 2B). DNA homologous to *otnAB* was not detected in O1 strains, neither the classical nor the El Tor biotype. Homologous DNA was detected, however, in a number of non-O1 strains, of serotype O69 and O141. The O69 strain is an

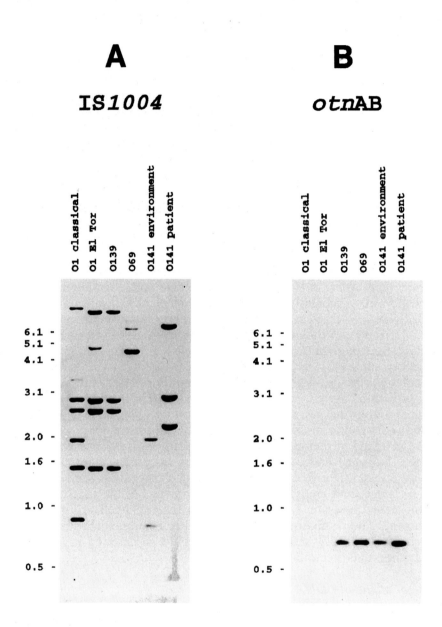

Fig. 2. Occurrence of *otnAB* DNA among *V. cholerae* O1 and non-O1 strains. (A) RFLP patterns of *V. cholerae* O1 and non-O1 strains. Chromosomal DNA was digested with *Hpa*II, and hybridized with IS*1004* DNA. (B) The membrane used in A was reprobed with *otnAB* DNA. Analyzed strains are indicated above the lanes. Molecular weight markers are indicated on the left (in kilo-bp). Reprinted by permission of Oxford University Press from Bik *et al.*, 1995.

Analysis of a genetic event

Indian patient isolate, while the O141 strains were isolated from a patient and the environment in the USA, respectively. Thus the *otnAB* DNA has a global distribution. Sequence analysis revealed that there was approximately 5% sequence divergence between the *otnAB* genes derived from the O139, O69 and O141 strains.

To study the genetic relatedness between these strains, we reprobed the same blot with an insertion sequence element which we have identified, and which can be used to differentiate *V. cholerae* strains (Fig 2A). The O1 and O139 strains showed very similar RFLP patterns. In fact the patterns of the El Tor and O139 strain were identical, with the exception of a 4,500 bp band. This band is derived from the part of O1-antigen gene cluster which was deleted from the O139 strain. The patterns of the O69 and O141 strains were totally unrelated. Interestingly, the RFLP patterns of the two O141 strains were are also unrelated. Thus there are genotypically unrelated strains with the same serotype (i.e. the O141 strains), and conversely, genotypically related strains with the different serotypes (i.e. the O1 and O139 strains). Using the RFLP analysis on a large number of non-O1 strains we have found more examples of this phenomenon, and it suggests a gene flow within the *V. cholerae* species through which strains may acquire the ability to synthesize new cell wall polysaccharides. This raises the possibility that there was a succession of different serotypes in the history of cholera, of which the O1 and O139 serotypes represent recent examples.

Acknowledgements

This work was supported by the Dutch Organization for Scientific Research (NWO), grant number 900-515-022.

References

Albert, M.J., A.K. Siddique, M.S. Islam, A.S. Faruque, M. Ansaruzzaman, S.M. Faruque and R.B. Sack, 1993 - Large outbreak of clinical cholera due to *Vibrio cholerae* non-O1 in Bangladesh, *Lancet* **341**, p. 704.

Albert, M.J., K. Alam, A.S. Rahman, S. Huda and R.B. Sack, 1994 - Lack of cross-protection against diarrhea due to *Vibrio cholerae* O1 after oral immunization of rabbits with *V. cholerae* O139 Bengal, *J. Infect. Dis.* **169**, 709–710.

Barua, D., 1992 - History of cholera, in, Barua, D. and W.B. Greenough III (eds), *Cholera*, Plenum Publishing Company, 1–35.

Batchelor, R.A., P. Alfino, E. Biffali, S.I. Hull and R.A. Hull, 1992 - Nucleotide sequences of the genes regulating O-polysaccharide antigen length (*rol*) from *Escherichia coli* and *Salmonella typhimurium*: protein homology and functional complementation, *J. Bacteriol.* **174**, 5228–5236.

Bhattacharya, M.K., S.K. Bhattacharya, S. Garg, P.K. Saha, D. Dutta, G.B. Nair, B.C. Deb and K.P. Das, 1993 - Outbreak of *Vibrio cholerae* non-O1 in India and Bangladesh, *Lancet* **341**, 1346–1347.

Bik, E.M., A.E. Bunschoten, R.D. Gouw and F.R. Mooi, 1995 - Genesis of the novel epidemic *Vibrio cholerae* O139 strain: evidence for horizontal transfer of genes involved in polysaccharide synthesis, *EMBO J.* **14**, 101–108.

Bronner, D., V. Sieberth, C. Pazzani, I.S. Roberts, G.J. Boulnois, B. Jann and K. Jann, 1993 - Expression of the capsular K5 polysaccharide of *Escherichia coli*: biochemical and electron microscope analyses of mutants with defects in region 1 of the K5 gene cluster, *J. Bacteriol.* **175**, 5984–5992.

Colwell, R.R. and A. Huq, 1994 - Vibrios in the environment: viable but non-culturable *Vibrio cholerae*, in, Wachsmuth, I.K., P.A. Blake and O. Olsvik (eds), *Vibrio cholerae and cholera - Molecular to Global perspectives*, Washington, DC, ASM Press, pp. 117–134.

Johnson, J.A., C.A. Salles, P. Panigrahi, M.J. Albert, A.C. Wright, R.J. Johnson and J.G. Morris, 1994 - *Vibrio cholerae* O139 synonym bengal is closely related to *Vibrio cholerae* El Tor but has important differences, *Infect. Immun.* **62**, 2108–2110.

Morris, J.G., 1994 - *Vibrio cholerae* 0139 Bengal, in, Wachsmuth, I.K., P.A. Blake and O. Olsvik (eds), *Vibrio cholerae and cholera - Molecular to Global perspectives*, Washington, DC, ASM Press, pp. 95-102.

Ramamurthy, T., S. Garg, R. Sharma, S.K. Bhattacharya, G.B. Nair, T. Shimada, T. Takeda, T. Karasawa, H. Kurazano, A. Pal, *et al.*, 1993 - Emergence of novel strain of *Vibrio cholerae* with epidemic potential in southern and eastern India, *Lancet* **341**, 703–704.

Sanyal, S.C., 1992 - Epidemiology and pathogenicity of non-O1 vibrio species and related organisms, in, Barua, D. and W.B. Greenough III (eds), *Cholera*, Plenum Publishing Company, pp. 57–65.

Stroeher, U.H., L.E. Karageorgos, R. Morona and P.A. Manning, 1992 - Serotype conversion in *Vibrio cholerae* O1, *Proc. Nat. Acad. Sci. USA* **89**, 2566–2570.

Waldor, M.K., R. Colwell and J.J. Mekalanos, 1995 - The *Vibrio cholerae* O139 serogroup antigen includes an O-antigen capsule and lipopolysaccharide virulence determinants, *Proc. Nat. Acad. Sci. USA* **91**, 11388-11392.

Weintraub, A., G. Widmalm, P.E. Jansson, M. Jansson, K. Hultenby and M.J. Albert, 1994 - *Vibrio cholerae* O139 Bengal possesses a capsular polysaccharide which may confer increased virulence, *Microb. Pathog.* **16**, 235–241.

Xiang, S., M. Hobbs and P.R. Reeves, 1994 - Molecular analysis of the *rfb* gene cluster of a group of D2 *Salmonella enterica* strain: evidence for its origin from an insertion sequence-mediated recombination event between group E and D1 strains, *J. Bacteriol.* **176**, 4357–4365.

Zhao, S., C.H. Sandt, G. Feulner, D.A. Vlazny, J.A. Gray and C.W. Hill, 1993 - *Rhs* elements in *Escherichia coli* K-12: complex composites of shared and unique components that have different evolutionary histories, *J. Bacteriol.* **175**, 2799–2808.

F. Rodríguez-Valera[1][*], J. García-Martínez[1], A. Zorraquino[2] and A.J. Martínez-Murcial

Genetic Diversity in Uropathogenic *Escherichia coli* as Shown by RAPD
(Random Amplified Polymorphic DNA), 16S-23S rDNA spacers and adhesin gene restriction patterns

Abstract

A collection of *Escherichia coli* strains isolated from urinary tract infections (UTI) and some representatives of the ECOR collection were characterized by using three different types of molecular markers. The strains were typed by RAPD (Random Amplified Polymorphic DNA). The 16S rDNA-23S rDNA spacers were amplified by PCR and subjected to restriction analysis. The presence or absence of G adhesins type II and/or III have also been assayed. Analysis of the spacers restriction patterns showed two markedly differentiated clusters designated α and β. Both RAPD and spacer restriction patterns originated similar clusters of strains showing a consistency in the evolution of the global genome with the sequence variation of the ribosomal spacers. Furthermore, the G adhesin type (and involvement in upper urinary tract infection) correlated well with the spacer groupings. The α and β clusters could be intraspecific groups produced by partial sexual isolation or other barriers that are originating a divergent evolution.

Molecular methods allow an extremely fine strain typing that can be used to establish the population structure of bacterial species. Here we have used three molecular approaches to characterize a collection of uropathogenic *Escherichia coli* (74 strains) obtained from three hospitals located in geographically distant towns in Spain, six representatives of the ECOR collection and other reference strains. The three markers investigated represent different levels of extension and, theoretically at least, of conservation of the genome. RAPD (Random Amplified Polymorphic DNA) can characterize a bacterial strain to the level of defining individual clones (only individuals sharing a very close common ancestor show identical RAPD patterns). To study intraspecies genomic diver-

[1] Departamento de Genética y Microbiología, Universidad de Alicante, Campus de San Juan, Apartado 374, 03080 Alicante, Spain.
[2] Hospital Universitario San Juan de Alicante, Carretera de Valencia s/n, San Juan de Alicante, Alicante, Spain.

sity, a RAPD band (characterized by size, but if required it can be hybridized or sequenced) can be used as a genetic marker, the absence of the band in one strain is a polymorphism affecting this locus (a different allele). If the band is present in two strains they share the same allele at this locus (Tibayrenc *et al.*, 1993). The amount of information obtained in a short time is enormous since an unlimited number of primers can be used and it requires very little time or investment. In addition RAPD allows a typing of the total genome with no distinction of the gene type or sequence.

The 16S rDNA-23S rDNA spacers were amplified by PCR and subjected to restriction analysis. Parts of them are stretches of non-coding DNA, presumably non-functional, and should exhibit a considerable degree of sequence variation by genetic drift. These sequence polymorphisms could make the spacer a fast molecular chronometer to measure short term phylogeny, i.e. a good marker of major intraspecies lineages. Recently, length and sequence variation of 16S-23S rRNA spacers have been used to discriminate between different species and strains of bacteria (Barry *et al.*, 1991; Jensen *et al.*, 1993, Kostman *et al.*, 1992; Dolzani *et al.*, 1994).

Finally, the presence and type of G adhesins in *Escherichia coli* were determined by PCR amplification followed by digestion with restriction enzymes. The presence of adhesins and P fimbriae are virulence factors that facilitate the colonization by *E. coli* of the upper urinary tract (Ikäheimo *et al.*, 1994). Three types (I, II and III) are known, with different binding specificities (Hultgren *et al.*, 1993). The possession of one type or other of adhesin genes has been considered as a trait that can be easily won or lost and horizontally transferred (Plos *et al.*, 1989).

All 16S-23S spacers amplified with 16S14F-231R were digested with endonucleases *Alu*I, *Cfo*I, *Dde*I, *Hae*III, *Hinf*I, *Rsa*I and *Taq*I, but polymorphisms were only obtained with *Hinf*I, *Rsa*I and *Taq*I, which were selected for comprehensive analysis. Twenty-six different patterns were distinguished from the 16S-23S spacer RFLPs. The data were analyzed by calculating the Jaccard coefficient of each pairwise comparison, the profile relationships were analyzed by generating the UPGMA dendrogram. The strains clustered in two large groups, named Groups α and β, with similarity levels below 70%. Group α contained 48 strains including ATCC25922, ECOR35, ECOR52 and ECOR58. Twenty-four (50%) of the strains within this group had identical RFLP patterns, conforming a sub-group, α2, represented by ECOR52. Group β comprised 33 strains including K12 (CECT102), DHSα, ECOR10, ECOR49 and ECOR44. Strains K12 and ECOR10 had identical patterns. Strains in Group α are frequently negative for sucrose (81%) and raffinose (95%), while those in Group β are positive (60% and 52% respectively).

Twelve primers out of 28 assayed generated informative RAPD prints (ranging from 200 to 2700 bp) that were reproducible and they were selected. As expected a wide diversity was shown by RAPD and only in the case of strains isolated from the same individual, an obvious case of relapse, were identical patterns found. A total of 107 RAPD prints obtained with eleven primers were used as markers for pattern comparison, and UPGMA relationships were calculated. The dendrogram of RAPD showed that most of the strains clustered with less than 80% similarity level which can be interpreted as having less than 80% common alleles for the loci studied. In spite of this high diversity two groups appear clearly separated with similarities around 40%. These two RAPD clusters precisely fit with the two groups (α and β) detected by RFLP of the spacers: 96% of the strains of one RAPD cluster belong to Group α and 90% of the other cluster to Group β of the spacer RFLP. Clustering by the UPGMA method has been carried out using the RAPD-prints of different primer combinations: primers A1, A2, A7, A8, A10 and A12; primers A16, A18, A28 and A29; and primers A2, A8, A12, A18 and A28. The clustering was well consistent in the four dendrograms obtained with different RAPD-print combinations and fits with Groups α and β at a similar level. It is noteworthy that reference strains clustered together in the same group in both spacer RFLP and RAPD dendrograms: ATCC25922, ECOR52, ECOR35 and ECOR58 in Group α and strains DH5α, R12 (CECT102), ECOR10, ECOR49 and ECOR44 in Group β. The fact that both RAPD and spacer restriction patterns originated similar clusters of strains showed a consistency of the evolution of the global genome and the sequence variation of the ribosomal spacers. The stability of the two groups, regardless of the number/type of genetic markers or group of strains used, is very high indicating that this grouping actually reflects a natural subdivision of the species.

A total of 32 strains contained one or more copies of the G adhesin gene, 21 of which were class II, 4 were class III and 7 strains contained both classes. The presence of adhesins was widely distributed among the strains of Group α: 50% of strains within this group showed patterns corresponding to classes II or/and III. Only 18% of Group β strains contained G adhesin Class II (6 out of 32) and none had type III. Although it is known that these genes are horizontally transferred (Plos *et al.*, 1989), the presence of G-adhesin was found to be more associated to Group α of UTI *E. coli* strains. Also the involvement in upper urinary tract infection correlated well with the spacer polymorphism, most of the strains isolated from pyelonephritis (6 out of 7) corresponded to the α rRNA spacer Group. This illustrates that in spite of the proven transferability of the adhesin genes, this happens rarely between strains of the α and β groups and this could also be true for other horizontally transferable markers.

The differences found between α and β Groups could be explained by a barrier to horizontal genetic transfer between the two groups, for example, due to a different restriction modification system, sensitivity to phages or recognition by sexual fimbriae. In fact, α and β groups could well be populations on their way to becoming new species, or they must be considered as such, if the establishment of recombinative barriers is part of the speciation process in bacteria as has been suggested (Dykhuizen *et al.*, 1991). The α and β clusters could be intraspecific groups produced by partial sexual isolation or other barriers that are originating a divergent evolution.

References

Barry, T., G. Colleran, M. Glennon, L.K. Dunican and F. Gannon, 1991 - The 16S/23S ribosomal spacer region as a target for DNA probes to identify eubacteria. *PCR Meth. Appl.* **1**, 51–56.

Dolzani, L., E. Tonin, C. Lagatolla and C. Monti-Bragadin, 1994 - Typing of *Staphylococcus aureus* by amplification of the 16S-23S rRNA intergenic spacer sequences. *FEMS Microb. Lett.* **119**, 167–174.

Dykhuizen, D.E. and L. Green, 1991 - Recombination in *Escherichia coli* and the definition of biological species. *J. Bacteriol.* **173**, 7257–7268.

Hultgren, S.J., F. Jacob-Dubuisson, C.H. Jones and C.-I. Bränden, 1993 - PapD and superfamily of periplasmic immunoglobulin-like pilus chaperones. *Adv. Protein Chem.* **44**, 99–123.

Ikäheimo, R., A. Siitonen, U. Karkkäinen, J. Mustonen, T. Heiskanen and P.H. Mäkela, 1994 - Community-acquired pyelonephritis in adults: characteristics of *E. coli* isolates in bacteremic and non-bacteremic patients. *Scandinavian J. Infect. Dis.* **26**, 289–296.

Jensen, M.A., J.A. Webster and N. Straus, 1993 - Rapid identification of bacteria on the basis of polymerase chain reaction-amplified ribosomal DNA spacer polymorphisms. *Appl. Environ. Microbiol.* **59**, 945–952.

Kostman, J.R., T.D. Edlind, J.J. LiPuma and T.L. Stull, 1992 - Molecular epidemiology of *Pseudomonas cepacia* determined by polymerase chain reaction ribotyping. *J. Clin. Microbiol.* **30**, 2084–2087.

Plos, K., S.I. Hull, R.A. Hull, B.R. Levin, F. Orskov and C. Suanborg-Eden, 1989 - Distribution of the P-associated-pilus (pap) region among *Escherichia coli* from natural sources: evidence for horizontal gene transfer. *Infect. Immun.* **57**, 1604–1611.

Tibayrenc, M., K. Neubauer, C. Barnabé, F. Guerrini, D. Skarecky and F.J. Ayala, 1993 - Genetic characterization of six parasitic protozoa: Parity between random-primer DNA typing and multilocus enzyme electrophoresis. *Proc. Nat. Acad. Sci., USA* **90**, 1335–1339.

F. Schut

16S rRNA Hybridization Probes for the Major Groups of Intestinal Bacteria: Development and *in situ* Application

> *'Whenever a man gets the idea that he is going to work out the bacteriology of the intestinal tract of any mammal, the time has come to have him quietly removed to some suitable institution'.* Jordan, *In*: Gorbach *et al.*, 1967.

Abstract

Investigations into the role of the gut microflora in pathogenesis are continuously frustrated by technical limitations. We are currently developing 16S rRNA targeted oligonucleotide probes for the enumeration of various phylogenetic groups of intestinal bacteria. Preliminary results show that bifidobacteria are grossly overestimated by cultural methods, and that members of the *Bacteroides vulgatus* cluster are underestimated. Microscopic image analysis in combination with 16S rRNA hybridization probes has proven to be a very powerful technique in ecological studies of intestinal flora.

The intestinal microflora

The richest and most complex part of the human intestinal microflora resides in the colon. Normal populations exceed 10^{11} per gram of stool and consist of a mixed culture of an estimated 100–400 species of bacteria (Moore and Holdeman, 1974). The initial inoculum is derived from the mother at the time of birth and although the climax flora alters as the subject ages (Mitsuoka, 1992) it is fairly constant in composition with *Bacteroides* and *Eubacterium* spp. dominating in adults. The stability of the gut flora can be appreciated when bearing in mind that food and drinks are in actuality minor components of the intestinal contents. Saliva (1.0 litre/day), gastric (1.5 l/d) and pancreatic (1.2 l/d) secretions, bile (1.0 l/d) and secretions of the glands in small and large intestine (2.0 l/d) form the bulk of the estimated 7 litres of fluid that enters the intestinal tract daily (Guyton, 1986). These highly concentrated endogenous secretia ensure a constant intestinal environment thus enabling the digestive enzymes to operate under controlled conditions.

The composition of the diet, and the administration of specific food supplements such as fibre, has been suggested to influence the composition and activity of the flora (Benno *et al.*, 1989; Mitsuoka, 1992). However, direct evidence is difficult to obtain due to statistical inaccuracy of the cultural technique employed (Gorbach *et al.*, 1967; Finegold *et al.*, 1974), a high inter-subject variability (Minelli *et al.*, 1993), the relatively low numbers of subjects that can be investigated (Drasar *et al.*, 1986), and the difficulty in determining causative relationships from observed correlations (e.g. Benno *et al.*, 1989).

Over 95% of the bacteria encountered in faeces are non-sporulating, strict anaerobes and pre-reduced, anaerobically sterilized (PRAS) media or anaerobic chambers are essential for cultivation of these organisms (Holdeman *et al.*, 1977). Although it is relatively easy to obtain a total viable count, counting of individually identifiable bacterial species is laborious and time consuming. Viable counts of the various aerobic and facultatively anaerobic species can be obtained by using selective media. However, such media are not available for most of the strict anaerobes. Since some 30–40 species account for 99% of the flora, several hundred isolates from each sample should be identified for reliable statistics and end-product analysis of fermentation in pure cultures is essential for reliable identification. As a result, studies on population dynamics of the intestinal flora are often limited in the number of subjects or the number of species investigated and, as a consequence, the observed changes in composition are often not statistically significant.

Clinical relevance: intra-abdominal sepsis as a case

Due to the advances in medical technology and the significant elevation in live expectancy of the severely ill, an increasing number of patients in hospitals have compromised immune systems. Subjects undergoing major surgery (e.g. transplantations), chemotherapy as a treatment for cancer, and those with major trauma form the majority of such patients. Concurrently, the type of infection has changed from predominantly pathogenic to potentially pathogenic, or opportunistic. Furthermore, antibiotic resistance among nosocomial infections is becoming a world-wide threat and treatment may soon become ineffective. It is expected that alternative strategies for infection prevention will arise from knowledge on the natural physiological control of potential pathogens. However, up till now such studies have rarely been performed.

Although probably not as important on a world-wide scale as colon cancer, intra-abdominal infections are in this respect of significant interest due to the presumed involvement of normal host immunity, gut flora, and antibiotics. Almost all bacteria isolated from intra-abdominal infections are indigenous to the intestinal tract. Whether they have escaped from the intestine by 'naturally' occurring translocation or after perforation of the gut wall is the subject of debate (Sedman *et al.*, 1994), but the excessive accumulation of opportunistic microbes on the mucosal surface is believed to be very hazardous in this context (McClean *et al.*, 1994). The predominance of certain isolates does not always correlate with the use of antibiotics (Baron *et al.*, 1992; Sawyer *et al.*, 1992). It is probably through changes in the structure of the mucous colonizing community as a whole that certain opportunists gain a foothold (Kennedy and Volz, 1985; Van der Waaij, 1989). Antibiotics greatly affect the community structure and for both *Candida* and enterococcal intra-abdominal infections antimicrobial therapy has already been identified as a major risk factor (Kujath *et al.*, 1990; Boulanger *et al.*, 1991).

So, although immediate antimicrobial treatment during peritonitis is essential, especially in the case of *Candida* infections, the increased use of antimicrobial agents in immunocompromised hosts will promote changes in the normal intestinal flora and relatively harmless organisms can suddenly give rise to serious complications (McClean *et al.*, 1994).

The human intestinal flora is responsible for a number of other health disorders. Through the production of carcinogens, some species of the intestinal flora are believed to play a role in the development of colon cancer. Crohn's disease, rheumatoid arthritis and chronic diarrhoea, are all believed to be related to intestinal bacteria or their products. Furthermore, there are indications that graft versus host reactions after transplantation are also influenced by the gut flora. The development of fundamental insight in the interaction between the healthy host and its gut flora is of primary importance to the understanding of the pathogenesis of these diseases.

The use of 16S rRNA probes for enumeration

The above clinical examples serve to illustrate the need for detailed and rapid community-level screening of the composition of the intestinal flora. Only when changes in the composition are accurately described can relationships with pathogenesis be recognized. The possibility of using 16S rRNA hybridization probes for this purpose deserves investigation.

Each living cell contains ribosomes for protein synthesis. Several tens of thousands of ribosomes are present in growing cells. Because of evolutionary changes, the sequence of the nucleotides in the rRNA molecules is unique in each bacterial species. Therefore, the bacterial ribosome is uniquely suited as a phylogenetic (evolutionary) or taxonomic marker (Olsen *et al.*, 1986; Pace *et al.*, 1986). Synthetic deoxyoligonucleotide probes can be constructed which hybridize specifically to a certain sequence of nucleotides in the rRNA molecules. The specificity of the oligonucleotide probes can be adjusted to fit any taxonomic level, from kingdom to subspecies. If a fluorescent molecule is attached to the probe, individual bacterial cells can be identified by using an epifluorescence microscope. Since the 16S rRNA sequence of over 2,000 bacterial species is currently known (Larsen *et al.*, 1993), most bacterial groups can be included in searches for taxon specific 16S rRNA sequences.

Presently, species and group-specific hybridization probes can be developed on a rational basis, the essence of which lies in the identification of a unique sequence of approximately 20 nucleotides in the sequence of the target organism(s). Shorter stretches (10 bases) harbour the danger that the same sequence occurs at other (unforeseen) regions in one of the three ribosomal RNA's. Long sequences (50 bases) have the disadvantage that the mismatches - necessary for discrimination between target and non-target cells - do not result in a significant decrease of the dissociation temperature of the hybrid complex. This dissociation temperature can be estimated from the relationship

$T_d = 81.5 + 16.6 \log(Na^+) + 0.41(\%G + C)\text{-}820/\text{probelength}$
(Stahl and Amann, 1991).

The 16S rRNA contains various 'conserved' regions essential for the biochemical function of the ribosome. Such regions are used as annealing sites for primers used in PCR amplification and sequencing of the 16S (Lane, 1991). Other regions are hypervariable by nature and can serve as target regions for species and subspecies-specific hybridization probes. Sequences of intermediate specificity can also be found and these can be used to distinguish higher taxonomic groups.

During an extensive study, using cultural methods of enumeration, some 200 species of bacteria have been isolated from human faecal samples (Finegold *et al.*, 1974). Approximately 30 of these are numerically important and represent 10 distinct genera. Genus specific probes could thus prove appropriate in describing community structures at large. However, the natural classification system for bacteria, based on phenetic characteristics, is known not to comply fully with genetically based methods: not all taxonomic genera are monophyletic on the basis of their 16S rRNA sequence. *Eubacterium* spp., for example, are clustered with several *Clostridium* and *Peptostreptococcus* spp. and peptostreptococci themselves are spread over several distinct phylogenetic clusters (fig. 1). Within these phylogenetic clusters, however, conserved regions can be identified and 16S rRNA probes designed for such regions can be used to identify the majority of the population to a well defined taxonomic level. Only a dozen probes is thus required for the enumeration of the various phylogenetic groups of the gut flora (fig. 1).

Although many copies of the ribosome should ensure sufficient signal, reality is often far from ideal. The accessibility of the target region, the number of fluorochromes attached to the probe, the hybridization temperature, the metabolic status of the cells and the level of autofluorescence of non-target cells are important factors in obtaining sufficient specific fluorescent signal. Optical aid in the form of CCD-camera's is often required for small and slowly growing cells with little rRNA. Image analysis can be very helpful in discriminating between non-fading autofluorescence and rapidly fading fluorochrome

Fig. 1. (opposite page) Unrooted distance tree obtained after Kimura-2 parameter analysis and neighbour joining of 200 nucleotides of the 16S rRNA sequence of some bacterial species isolated from human faecal samples. Analysis was performed using MEGA software. The assignment of the twelve large phylogenetic clusters is supported by findings of the RDP project (Larsen *et al.*, 1993). Fluorescent oligonucleotide probes have been developed for all clusters assigned.

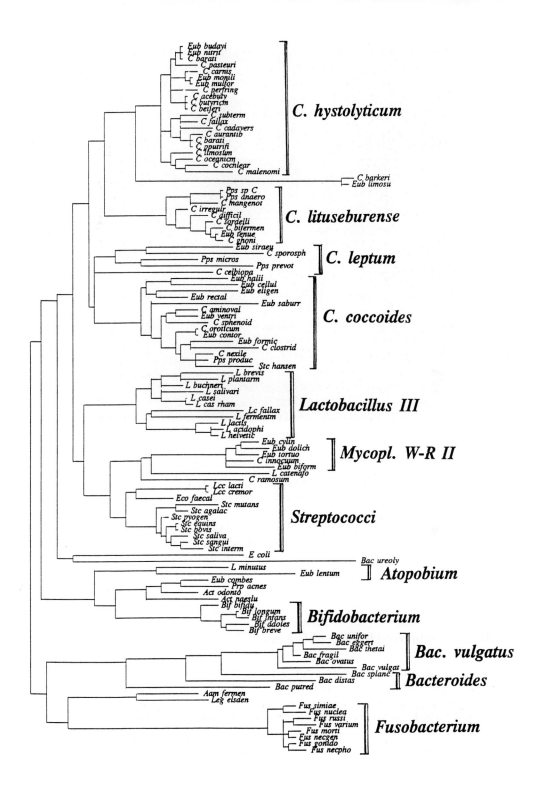

C. hystolyticum

C. lituseburense

C. leptum

C. coccoides

Lactobacillus III

Mycopl. W-R II

Streptococci

Atopobium

Bifidobacterium

Bac. vulgatus

Bacteroides

Fusobacterium

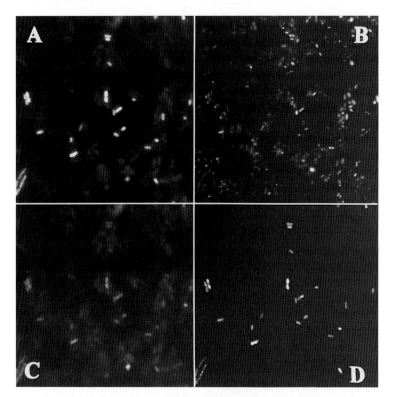

Fig. 2.   Fluorescence lifetime imaging of walled mycoplasmas subgr. II in human faecal flora using 16S rRNA hybridization probes. For a period of 8 sec FITC fluorescence is recorded (panel A). Subsequently, a DAPI image is recorded under UV illumination (panel B). After 20 sec of UV illumination during which FITC fluorescence but not autofluorescence fades significantly, a second FITC image is recorded (panel C). Graphical subtraction of the image in panel C from that in panel A produces the frame in panel D with clearly distinguishable hybridized cells.

fluorescence (fig. 2). Using such fluorescence lifetime imaging techniques, only a few positively hybridized cells can be distinguished among several thousand non-target cells in a microscope field (manuscript in preparation). This is necessary to enumerate those bacterial clusters that form a minority of the population, (*e.g.* streptococci).

Whole cell in situ hybridization of faeces

We have developed a relatively simple protocol for the enumeration of hybridized cells in faecal samples (fig. 3): A known quantity of homogenized faeces is resuspended in phosphate buffered saline (PBS). For cultivation, appropriate dilutions are made and cells are inoculated on the surface of selective and non-selective agar media. Plates are incubated anaerobically at 37°C. For microscopic enumeration and probe hybridization, cells are fixed for a mini-

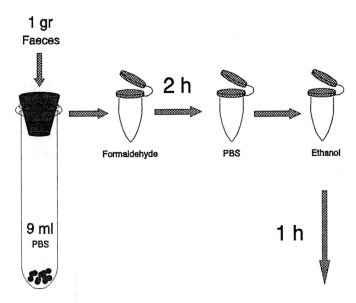

Fig. 3. Protocol for the hybridization and enumeration of faecal bacteria.

mum of 2 hrs in 4% paraformaldehyde. Debris is separated from bacterial cells by low-spin centrifugation. Cells are pelleted, washed in PBS and suspended in gradually increasing concentrations of ethanol (to 75%). After pelleting, the cells are resuspended in hybridization buffer and FITC-labelled probe is added. Hybridization is carried out at a temperature 2°C below the dissociation temperature of the probe for a minimum of 2 hrs. After hybridization, cells are stained with 4′,6-diamidino-2-phenylindole (DAPI), filtered onto a 0.2 μm pore-size polycarbonate filter and washed with hybridization buffer at hybridization temperatures. The filter is mounted on a microscope slide and viewed under an epifluorescence microscope equipped with the appropriate excitation and emission filters for FITC and DAPI. An image analysis system (Wilkinson, 1995) is used when fluorescence signals of target cells are too low to allow proper enumeration by eye.

Laboratory trials

We investigated the population of bifidobacteria in the faecal samples of ten volunteers. During this study, cultural methods were compared with the 16S hybridization method. A genus-specific *Bifidobacterium* probe targeted for position 164 (Bif164) was used (Langendijk *et al.*, submitted). The mean number of culturable bifidobacteria ($\pm$S.E.) from all samples was 2.45 ($\pm$1.40)x10^9 per gram of wet faeces. The mean number of total culturable anaerobes on BBA from all samples was 3.87 ($\pm$1.73)x10^{10} per gram of wet faeces. On average, bifidobacteria accounted for 6.9% $\pm$ 3.3% of the total culturable population. For all ten individuals investigated, the total counts of faecal bacteria as obtained on non-selective anaerobic brucella blood agar were significantly lower than the total microscopic counts on membrane filters with DAPI as a nuclear stain.

The membrane filter technique was also used to enumerate the number of bacteria that hybridized with probe Bif164. In theory, all bifidobacteria present in faeces, including those that are nonculturable on agar media, should be detected when using this probe hybridization technique. In analogy to the discrepancy between cultural counts and DAPI total counts, we expected the cultural counts of bifidobacteria to be considerably below probe hybridization counts. By contrast, the number of culturable bifidobacteria enumerated on BIF agar (Sutter et al., 1985) was not significantly different from the microscopic count using the *Bifidobacterium* probe Bif164 (av. 2.38×10^9 per g wet faeces). Based on DAPI total counts, *Bifidobacterium* spp., on average, accounted for 0.8% $\pm$ 0.4% of the total population. This implies that nearly all bifidobacteria in human faeces are culturable, possibly as a result of their oxygen tolerance and that the contribution of bifidobacteria to the total intestinal microflora is largely overestimated when using cultural methods as sole method of enumeration. Such overestimations can approach an order of magnitude.

In a second study, we have enumerated members of the *Bacteroides vulgatus* subgroup (*Bacteroides fragilis* group). Cultural methods of enumeration result in counts half of those obtained when using a subgroup-specific hybridization probe. Currently we are developing and testing other phylogenetic group-specific probes for detection of major subpopulations of bacteria in human faeces. Included are probes specific for streptococci, the *Clostridium coccoides* subgroup, *Bacteroides distasonis* (species-specific), and subgroup II of the walled mycoplasmas (Larsen et al., 1993) (see also fig. 2). Together these probes 'cover' around 50% of the total microscopic count in faecal samples.

Conclusions and prospects

Phylogenetic group-specific 16S rRNA hybridization probes can successfully be used for the enumeration of the major subpopulations of bacteria in human faeces. This method has several advantages to the classic cultural method for enumeration. The most important one is the relative ease and speed of the technique. With FITC-labelled 16S probes several samples can be processed per day. Once large-scale dynamics in composition of major subpopulations have been established species-specific probes can be used to elucidate the more detailed dynamics within such phylogenetic clusters. Before this can be achieved, the sensitivity of the technique is limited to threshold population densities of 1 positive cell per 500 negative cells, i.e. around 0.2% of the population. Several species of the intestinal flora, specifically the aerobic and facultatively anaerobic potentially pathogenic bacteria, drop well below this level. This is where the cultural technique is superior.

The use of flow cytometers, in which several tens of thousands of cells can be analyzed within minutes, will prove useful in the future. Flow cytometry in combination with 16S probe hybridization dramatically increases the number of samples that can be analyzed per study. In preliminary trials we have enumerated six phylogenetic clusters of intestinal bacteria in a single sample, some with good precision when compared with microscopic counts, in less than a day. The hybridization time being the rate limiting step. Although several problems related to signal to noise ratio still have to be overcome, 16S rRNA hybridization has already proven to be a very powerful technique in ecological studies of intestinal flora. Investigations into the dynamics of the community structure will help to fill the gaps in knowledge on the interaction between the host immunity and gut microflora. Such knowledge is crucial to the understanding of gut flora related pathogenesis.

References

Baron, E.J., R. Bennion, J. Thompson, C. Strong, P. Summanen, M. McTeague and S.M. Finegold, 1992 - A microbiological comparison between acute and complicated appendicitis, *Clin. Infect. Dis.* **14**, 227–231.

Benno, Y., K. Endo, T. Mizutani, Y. Namba, T. Komori and T. Mitsuoka, 1989 - Comparison of faecal microflora of elderly persons in rural and urban areas of Japan, *Appl. Environ. Microbiol.* **55**, 1100–1105.

Boulanger, J.M., E.L. Ford-Jones and A.G. Matlow, 1991 – Enterococcal bacteraemia in a paediatric institution: a four year review, *Rev. Infectious Dis.* **13**, 847–856.

Drasar, B.S. and P.A Barrow, 1985 - Intestinal Microbiology, *Aspects of Microbiology*, **10**. American Society for Microbiology, Washington, USA.

Drasar, B.S., F. Montgomery and A.M. Tomkins, 1986 - Diet and faecal flora in three dietary groups in rural northern Nigeria, *J. Hyg. Camb.* **96**, 59–65.

Finegold, S.M., H.R. Attebery and V.L. Sutter, 1974 - Effect of diet on human fecal flora: comparison of Japanese and American diets, *Am. J. Clin. Nutr.* **27**, 1456–1469.

Gorbach, S.L., L. Nahas, P.I. Lerner and L. Weinstein, 1967 - Studies of intestinal microflora. I. Effects of diet, age, and periodic sampling on numbers of fecal microorganisms in man, *Gastroenterology* **53**, 845–855.

Guyton, A.C., 1986 - *Textbook of medical physiology*, 7th ed., pp. 770–786, W.B. Saunders Comp. Philadelphia, PA, USA.

Holdeman, L.V., E.P. Cato and W.E.C. Moore, 1977 - *Anaerobe Laboratory Manual*, 4th ed., Virginia Polytechnic Institute and State University, Blacksburg, VA.

Kennedy, M.J. and P.A. Volz, 1985 - Ecology of *Candida albicans* gut colonization: inhibition of *Candida* adhesion, colonization and dissemination from the gastrointestinal tract by bacterial antagonism, *Infect. Immun.* **49**, 654–663.

Kujath, P., K. Lerch and J. Dämmrich, 1990 - Fluconazole monitoring in *Candida* peritonitis based on histological control, *Mycoses* **33**, 441–448.

Lane, D.J., 1991 - 16S/23S rRNA sequencing, in, E. Stackebrandt and M. Goodfellow (eds), *Nucleic acid techniques in bacterial systematics*, Wiley and Sons, Chichester, England, pp. 115–175.

Langendijk, P.S., F. Schut, G.J. Jansen, G.C. Raangs, G.R. Kamphuis, M.H.F. Wilkinson and G.W. Welling, 1995 - Quantitative fluorescence in situ hybridization of *Bifidobacterium* spp. with genus-specific 16S rRNA targeted probes and its application in faecal samples. *Appl. Environ. Microbiol.* **61**, 3069–3075.

Larsen, N., G.J. Olsen, B.L. Maidak, M.J. McCaughey, R. Overbeek, T.J. Macke, T.L. Marsh and C.R. Woese, 1993 - The ribosomal database project, *Nucleic Acids Res.* **21**, 3021–3023.

McClean, K.L., G.J. Sheehan and G.K.M. Harding, 1994 - Intraabdominal Infection: A review, *Clin. Infect. Dis.* **19**, 100–116.

Minelli, E.B., A. Benini, A.M. Beghini, R. Cerutti and G. Nardo, 1993 - Bacterial faecal flora in healthy woman of different ages, *Microb. Ecol. Health Dis.* **6**, 43–51.

Mitsuoka, T., 1992 - Intestinal flora and aging, *Nutrition Rev.* **50**, 438–446.

Moore, W.E.C. and L.V. Holdeman, 1974 - Human fecal flora: The normal flora of 20 Japanese-Hawaiians, *Appl. Microbiol.* **27**, 961–979.

Olsen, G.J., D.J. Lane, S.J. Giovannoni and N.R. Pace, 1986 - Microbial ecology and evolution: A ribosomal RNA approach, *Ann. Rev. Microbiol.* **40**, 337–365.

Pace, N.R., D.A. Stahl, D.J. Lane and G.J. Olsen, 1986 - The analysis of microbial populations by ribosomal RNA sequences, *Adv. Microbial Ecol.* **9**, 1–55.

Sawyer, R.G., L.K. Rosenlof, R.B. Adams, A.K. May, M.D. Spengler and T.L. Pruett, 1992 - Peritonitis into the 90s: Changing pathogens and changing strategies in the critically ill, *Am. Surg.* **58**, 82–87.

Sedman, P.C., J. Macfie, P. Sagar, C.J. Mitchell, J. May, B. Mancey-Jones and D. Johnstone, 1994 - The prevalence of gut translocation in humans, *Gastroenterology* **107**, 643–649.

Stahl, D.A. and R. Amann, 1991 - Development and application of nucleic acid probes, pp. 205–248, in, E. Stackebrandt and M. Goodfellow (eds), *Nucleic acid techniques in bacterial systematics*, Wiley and Sons, Chichester, England.

Sutter, V.L., D.M. Citron, M.A.C. Edelstein and S.M. Finegold, 1985 - *Wadsworth Anaerobic Bacteriology Manual*, 4th ed., Star Publ. Corp., Belmont, CA.

Van der Waaij, D., 1989 - The ecology of the human intestine and its consequences for overgrowth by pathogens such as *Clostridium difficile*, *Ann. Rev. Microbiol.* **43**, 67–87.

Wilkinson, M.H.F., 1995 - *Fluoro-morphometry. Adding fluorimetry to an image processing system for bacterial morphometry.* Academic thesis. University of Groningen, the Netherlands.

F. Schut
Department of Medical Microbiology
University of Groningen
Oostersingel 59
9713 EZ Groningen
The Netherlands
Tel: +31 50633507
Fax: +31 50633528
E-mail: f.schut@med.rug.nl

T.R. Licht, L.K. Poulsen, S. Molin and K.A. Krogfelt

Applications of Ribosomal *in situ* Hybridization for the Study of Bacterial Cells in the Mouse Intestine

Abstract

Localization of *E. coli* and *S. typhimurium* in the large and small intestine of streptomycin-treated mice was visualized by *in situ* hybridization with specific rRNA target probes and epi-fluorescence microscopy. Growth rates of *E. coli* BJ4 colonizing the large intestine of streptomycin treated mice were estimated by quantitative hybridization. The ribosomal contents were measured in bacteria isolated from cecal mucus, cecal contents and feces and correlated with the ribosomal contents of bacteria growing in vitro with defined rates. The data suggest that *E. coli* BJ4 grows with an apparent doubling time of 40–80 minutes in the intestinal mucosa.

Introduction

The large intestine is the most heavily colonized part of the gastrointestinal tract of mammals. At least 500 different bacterial species are thought to be present at any time in the healthy human intestinal tract and up to 10^{12} bacteria are found in every gram of feces. In this complex ecosystem the microorganisms co-exist in a fine balance. They must grow slowly enough not to overgrow the host, but fast enough not to be flushed out by the host's intestinal activities, e.g. peristaltic movements, fluid flow etc. (Borriello, 1986; Finegold *et al.*, 1983).

Most work performed on the bacterial flora of the gut has concentrated on the analysis of fecal specimens. Much less information is found about the flora of the cecum or that associated with the intestinal mucosa. *In situ* investigations of the growth physiology of intestinal bacteria are therefore of great interest. In the past, calculations of the rates of bacterial proliferation in the intestine have been based on average estimates at the level of populations. For example, the growth rate of *E. coli* in the mouse intestine has been estimated *in vivo* using radioisotope techniques, dilution by growth of a non-replicating genetic marker and simply by counting the number of viable cells (Meynell, 1959, Hiram *et al.*, 1971, Eudy and Burros, 1973, Gibbons and Kapsimalis, 1967, Freter *et al.*, 1983). Using these techniques, generation times ranging from 30 minutes to 40 hours of *E. coli* have been estimated. These systems, however, do not reflect the physiological conditions in the gut, where entrapment of the bacteria in the mucus gel plays an important role. Furthermore, in the intestine, the bacterial cell morphology, protein profiles and growth physiology have been described to differ from what is observed during growth in laboratory media (Krogfelt *et al.*, 1993; Panigrahi *et al.*, 1992).

Bacterial growth rates can be estimated from the cellular RNA concentrations, since RNA content is dependent on the growth rate (Schaechter *et al.*, 1958; Neidhart and Magasanik, 1960; Kjelgaard and Kurland, 1963). Recently developed methods based on hybridization to whole cells with fluorophore-labelled oligonucleotide probe targeting the ribosomal RNA (rRNA) and epi-fluorescence microscopy coupled to digital image analysis allow estimations of concentration of rRNA in single cells. The ribosomal contents of the bacteria isolated from the environment can then be compared to the ribosomal contents of bacteria growing with defined rates. (DeLong *et al.*, 1989; Poulsen *et al.*, 1993). In this study, the total indigenous flora, as well as introduced streptomycin resistant strains of *E. coli* and *S. typhimurium*, were visualized and the apparent growth of *E. coli* BJ4 in the large intestine of streptomycin treated mice was estimated (Poulsen *et al.*, 1995).

In situ hybridization: The method

Sectioning and fixation

Tissue specimens from the mouse large and small intestine were prepared either by embedding in tissue glue and freezing in liquid nitrogen for cryostat sections, or by embedding in paraffin for microtome sections. Cryostate sections were fixed in 3% paraformaldehyde immediately after cryostat cutting. Tissue for microtome sections was fixed in formalin prior to embedding.

The sections on slides were air dried and stored at 4°C until they were either stained with Alcian blue PAS and Meyers Hematoxylin, or used for *in situ* rRNA-hybridization.

Bacterial cells growing in laboratory cultures and bacterial cell smears from the ceca of colonized mice were fixed in 3% paraformaldehyde. Fixed cells were stored in storage buffer (Poulsen *et al.*, 1994). Hybridizations were carried out as described by Poulsen 1994. Briefly, the speciments on slides were hybridized at 37°C in a hybridization solution containing various concentrations of formamide, depending on the melting point of the probe and on the desired specificity. The slides were then washed twice in washing solutions with decreasing specificity, rinsed quickly in distilled water and air dried.

Probes

Specific probes to *E. coli* 23S rRNA (Poulsen *et al.*, 1994) and *S. typhimurium* (Poulsen, unpublished) were designed in order to perform *in situ* hybridization of bacteria in the mouse gut. The specificity of the probes was tested by use of the CHECK-PROBE program (Larsen *et al.*, 1993).

Probe EUB338 (Stahl *et al.*, 1991), specific to the Eubacterial domain was used to visualize the total bacterial population in the intestine of streptomycin treated mice. The probes were labeled with various fluorocromes, i.e. fluorescein, Lissamin Rhodamine B or CY3 as previously described (Poulsen *et al.*, 1994).

Different fluorochromes were assessed for labeling the probes in order to obtain the lowest background binding to the tissue. The use of hydrophobic fluorochromes sometimes resulted in high nonspecific binding of the probe to hydrophobic compartments of the mouse epithelial cells. When the hydrophilic fluorochromes were tested, a higher signal to noise ratio was obtained. In order to overcome the inherent fluorescence of epithelial cells and material trapped in the mucosal layer, we used narrow band by-pass filters for the emission.

Microscopy and Image analysis

The hybridizations were visualized as described in detail by Poulsen *et al.*, 1994. An Axioplan epi-fluorescence microscope was equipped with filter sets and narrow band by-pass filters depending on the exitation and emision wavelengths of the fluorocromes.

A slow scan CCD (Charged Coupled Device) camera was used for capturing digitalized images. The camera was operated at $-40C$. The integration time for the CCD camera varied between 500 msec and 3–6 sec depending on the intensity of the hybridized probe and on the use of narrow band by pass filters.

Image analysis was performed in order to determine the amount of fluorescence per bacterial cell volume. This ratio corresponds to the ribosomal concentration in individual bacterial cells. The applied software has previously been described (Poulsen *et al.*, 1994).

In order not to bleach the fluorocromes prior to capturing images, cells were counter stained with DAPI (4',6'-DiAmidino-2'-PhenylIndole) which was used for focusing the camera. At least 3 different images of 200–400 cells at each growth rate were quantified. The standard deviations of these measurements were 8–25%

The streptomycin treated mouse model

Treatment of conventional mice with streptomycin-containing drinking water removes the indigenous facultative flora, and thereby allows orally introduced streptomycin resistant strains of *S. typhimurium* SL5319 (Franklin *et al.*, 1990) or *E. coli* (Krogfelt *et al.*, 1993) to colonize.

This animal model has been studied in great detail (Franklin *et al.*, 1990; Krivan *et al.*, 1992; Myhal *et al.*, 1982 and Wadolkowsky *et al.*, 1988), and was therefore chosen for the present work.

Visualization of specific bacterial strains in the intestine

As an example of the application of the hybridization method to *S. typhimurium* SL5319, in figure 1 we show a hybridized section of the ileum of a mouse colonized with this strain. Panels A and B show the section stained with Mayers Hematoxylin and Alcian blue. In Panel C one single bacterial cell caught by the

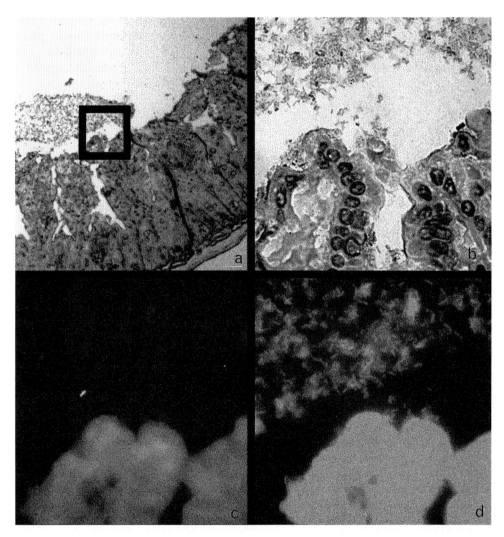

Fig. 1.   5 μm thin microtome section of the ileum of a mouse colonized with *Salmonella typhimurium* SL5319. In panels A) and B) are shown the staining of the section with Meyers heamatoxylin and Alcian blue, enlarged 100X and 630X respectively. The simultaneous probing of the same section with a probe specific for *Salmonella* (C) and a probe targeting the eubacterial domain (D) are also shown.

Salmonella specific probe is visualized, while in panel D bacteria responding to the universal probe, targeting all the eubacteria, are shown.

In this experiment, *S. typhimurium* colonized the mouse cecum at levels of 10^8 to 10^{10} CFU per gram, while the concentration of CFU found in the ileum was four orders of magnitude lower.

E. coli BJ4 was found to colonize the gut at levels of 10^8 to 10^9 CFU per gram feces. In cecal contents the same levels of 10^9 CFU per gram were observed, while in cecal mucus the concentration of CFU was an order of magnitude lower, i.e. 10^8 CFU per gram of mucus (Poulsen *et al.*, 1995).

E. coli BJ4 (Krogfelt *et al.*, 1993) was easily detected on sections from the large intestine of the colonized mice. The bacterial cells were embedded in the mucosal material and were never observed to bind to the intestinal epithelium (Poulsen *et al.*, 1994)

Unchallenged streptomycin-treated mice were used as controls. No *E. coli* or *S. typhimurium cells* were detected in sections from their intestines.

Determination of ribosomal cell content of bacteria growing *in vitro* and *in vivo*, and correlation between growth rates and ribosomal concentrations

In vitro measurements upon growth in defined laboratory media.

Pure cultures were grown in minimal media with different carbon sources, resulting in a series of different generation times. Growth rates were measured by following the optical density at 450 nm. The ribosomal contents of *E. coli* BJ4 cells growing under different conditions in various media supporting various growth rates were determined by whole cell rRNA hybridization.

A linear correlation between bacterial growth rate and ribosomal concentration was observed (Poulsen *et al.*, 1995).

In vivo measurements upon growth in the mouse intestine.

Growth rates of *E. coli* BJ4 were estimated in samples from feces, cecal contents, and cecal mucus taken from mice colonized with this strain. The samples were fixed, spread in a monolayer on a hybridization slide, and hybridized as described above. Digital images were captured for image analysis and the mean signal intensity measured. By use of a linear standard curve obtained from cultures grown in defined laboratory media, the mean signal intensities could be converted into apparent growth rates.

The initial stages of bacterial colonization were investigated by administering a low amount of bacteria to the mice. Two mice were sacrificed at 1, 3, 5, 24, 40, 96 and 120 hours after challenge and mucus samples were taken for CFU determinations and hybridization. *E. coli* BJ4 colonization of the intestinal mucus increased rapidly as shown in Figure 2A. Intensity measurements followed by hybridization showed ribosomal contents corresponding to genera-

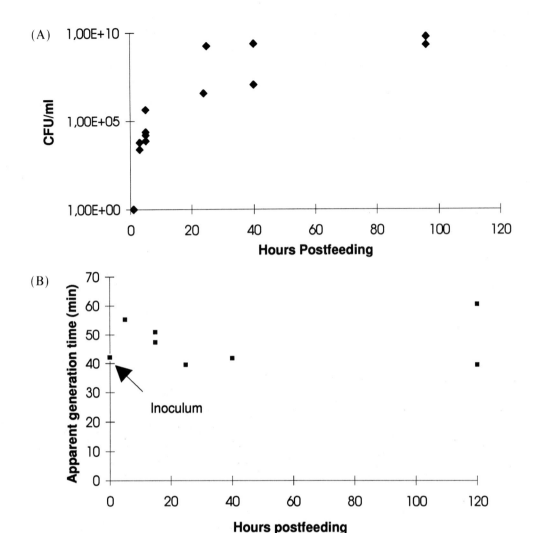

Fig. 2. Colonization of the mouse large intestine by *E. coli* BJ4 during the first 120 hours post inoculation. A) *E. coli* BJ4 CFU/ml in mucus. B) Generation times in cecal mucus inferred by ribosomal hybridization.

tion times of 40–80 minutes for all samples taken between 1 and 120 hours after challenge (Fig.–2B). The apparent generation times of 40–80 minutes remained constant throughout the 20 days investigated (not shown). Colony forming units of *E. coli* BJ4 remained constant throughout the experiment at the levels of 10^9 and 10^8 CFU/ml in cecal contents and cecal mucus respectively, and 10^9 CFU/g in the fecal samples.

Cecal mucus and cecal contents from two streptomycin treated unchallenged mice were hybridized with the *E. coli* specific probe. No hybridization was observed, thereby confirming the specificity of the probe used.

Discussion

Studies on the growth of bacterial cells have usually been performed with pure cultures growing in well defined liquid laboratory media under well controlled conditions. In natural environments bacterial growth is influenced by a number of factors that are often unknown. The complexity of the natural ecosystems makes it difficult to mimic the conditions *in vitro*. Therefore, it is important to develop methods by which bacterial growth physiology can be studied *in situ*.

The method of *in situ* rRNA hybridization in whole fixed cells has proven very useful in several complex environmental contexts for specific identification of single bacterial species. Moreover, quantification of the hybridization signal may be achived by the aid of digitilized video cameras (CCD-cameras) and fluorescence microscopy. Through such measurements ribosomal concentrations in bacteria can be determined (Poulsen *et al.*, 1993).

In the present study, we have applied rRNA hybridization to detect the spatial distribution of bacterial cells in the small and large intestines of mice. Furthermore, by use of this method we have measured the cellular ribosomal concentration and thereby estimated the bacterial growth rates in the large intestine.

In a series of growth experiments supporting growth rates of *E. coli* BJ4 betweeen 30 and 180 min. followed by rRNA hybridizations, a linear relationship between growth rate and ribosomal contents was observed. Having this standard curve, *E. coli* BJ4 cells isolated from the cecal mucus of mice colonized for 20 days with this strain showed a rRNA content corresponding to a generation time of 40–80 minutes. Hybridizations on *E. coli* BJ4 isolated from cecal contents and feces showed approximately the same rRNA content (intensity/ bacterial volume) as cells isolated from mucus, indicating the same doubling times. However, we observed that *E. coli* BJ4 did not grow in fecal pellets after excretion during a period of 24 hours at room temperature (data not shown), and it is also unlikely that *E. coli* grows in the intestinal contents (Wadolkowski *et al.*, 1988). We therefore assume that the high ribosome content observed in the *E. coli* BJ4 cells isolated from cecal contents and fecal pellets reflects that the bacteria have been growing rapidly while associated with the mucosal layer, and that the ribosomes needed to maintain this high growth rate stay intact in cecal contents and feces (Poulsen *et al.*, 1995).

That fast growth does indeed occur in the mucosal layer is supported by the increase in CFU counts observed during the initial stages of colonization (figure 2A). Even if factors such as washout, mucosal turnover and release of bacteria from the mucosal layer are not taken into consideration, the bacteria must grow with a generation time of at least 80 minutes to achieve the increase in CFU's observed in the period between 3 and 24 hours after challenge.

Later, when the number of CFU in the intestine stays at a constant high level, the low bacterial generation times in mucus estimated by *in situ* hybridization are supported further by the following considerations:

Since the total mucosal population stays constant, the mean stay of bacteria in mucus must be equal to the mean growth rate of the mucosal population. The hybridization data suggest an average generation time of about one hour, and thus the bacteria must stay associated with the mucosal layer for a similar period. If we assume that no bacterial growth occurs neither in luminal contents, nor in feces, the minimum size of the population in mucus needed to produce the 10^9 BJ4 cells counted in faeces from 24 hours is $10^9/24 = 4*10^7$ CFU. This correlates well with the actual plate counts showing a total cecal mucosal BJ4 population of about 10^7 CFU (Poulsen et al., 1995).

Thus, the generation time of 40–80 min for E. coli BJ4 in the mucus of the large intestine of mice estimated by in situ hybridization is in agreeement with the counted colony forming units, if we assume that growth mainly takes place in mucus.

In summary, it is clear that in situ rRNA hybridization can be applied in the complex environment of the intestine, and reveal useful information about bacterial distribution. In addition, the concentration of ribosomal RNA in a given bacterial cell as measured by in situ hybridization can provide further information about the physiological state of the cell.

Affiliations

T.R. Licht and K.A. Krogfelt*:
Department of Clinical Microbiology, Statens Seruminstitut, DK-2300
Copenhagen S, Denmark.
T.R. Licht, L.K. Poulsen, and S. Molin:
Department of Microbiology, Technical University of Denmark, DK-2800
Lyngby, Denmark.
*Corresponding

References

Borriello, S.P., 1986 - Microbial flora of the gastrointestinal tract, pp. 2–16. in M.J. Hill (ed.), Microbial metabolism in the digestive tract. CRC Press, Inc. Roca Raton, FL.

DeLong, E.F., G.S. Wickham and N.R. Pace, 1989 - Phylogenetic stains: Ribosomal RNA-based probes for identification of single cells. Science 243, 1360–1363.

Eudy, W.W. and S.E. Burrous, 1973 - Generation times of Proteus mirabilis and Escherichia coli in experimental infections. Chemotherapy 19, 161–170.

Finegold, S.M., V.L. Sutter and G.E. Mathisen, 1983 - Normal indigenous intestinal flora, pp. 3–31. in D.J. Hentges (ed.), Human intestinal microflora in health and disease. Academic Press, New York.

Franklin, D.P., D.C. Laux, T.J. Williams, M.C. Falk and P.S. Cohen, 1990 - Growth of Salmonella typhimurium SL5319 and Escherichia coli F-18 in mouse cecal mucus: role of peptides and iron. *FEMS Microbiol. Ecol.* **74**, 229–240.

Freter, R., H. Brickner, J. Fenkete, M.M. Vickerman and K.E. Carey, 1983 - Survival and implantation of *Escherichia coli* in the intestinal tract. *Infect. Immun.* **39**, 686–703.

Gibbons, R.J. and B. Kapsimalis, 1967 - Estimates of the overall rate of growth of the intestinal microflora of hamsters, guinea pigs, and mice. *J. Bacteriol.* **93**, 510–512.

Hiram, C.P., M.S. Mallone, P.F. Denunzio and R.F. Auclair, 1971 - Bacterial growth rates in crushed and devascularized skeletal muscle. *J. Trauma* **11**, 919–922.

Kjeldgaard, N.O. and C.G. Kurland, 1963 - The distribution of soluble and ribosomal RNA as a function of growth rate. *J. Mol. Biol.* **6**, 341–348.

Krivan, H.C., D.P. Franklin, W. Wang, D.C. Laux and P.S. Cohen, 1992 - Phosphatidylserine found in intestinal mucus serves as a sole source of carbon and nitrogen for salmonellae and *Escherichia coli*. *Infect. Immun.* **60**, 3943–3946.

Krogfelt, K.A., L.K. Poulsen and S. Molin, 1993 - Identification of coccoid *Escherichia coli* BJ4 cells in the large intestine of streptomycin-treated mice. *Infect. Immun.* **61**, 5029–5034.

Larsen, N., G.J. Olsen, B.L. Maidak, M.J. McCaughey, R. Overbeek, T.J. Macke, T.L. Marsh and C.R. Woese, 1993 - The ribosomal RNA database project. *Nucleic Acids Res.* **21**, 3021–3023.

Meynell, G.G., 1959 - Use of superinfecting phage for estimating the division rate of lysogenic bacteria in infected animals. *J. Gen. Microbiol.* **21**, 421–437.

Myhal, M.L., D.C. Laux and P.S. Cohen, 1982 - Relative colonizing abilities of human fecal and K12 strains of *Escherichia coli* in the large intestines of streptomycin-treated mice. *Eur. J. Clin. Microbiol.* **1**, 186–192.

Neidhardt, F.C. and B. Magasanik, 1960 - Studies on the role of ribonucleic acid in the growth of bacteria. *Biochem. Biophys. Acta* **42**, 99–116.

Panigrahi, P., G. Lovonsky, L.J. DeTolla and J.G. Morris, Jr., 1992 - Human immune response to *Campylobacter jejuni* proteins expressed in vivo. *Infect. Immun.* **60**, 4938–4944.

Poulsen, L.K., G. Ballard and D.A. Stahl, 1993 - Use of rRNA fluorescence in situ hybridization for measuring the activity of single cells in young and established biofilms. *Appl. Environ. Microbiol.* **59**, 1354–1360.

Poulsen L.K., F. Lan, C.S. Kristensen, P. Hobolth, S. Molin and K.A. Krogfelt, 1994 - Spatial distribution of *Escherichia coli* in the mouse large intestine inferred from rRNA *in situ* hybridization. *Infect. Immun.* **62**, 5191–5194.

Poulsen L.K., T.R. Licht, C. Rang, K.A. Krogfelt and S. Molin, 1995 - The physiological state of *E. coli* BJ4 growing in the large intestine of streptomycin-treated mice. *J. Bacteriol.* **177**, 5840–5845.

Schaechter, M., O. Maaløe and N.O. Kjeldgaard, 1958 - Dependency on medium and temperature of cell size and chemical composition during balanced growth of *Salmonella typhimurium J. Gen. Microbiol.* **19**, 592–606.

Stahl, D.A. and R.I. Amann, 1991 - Development and application of nucleic acid probes, pp. 205–248. in E. Stackebrandt and M. Goodfellow (ed.), *Nucleic acid techniques in bacterial systematics.* John Wiley and Sons, New York.

Wadolkowski, E.A., D.C. Laux and P.S. Cohen, 1988 - Colonization of streptomycin-treated mouse large intestine by a human fecal *Escherichia coli* strain: Role of growth in mucus. *Infect. Immun.* **56**, 1030–1035.

Host parasite interactions

Alexander E. Hromockyj[1] and Stanley Falkow[1, 2]

Bacterial Resistance to Macrophage Killing.
An evolutionary perspective

Introduction

Pathogens have evolved elaborate mechanisms that allow them to survive environmental conditions inside and outside of their hosts. A bacterial pathogen's adaptation to adverse surroundings within a host is manifested in the expression of virulence factors. Virulence genes encoding these factors are located both on the bacterial chromosome and on extrachromosomal elements. Bacterial pathogens enhance their capacity for survival through the expression of protein regulatory networks which ensure the coordinate expression of virulence genes in response to changes in environmental cues such as temperature, osmolarity, pH, aerobic conditions, and nutrient availability. Thus, bacteria that cause human disease are fully armed to confront the physical and biochemical barriers they face while entering and establishing a niche within their host.

Among the barriers first encountered by most pathogenic bacteria are the human mucosal epithelial surfaces found in the gastrointestinal and respiratory tracts. Bacteria are trapped within mucus and are subject to the effects of proteolytic enzymes and secretory antibody. Alternatively, they may be expelled by the action of gut peristalsis or the motion of the lung's ciliated epithelium. Bacterial attachment to and colonization of these locations is impeded by competition for attachment sites and nutrients from the resident microflora.

Pathogens that penetrate into the submucosa next face the hosts non-specific immune defenses in the form of macrophages. Since the first time bacteria met predatory protozoans, they have evolved of necessity, adaptive mechanisms to thwart phagocytic mechanisms. Arguably, the human pathogenic species are among the descendants of this ancient encounter. The bacterial mechanisms that have evolved to neutralize macrophage function and the genetic basis of these mechanisms will be the focus of this review.

Macrophages reside in all tissues of the body and play a critical role in the suppression of bacterial spread into deeper tissues. Phagocytosis is triggered by

[1] Department of Microbiology and Immunology, Stanford University School of Medicine, Stanford, California 94305-5402
[2] Microsocopy Branch, Rocky Mountain Laboratories, National Institutes of Health, Hamilton, MT 59840

bacteria bound either directly or indirectly to macrophage surface components. Bacterial outer membrane proteins, sugars and lectins directly bind the macrophage surface, while the host serum complement components or anti-bacterial antibodies enhance indirect bacterial binding to macrophages. Pathogens opsonized with complement or immunoglobulins on their surfaces are then bound to complement or immunoglobulin Fc receptors. As additional receptors are engaged, the macrophage membrane extends pseudopods around the bound bacterium in what is referred to as the 'zipper' model of phagocytosis (Griffin and Silverstein, 1974). Eventually, the pseudopods completely envelop the bacterium into a phagosome where the acidic pH is lethal for most non-pathogenic and many pathogenic bacteria. Fusion of the phagosome with lysosomes, modifies the phagosome into a phagolysosome. The phagolysosome is filled with bactericidal hydrolytic enzymes, defensins (small cationic peptides), and oxygen radical and nitrogen radical intermediates, all of which reduce bacteria into their component parts. Ultimately, phagocytosis results in the processing and expression of these bacterial components or 'antigens' on the macrophage cell surface in conjunction with MHC class II molecules. T-cell recognition of this macrophage surface complex leads to activation of the cellular and humoral arms of the immune system. Also during phagocytosis, macrophages become 'activated' and secrete immune modulating factors known as cytokines which regulate the host immune response by activating T-cell populations. Macrophage functions are therefore, central in expanding the immune response to restrict possible secondary infections.

Clearly, in order to replicate beyond the mucosal borders pathogenic bacteria must either avoid or somehow subvert phagocytosis. Mechanisms by which bacterial pathogens evade macrophage killing generally fall into two categories: those which inhibit phagocytosis, and those that alter the normal phagocytic pathway. Pathogens that alter the phagocytic pathway do so by employing one or more of the following strategies (i) triggering an alternate entry (invasion) process, thereby circumventing phagolysosome formation, (ii) modifying the phagosome and/or phagolysosome into a compartment more suitable for growth, (iii) directly neutralizing bactericidal components in the phagolysosome, and (iv) breaking out of the phagosome and replicating in the macrophage cytoplasm.

The organisms discussed in this review do not encompass the entire spectrum of anti-macrophage mechanisms expressed by human pathogenic bacteria. However, the *Salmonella* and enteropathogenic *Yersinia* species represent bacterial pathogens that infect identical anatomic sites while using completely different strategies for resisting macrophage function. As such, these organisms exemplify a number of themes common to bacterial pathogens and their evolution.

Enteropathogenic *Yersinia*

Yersiniae cause zoonotic infections in birds, pigs, and rodents. Humans are not the normal reservoir of *Yersinia* in nature. Bubonic plague caused by *Y. pestis* is transmitted to humans by the bite of an infected flea although human-to-human transmission can follow subsequently by aerosol droplet infection. Gastroenteritis and mesenteric lymphadenitis caused by *Y. enterocolitica* and *Y. pseudotuberculosis* result from the ingestion of contaminated food. Despite the varied means of transmission and diseases elicited by these *Yersinia* species, they all exhibit a predilection for colonization of the human reticuloendothelial system (RES) during infection.

Peyer's patch (PP) lymphoid follicles of the small intestine are the primary site of enteric *Yersinia* infection. On the basis of the murine model of infection (Carter, 1975), the following scenario of events seems likely. First, organisms selectively bind to and transcytose the specialized epitheloid M-cells located in the PP follicle-associated epithelium (FAE; Grutzkau, et al., 1990). M-cells normally sample the intestinal lumen and introduce antigens to the immune cells beneath the FAE (Owen and Ermak, 1990). *Yersinia* appear to exploit this sampling system to access a site more permissive for their growth. Within the PP, *Yersinia* are thought to first encounter macrophages. Whether or not this putative interaction triggers the subsequent events that lead to a systemic infection is unclear. However, 48–72 hours after oral inoculation, large numbers of bacteria are seen in the PP's and they are exclusively extracellular, despite the presence of macrophages and neutrophils (Hanski, et al., 1989). Similar observations have been made in other tissues later in infection (Simonet, et al., 1990). Thus, one essential strategy used by the enteropathogenic *Yersinia* is to avoid macrophage phagocytosis.

A number of *Yersinia* virulence factors have been identified, which include several surface proteins that promote efficient bacterial adherence to mammalian cells and other secreted proteins that inhibit macrophage and neutrophil phagocytic functions. Recent studies suggest how these determinants may act in concert to prevent phagocytosis (Hromockyj and Falkow personal observations).

At least three distinct adherence and entry pathways are potentially involved in enteric-*Yersinia* pathogenesis. Two of these pathways involve bacterial interaction with the integrin family of mammalian cell surface receptors. Integrins are heterodimeric receptors, composed of an α and β chain, that mediate cell-to-cell and cell-to-extracellular matrix protein interactions through both a signalling mechanism and possibly direct linkage with the eukaryotic cell cytoskeleton (Hynes, 1992). The 103-kDa invasin protein (Inv) encoded by a chromosomal gene is the best studied of *Yersinia* proteins and mediates adherence to a wide variety of cultured mammalian cells (Isberg, *et al.*, 1987; Isberg and Leong, 1990). The 45-kDa YadA protein, is also thought to mediate attachment and invasion of *Yersinia* mammalian cells via a β_1 integrin receptor (Bliska, *et al.*, 1993; Yang and Isberg, 1993). In contrast to *inv*, the *yadA* gene is located on the ~70 kilobase virulence plasmid common to all the pathogenic *Yersinia* species (Skurnik and Wolf-Watz, 1989). Ail mediates a third mechanism of *Yersinia* adherence into mammalian cells. Encoded by a chromosomal gene, this 17-kDa protein facilitates *Yersinia* entry into several mammalian cell types *in vitro* through an unknown host cell receptor (Miller and Falkow, 1988). However, Ail also mediates resistance to serum complement killing (Bliska and Falkow, 1992; Pierson and Falkow, 1993). This latter function may reflect Ail's major role during infection, as Ail shares protein sequence homology with *Salmonella* serum resistance proteins Rck and PagC which also mediate resistance to defensins (Heffernan, *et al.*, 1992; Heffernan, *et al.*, 1992; Heffernan, *et al.*, 1994; Miller, 1991; Pulkkinen and Miller, 1991). Inv, YadA and Ail expression is regulated by temperature. Inv is maximally expressed at 26°C although recent studies reveal that Inv is also highly expressed at 37°C in low pH conditions (Isberg, *et al.*, 1988; Pepe, *et al.*, 1994). YadA and Ail are primarily expressed at 37°C (Martinez, 1989; Bliska and Falkow, 1992). Thus, when *Yersinia* enter the host, they immediately respond to environmental signals that could affect the expression of the adherence proteins, and permit interaction with specific host cell surface receptors.

The ability of *Yersinia* to inhibit macrophage phagocytosis is mediated by the direct action of two plasmid-mediated *Yersinia* outer membrane proteins (Yops), YopH and YopE. YopH and YopE along with 14 other Yops that have been identifed, are coded for by genes located on the *Yersinia* virulence plasmid. The Yop's are exclusively synthesized at 37°C and secreted under growth conditions of low calcium concentration ($[Ca^{2+}] < 100$mM; Pollack, *et al.*, 1986). Yop expression in response to these signals is tightly controlled by two independent transcriptional regulatory loops. A positive regulatory loop requires the activity of the temperature-regulated transcriptional activator protein VirF (Lambert de Rouvroit, *et al.*, 1992). The Lcr (low calcium response) proteins constitute a negative regulatory loop which repress Yop expression in conditions of high $[Ca^{2+}]$ (Straley, *et al.*, 1993). Yop export requires the specialized function of the Ysc (Yersinia secretion)/Lcr proteins (Straley, *et al.*, 1993; Forsberg, *et al.*, 1994). Transcription of the *ysc/lcr* genes is also regulated by the positive-temperature and negative-$[Ca^{2+}]$ regulatory loops (Straley, *et al.*, 1993; Forsberg, *et al.*, 1994). The Ysc/Lcr proteins are members of a growing family of specialized bacterial proteins involved in the specific secretion and export of bacterial virulence proteins. Several of the Lcr and Ysc proteins share sequence homology with proteins essential for surface expression of bacterial flagellar proteins in the *Erwinia* and *Caulobacter* spp. as well as *Salmonella* invasion proteins (Erickson, *et al.*, 1994; Forsberg, *et al.*, 1994). Moreover, LcrD functionally complements the specialized secretory protein InvA of *Salmonella* (Ginocchio and Galan, 1995). In order for YopH and YopE to elicit their antiphagocytic effects on target macrophages, they must be delivered into the target cell cytoplasm (Rosqvist, *et al.*, 1994). Three additional Yops, YopD, YopN, and YopB, have been described as essential for YopH and YopE delivery into the host cell cytoplasm by an undetermined mechanism (Forsberg, *et al.*, 1994). Once exported out of the bacterial cytoplasm into the surrounding environment, the Yops are capable of acting on target cells. YopH, while sharing no significant homology with other bacterial proteins, contains an amino acid sequence highly homologous to the catalytic site of eukaryotic tyrosine phosphatases (Guan and Dixon, 1990). In vitro, YopH exhibits protein tyrosine phosphatase activity and at least two macrophage proteins of 120-kDa and 55-kDa in size have been identified as YopH targets (Bliska, *et al.*, 1991). The identity and function of these proteins is unknown, although preliminary evidence suggests that they are protein tyrosine kinases (Bliska, *et al.*, 1992). YopE mediates a contact-dependent cytotoxicity, which results in host-cell actin depolymerization (Rosqvist, *et al.*, 1991). The actual macrophage cell targets of YopE remain to be identified. *Yersinia* employs the concerted effects of the YopH tyrosine phosphatase activity and YopE actin depolymerization as part of a sophisticated, specialized, multi-faced strategy to inhibit phagocytosis.

The relationship between *Yersinia* adherence to mammalian cells and the inhibition of macrophage phagocytosis is not readily apparent when these mechanisms are viewed independently. However, when evaluated together in the context of bacterial-macrophage interactions a clearer picture emerges. Expression of Inv and YadA in the absence of YopH and YopE mediate a highly efficient adherence and entry into murine macrophages *in vitro*. In turn, wild-type *Y. pseudotuberculosis* expressing a full complement of Yops, quickly neutralizes a target macrophage's phagocytic capacity. Yet, in the absence of Inv and YadA expression the ability of yersiniae to inhibit macrophage phagocytosis is markedly reduced. Thus, the interaction of enteropathogenic *Yersinia* with macrophage β_1 integrins either via Inv or YadA is the requisite first step in facilitating YopH and YopE mediated inhibition of phagocytosis (Hromockyj and Falkow personal observations). It appears then that the enteropathogenic *Yersinia* spp. following M-cell transytosis are capable of intimately associating with PP macrophages, neutralizing their phagocytic capacity and colonizing the macrophage surface.

Salmonellae

The *Salmonella* spp. are a diverse group of pathogenic bacteria that have been isolated from birds, mammals and reptiles. Salmonellae cause human disease ranging from a self-limiting gastroenteritis to a severe systemic infection, typhoid fever. Infections in animals constitute the principal reservoir of non-typhoidal infection in humans. Humans are the only known reservoir of the typhoid bacillus. However, murine salmonellosis caused by *S. typhimurium* resembles human typhoid. This model demonstrates that like the enteropathogenic *Yersinia* species, PP's of the small intestine are the primary site of *Salmonella* infection and that Salmonella colonize the hosts RES (Carter and Collins, 1974). *Salmonella* appears to specifically target M-cells in order to trancytose the mucosal epithelium and enter the PP (Kohbata, *et al.*, 1986; Clark, *et al.*, 1994; Jones, *et al.*, 1994). Once inside the PP and later in infection these bacteria are thought to survive within macrophages. *Salmonella* survival within macrophages during infection has never been conclusively demonstrated. However, macrophage studies *in vitro* provide circumstantial evidence to support this contention.

Most notably, genetic mutants of *Salmonella* unable to survive within macrophages are less virulent in the murine model of infection.

The study of *Salmonella* pathogenesis has focused on the genetic basis of mammalian cell invasion and survival within macrophages with an emphasis on the host cell signals that might trigger virulence gene expression. More recent work has examined the cell biology of *Salmonella*-host cell interaction during and following invasion.

The genetic basis of *Salmonella* invasion of mammalian cells requires the expression of numerous invasion associated loci. These loci have been mapped to several positions on the *Salmonella* chromosome and include genes required for LPS expression and chemotaxis (Finlay, *et al.*, 1988; Jones, *et al.*, 1992). In *S. typhimurium* a chromosomal region of approximately 40 to 50 kilobases contains the key invasion genes and likely constitute a 'pathogenicity island' (Blum, *et al.*, 1994). Within this region at least 15 different genes, *invA-D* and *H*, *spaM-T*, *hil*, *prgH* and *orgA* have been mapped (Galan and Curtiss III, 1989; Ginocchio, *et al.*, 1992; Groisman and Ochman, 1993; Lee, *et al.*, 1992; Behlau and Miller, 1993; Jones and S. Falkow, 1994). The function of many of these loci in invasion is still unclear. InvA and E along with SpaM and N display sequence homology with the Lcr/Ysc proteins of *Yersinia* and virulence protein secretion mechanisms of other human and plant pathogens (Groisman and Ochman, 1993; Collazo, *et al.*, 1995). Also, mutant InvA protein can be functionally complemented by both a portion of the *Yersinia* LcrD protein and the MixA protein from human pathogenic *Shigella* spp. (Ginocchio and Galan, 1995). This evidence indicates that *S. typhimurium* harbours a specialized secretory mechanism for surface expression of invasion proteins. Additional invasion loci have been identified in *S. typhi* and *S. cholerasuis* that are distinct from those found in *S. typhimurium* (Finlay, *et al.*, 1988; Elsinghorst, *et al.*, 1989). In the human pathogenic species *S. typhi* invasion associated genes, also designated *invA-D*, *H*, have been identified (Elsinghorst, *et al.*, 1989). This region of DNA is present in *S. typhimurium*, yet, it appears to serve a function different from that of *S. typhi*. Environmental growth conditions of low oxygen tension and high osmolarity enhance epithelial cell invasion by *S. typhimurium* and *S. typhi*, respectively (Lee and Falkow, 1990; Tartera and Metcalf, 1993) and accordingly transcription of several *S. typhimurium* invasion-associated genetic loci and specifically *orgA* are enhanced by low-oxygen growth conditions (Jones and S. Falkow, 1994).

Coincident with *Salmonella* invasion dramatic morphological changes occur in target mammalian cell membranes and cytoskeletal proteins. In epithelial cells, brush border microvilli on the apical surface are destroyed followed by entry of the bacterium within a membrane bound vacuole (Takeuchi, 1967; Finlay, *et al.*, 1991). These morphological changes occur rapidly, and entry begins within a few minutes of the salmonellae-host cell interaction (Francis, *et al.*, 1992). At the site of bacterial entry there is a profound but transient rearrangement of the host cell cytoskeletal protein actin, along with the accumulation of actin-associated proteins talin, ezrin, a-actinin, tropomysin, and tubulin (Finlay, *et al.*, 1991). The morphological and cytoskeletal alterations of the host cell plasma membrane induced by *Salmonella* invasion closely resemble normal eukaryotic cell ruffling. Ruffles are specialized plasma membrane ultrastructures of mammalian cells (Kadowaki, *et al.*, 1986). These structures are composed in part of rearranged filamentous actin and temporally associated with increased pinocytosis (Kadowaki, *et al.*, 1986). Considered to be an integral part of mammalian cell growth, development, and locomotion, ruffles are triggered by signaling events mediated by growth factors, mitogens, and oncogene expression (Bar-Sagi and Feramisco, 1986; Kadowaki, *et al.*, 1986; Miyata, *et al.*, 1989; Ridley, *et al.*, 1992). Ruffles induced by invasive salmonellae or other stimuli also facilitate epithelial cell internalization of non-invasive bacteria. Following *Salmonella* entry, target cells are induced to form large numbers of macropinosomes (Garcia-del Portillo and Finlay, 1994). Together, these data suggest that *Salmonella* invasion of epithelial cells may represent an exploitation of the host cell pinocytic machinery (Francis, *et al.*, 1993). In contrast, *Salmonella* entry into macrophages appears in two forms. In cultured murine macrophages, as in epithelial cells, *Salmonella* can induce membrane ruffles and increase macropinosome formation (Alpuche-Aranda, *et al.*, 1994). Following entry, these bacteria are localized in a characteristic 'spacious phagosome' (Alpuche-Aranda, *et al.*, 1994). Within the same population of bacteria, however, Salmonella are also phagocytosed by a process involving pseudopod formation as described for the 'zipper model' (Monack and Falkow personal observations). Bacteria internalized by this mechanism are subsequently found in tightly opposed rather than spacious phagosomes. Once inside the macrophage at least two seperate populations of *Salmonella* have been identified based on their growth characteristics: one static and the other rapidly dividing (Abshire and Neidhardt, 1993; Rathman and Falkow personal observations). Do either of these intracellular populations represent organisms better able to survive the intracellular environment? Does the mechanism of *Salmonella* entry into macrophages correlate with the ability of the intracellular populations to grow rapidly or remain static? Moreover, does Salmonella invasion result in evasion of the constitutive phagocytic pathway by sending these bacteria along an alternative pathway critical to survival?

Salmonella survival within macrophages is speculated to involve some 200 bacterial genes. The best characterized of these genes are those expressed in response to the phagolysosomal environment. Oxygen radicals induce *Salmonella* synthesis of catalase and superoxide dismutase, enzymes which reduce oxygen radicals and their intermediates to water and and carbon dioxide. *Salmonella* resistance to defensins is dependent on the expression of the phoP/phoQ regulatory locus. The PhoP/PhoQ proteins constitute a two component regulatory system which coordinately regulates *Salmonella* virulence gene expression in response to conditions of low pH and exposure to defensins (Miller, 1991). At least 40 distinct proteins constitute the phoP/phoQ regulatory network. Genes which make up this regulatory network fall into the phoP/phoQ activated genes (*pag*'s) and phoP/phoQ repressed genes (*prg*'s) (Miller, 1991). Of the genes activated by phoP/phoQ, *pagC* is the best characterized. PagC is a single 188 amino acid envelope protein essential for survival within macrophages although the exact function of PagC is unknown (Miller, 1991). PagC exhibits protein homology with bacterial outer membrane proteins that include *Yersinia* Ail which suggests that PagC is a bacterial surface protein that may interact with some toxic intra-phagolysomal component (Miller, 1991; Pulkkinen and Miller, 1991). Eight *prg* loci have been identified and characterized to a limited extent. These loci are also thought to code for outer membrane associated but of an unknown function. One of these loci, *prgH*, is involved in invasion of epithelial cells (Behlau and Miller, 1993). The direct interaction of *Salmonella* with macrophages, therefore, may constitute a signal recognized by the phoP/phoQ system to repress the expression of proteins necessary for survival outside and invasion into the macrophage while activating the expression of proteins essential for survival within macrophages.

Conclusion & Perspectives

The enteropathogenic *Yersinia* and *Salmonella* spp. represent a divergent co-evolution of pathogens that neutralize one of the hosts first lines of immune defense, the macrophage. For these bacterial pathogens exploitation of the hosts natural antigen sampling system, the M-cell, and colonization of the host Peyer's patches are conserved virulence mechanisms. However, once the hosts immune system is accessed, the unique pathogenic strategies of these organisms emerge. *Yersinia* avoid macrophage killing by inhibiting phagocytosis while, *Salmonella* attain the same goal by modifying macrophages into suitable sites for survival. And yet, efficient expression of the *Yersinia* antiphagocytic Yop and the *Salmonella* invasion proteins requires specialized secretory proteins that are functionally conserved in these two bacterial genuses. The functional conservation of this virulence protein secretion pathway is not limited to the *Salmonella* and enteric *Yersinia* spp. The human enteropathogenic *Shigella* spp. also utilize this alternative secretory mechanism to express invasion genes on their surface. However, intracellular *Shigella*, unlike *Salmonella*, break out of their phagosome and kill the macrophage through apoptosis, programmed cell death (Zychlinsky, *et al.*, 1992).

Neutralization of macrophage function is not limited to enteric bacterial species. Alveolar macrophage phagosomes are sites of *Mycobacteria tuberculosis* and *Legionella pneumophila* persistance in the lung. Both of these human pathogens, like *Salmonella*, remodel their macrophage phagosomes. Mycobacterium-containing vacuoles lack a host cell proton-ATPase pump thought to facilitate vacuolar acidification (Sturgill-Koszycki, *et al.*, 1994). Thus, these organisms seem to enhance their chances for survival within the macrophage by inactivating a mechanism for phagolysosomal acidification. The etiologic agent of Legionaires disease, *L. pneumophila* invades macrophages by a unique coiling phagocytic mechanism and once inside the macrophage the *L. pneumophila* phagosome does not fuse with lysosomes (Horwitz, 1983; Horwitz, 1984). The

L. pneumophila phagosome thus, does not acidify and these organisms are safe within the macrophage. This phagosome is further modified through an apparent recruitment of ribosomes and mithochondria to the phagosomes outer surface (Horwitz, 1983; Berger and Isberg, 1993). As a result of this organelle localization *L. pneumophila* survival and growth may be further accomodated.

The evolution of bacterial pathogens' resistance to macrophage killing has taken a number of unique pathways. Still many common features exist. Does this suggest that the equation for success against macrophages has a finite number of solutions. Conversely, is there a common reservoir of genetic information used by the numerous pathogenic bacteria?

In this review we have touched upon only a small portion of the host-parasite interaction. The cooperative interaction between the *Yersinia* adherence/invasion and antiphagocytic effector proteins provides significant insight into the ability of these bacteria to avoid phagocytosis. While these events give a firm impression of the subtlety of the *Yersinia* strategy for survival within humans they do not address the total host-parasite interaction. We have not discussed other proteins such as YopM, which is homologous to the platelet receptor for vonWillebrand factor and inhibits platelet aggregation (Leung and Straley, 1989; Reisner and Straley, 1992) or YpkA which shares protein sequence homology with serine/threonine kinases and expresses kinase activity *in vitro* (Gaylov, *et al.*, 1993). Moreover, *Yersinia* survival within insects and rodents in nature adds further complexity to the understanding of bacterial adaptability to different host environments. Similarly, the *Salmonella* spp. take up residence in a number of vertebrate hosts. Yet, despite virtually identical genetic composition and pathogenic strategy for survival within macrophages *S. typhi* is exclusively a human pathogen, while *S. typhimurium* can cause disease in mice and humans. In addition, *S. typhimurium* as a mouse pathogen causes a typhoid infection and as a human pathogen causes gastroenteritis. Therefore, a more holistic approach to the study of bacterial pathogens both in the context of disease and a pathogen's life outside the human host should lead to a better understanding of the evolution of the host parasite relationship.

References

Abshire, K.Z. and F.C. Neidhardt, 1993 - Growth rate paradox of *Salmonella typhimurium* within host macrophages. *J. Bacteriol.* **175**, 3744–3748.

Alpuche-Aranda, C.M., E.L. Racoosin, J.A. Swanson and S.I. Miller, 1994 - *Salmonella* stimulate macrophage macropinocytosis and persist within spacious phagosomes. *J. Exp. Med.* **179**, 601–8.

Bar-Sagi, D. and J.R. Feramisco, 1986 - Induction of membrane ruffling and fluid phase pinocytosis in quiescent fibroblasts by *ras* proteins. *Science* **233**, 1061–1068.

Behlau, I. and S. Miller, 1993 - A *phoP*-repressed gene promotes *Salmonella typhimurium* invasion of epithelial cells. *J. Bacteriol.* **175**, 4475–4484.

Berger, K.H. and R.R. Isberg, 1993 - Two distinct defects in intracellular growth complemented by a single genetic locus in Legionella pneumophila. *Mol. Microbiol.* **7**, 7–19.

Bliska, J.B., J.C. Clemens, J.E. Dixon and S. Falkow, 1992 - The *Yersinia* tyrosine phosphatase: specificity of a bacerial virulence determinant for phosphoproteins in the J774A.1 macrophage. *J. Exp. Med.* **176**, 1625–1630.

Bliska, J.B., M.C. Copass and S. Falkow, 1993 - The *Yersinia pseudotuberculosis* adhesin YadA mediates intimate bacterial attachment to and entry into HEp-2 cells. *Infect. Immun.* **61**, 3914–3921.

Bliska, J.B. and S. Falkow, 1992 - Bacterial resistance to complement killing mediated by the Ail protein of *Yersinia enterocolitica. Proc. Natl. Acad. Sci. USA* **89**, 3561–3565.

Bliska, J.B., K. Guan, J.E. Dixon and S. Falkow, 1991 - Tyrosine phosphate hydrolysis of host proteins by an essential *Yersinia* virulence determinant. *Proc. Natl. Acad. Sci. USA* **88**, 1187–1191.

Blum, G., M. Ott, A. Lischewski, A. Ritter, H. Imrich, H. Tschape and J. Hacker, 1994 - Excision of large DNA regions termed pathogenicity islands from tRNA-specific loci in the chromosome of an *Escherichia coli* wild-type pathogen. *Infect. Immun.* **62**, 606–614.

Carter, P.B., 1975 - Pathogenicity of *Yersinia enterocolitica* for mice. *Infect. Immun.* **11**, 164–170.

Carter, P.S. and F.M. Collins, 1974 - The route of enteric infection in normal mice. *J. Exp. Med.* **139**, 1189–1203.

Clark, M.A., M.A. Jepson, N.L. Simmons and B.H. Hirst, 1994 - Preferential interaction of *Salmonella typhimurium* with mouse Peyer's patch M cells. *Res. Microbiol.* **145**, 543–552.

Collazo, C.M., M.K. Zierler and J.E. Galan, 1995 - Functional analysis of the Salmonella typhimurium invasion gene invI and invJ and identification of a target of the protein secretion apparatus encoded in the inv locus. *Mol. Microbiol.* **15**, 25–38.

Elsinghorst, E.A., L.S. Baron and D.J. Kopeko, 1989 - Penetration of human intestinal epithelial cells by *Salmonella*: molecular cloning and expression of *Salmonella typhi* invasion determinants in *Escherichia coli. Proc. Natl. Acad. Sci. USA* **86**, 5173–5177.

Erickson, K., E. Galyov, C. Persson and H. Wolf-Watz, 1994 - The *lcrB* (*yscB/U*) gene cluster of *Yersinia pseudotuberculosis* is involved in Yop secretion and shows high homology to the spa gene clusters of *Shigella flexneri* and *Salmonella typhimurium. J. Bacteriol.* **176**, 2619–26.

Finlay, B.B., S. Ruschkowski and S. Dedhar, 1991 - Cytoskeletal rearrangements accompanying Salmonella entry into eptihelial cells. *J. Cell Sci.* **99**, 283–296.

Finlay, B.B., M.N. Starnbach, C.L. Francis, B.A. Stocker, S. Chatfield, G. Dougan and S. Falkow, 1988 - Identification and characterization of TnphoA mutants of Salmonella that are unable to pass through a polarized MDCK epithelial cell monolayer. *Mol. Microbiol.* **2**, 757–766.

Forsberg, A., R. Rosqvist and H. Wolf-Watz, 1994 - Regulation and polarized transfer of the *Yersinia* outer proteins (Yops) involved in antiphagocytosis. *Trends Microbiol.* **2**, 14–19.

Francis, C.L., T.A. Ryan, B.D. Jones, S.J. Smith and S. Falkow, 1993 - Ruffles induced by *Salmonella* and other stimuli direct macropinocytosis of bacteria. *Nature* **364**, 639–642.

Francis, C.L., M.N. Starnbach and S. Falkow, 1992 - Morphological and cytoskeletal changes in epithelial cells occur immediately upon interaction with Salmonella typhimurium grown under low-oxygen conditions. *Mol. Microbiol.* **6**, 3077–3087.

Galan, J.E. and R. Curtiss III, 1989 - Cloning and molecular characteriazation of genes whose products allow *Salmonella typhimurium* to penetrate tissue culture cells. *Proc. Natl. Acad. Sci. USA* **86**, 6383–6387.

Garcia-del Portillo, F. and B.B. Finlay, 1994 - *Salmonella* invasion of non-phagocytic cells induces formation of macropinosomes in the host cell. *Infect. Immun.* **62**, 4641–4645.

Gaylov, E.E., S. Hakansson, A. Forsberg and H. Wolf-Watz, 1993 - A secreted protein kinase of *Yersinia pseudotuberculoss* is an indispensible virulence determinant. *Nature* **361**, 730–732.

Ginocchio, C., J. Pace and J.E. Galan, 1992 - Identification and molecular characterization of a *Salmonella typhimurium* gene involved in triggering the internalization of salmonellae into cultured eptithelial cells. *Proc. Natl. Acad. Sci. USA* **89**, 5976–5980.

Ginocchio, C.C. and J.E. Galan, 1995 - Functional conservation among members of the *Salmonella typhimurium* InvA family of proteins. *Infect. Immun.* **63**, 729–732.

Griffin, F.M. and S.C. Silverstein, 1974 - Segmental response of the macrophage plasma membrane to a phagocytic stimulus. *J. Exp. Med.* **139**, 323–336.

Groisman, E.A. and H. Ochman, 1993 - Cognate gene clusters govern invasion of host epithelial cells by Salmonella typhimurium and Shigella flexneri. *EMBO J.* **12**, 3779–87.

Grutzkau, A., C. Hanski, H. Hahn and E.O. Riecken, 1990 - Involvement of M cells in the bacterial invasion of Peyer's patches: a common mechanism shared by *Yersinia enterocolitica* and other enteroinvasive bacteria. *Gut* **31**, 1011–1015.

Guan, K. and J.E. Dixon, 1990 - Protein tyrosine phosphatase activity of an essential virulence determinant in *Yersinia*. *Science* **249**, 553-556.

Hanski, C., U. Kutschka, H.P. Schmoranzer, M. Naumann, A. Stallmach, H. Hahn, H. Menge and E.O. Riecken, 1989 - Immunohistochemical and electron microscopic study of interaction of *Yersinia enterocolitica* serotype O8 with intestinal mucosa during experimental eteritis. *Infect. Immun.* **57**, 673–678.

Heffernan, E.J., J. Harwood, J. Fierer and D. Guiney, 1992 - The Salmonella typhimurium virulence plasmid complement resistance gene *rck* is homologous to a family of virulence-related outer membrane protein genes, including *pagC* and *ail*. *J. Bacteriol.* **174**, 84–91.

Heffernan, E.J., S. Reed, J. Hackett, J. Fierer, C. Roudier and D. Guiney, 1992 - Mechanism of resistance to complement-mediated killing of bacteria encoded by the *Salmonella typhimurium* virulence plasmid gene *rck*. *J. Clin. Invest.* **90**, 953–64.

Heffernan, E.J., L. Wu, J. Louie, S. Okamoto, J. Fierer and D.G. Guiney, 1994 - Specificity of the complement resistance and cell association phenotypes encoded by the outer membrane protein genes *rck* from *Salmonella typhimurium* and ail from *Yersinia enterocolitica. Infect. Immun.* **62**, 5183–6.

Horwitz, M.A., 1983 - Formation of a novel phagosome by the Legionnaires' disease bacterium (Legionella pneumophila) in human monocytes. *J. Exp. Med.* **158**, 1319–31.

Horwitz, M.A., 1983 - The Legionnaires' disease bacterium (*Legionella pneumophila*) inhibits phagosome-lysosome fusion in human monocytes. *J. Exp. Med.* **158**, 2108–26.

Horwitz, M.A., 1984 - Phagocytosis of the Legionnaires' disease bacterium (*Legionella pneumophila*) occurs by a novel mechanism: engulfment within a pseudopod coil. *Cell* **36**, 27–33.

Hynes, R.O., 1992 - Integrins: versatility, modulation and signalling in cell adhesion. *Cell* **69**, 11–25.

Isberg, R.R. and J.M. Leong, 1990 - Multiple β1 chain integrins are receptors for invasin, a protein that promotes bacterial penetration into mammalian cells. *Cell* **60**, 861–871.

Isberg, R.R., A. Swain and S. Falkow, 1988 - Analysis of expression and thermoregulation of the *Yersinia pseudotuberculosis inv* gene with hybrid proteins. *Infect. Immun.* **56**, 2133–2138.

Isberg, R.R., D.L. Voorhis and S. Falkow, 1987 - Identification of invasin: a protein that allows enteric bacteria to penetrate cultured mammalian cells. *Cell* **50**, 769–778.

Jones, B.D., N. Ghori and S. Falkow, 1994 - Salmonella typhimurium initiates murine infection by penetrating and destroying the specialized epithelial M cells of the Peyer's patches. *J. Exp. Med.* **180**, 15–23.

Jones, B.D., C.A. Lee and S. Falkow, 1992 - Invasion by *Salmonella typhimurium* is affected by the direction of flagellar rotation. *Infect. Immun.* **60**, 2475–2480.

Jones, B.D. and S. Falkow, 1994 - Identification and characterization of a *Salmonella typhimurium* oxygen-regulated gene required for bacterial internalization. *Infect. Immun.* **62**, 3745–52.

Kadowaki, T., S. Kayasu, E. Nishida, H. Sakai, F. Takaku, I. Yahara and M. Kasuga, 1986 - Insulin-like growth factors, insulin, and epidermal growth factor cause rapid cytoskeletal reorganization in KB cells. *J. Biol. Chem.* **261**, 16141–16147.

Kohbata, S., H. Yokoyama and E. Yabuuchi, 1986 - Cytopathogenic effect of *Salmonella typhi* GIFU 10007 on M cells of murine ileal Peyer's Patches in ligated ileal loops: an ultrastructural study. *Microbiol. Immunol.* **30**, 1225–1237.

Lambert de Rouvroit, C., C. Sluiters and G.R. Cornelis, 1992 - Role of the transcriptional activator, VirF, and temperature in the expression of the pYV plasmid genes of Yersinia enterocolitica. *Mol. Microbiol.* **6**, 395–409.

Lee, C.A. and S. Falkow, 1990 - The ability of *Salmonella* to enter mammalian cells is affected by bacterial growth state. *Proc. Natl. Acad. Sci. USA* **87**, 4304–4308.

Lee, C.A., B.D. Jones and S. Falkow, 1992 - Identification of a Salmonella typhimurium invasion locus by selection of hyperinvasive mutants. *Proc. Natl. Acad. Sci.* **89**, 1847–1851.

Leung, K.Y. and S.C. Straley, 1989 - The *yopM* gene of *Yersinia pestis* encodes a released protein having homology with the human platelet surface protein GPIbα. *J. Bacteriol.* **171**, 4623–4632.

Martinez, R.J., 1989 - Thermoregulation-dependent expression of *Yersinia enterocolitica* protein 1 imparts serum resistance to *Escherichia coli* K-12. *Infect. Immun.* **61**, 3732–3739.

Miller, S.I., 1991 - PhoP/PhoQ: macrophage-specific modulators of Salmonella virulence? *Mol. Microbiol.* **5**, 2073–2078.

Miller, V.L. and S. Falkow, 1988 - Evidence for two genetic loci in *Yersinia enterocolitica* that can promote invasion of epithelial cells. *Infect. Immun.* **56**, 1242–8.

Miyata, Y., E. Nishida and H. Sakai, 1989 - Regulation of the intracellular Ca^{2+} and cyclic AMP of the growth factor-induced ruffling membrane fromation and stimulation of fluid-phase endocytosis. *Exp. Cell Res.* **175**, 286–297.

Owen, R.L. and T.H. Ermak, 1990 - Structural specializations for antigen uptake and processing in the digestive tract. *Springer Semin. Immunopathol.* **12**, 139–152.

Pepe, J.C., J.L. Badger and V.L. Miller, 1994 - Growth phase and low pH affect the thermal regulation of the Yersinia enterocolitica inv gene. *Mol. Microbiol.* **11**, 123–35.

Pierson, D.E. and S. Falkow, 1993 - The *ail* gene of *Yersinia enterocolitica* has a role in the ability of the organism to survive serum killing. *Infect. Immun.* **61**, 1846–1852.

Pollack, C., S.C. Straley and M.S. Klempner, 1986 - Probing the phagolysosomal environment of human macrphages with a Ca^{2+}-responsive operon fusion in *Yersinia pestis*. *Nature* **322**, 834–837.

Pulkkinen, W.S. and S.I. Miller, 1991 - A *Salmonella typhimurium* virulence protein is similar to a *Yersinia enterocolitica* invasion protein and a bacteriophage lambda outer membrane protein. *J. Bacteriol.* **173**, 86–93.

Reisner, B.S. and S.C. Straley, 1992 - *Yersinia pestis* YopM: throbin binding and overexpression. *Infect. Immun.* **60**, 5242–5252.

Ridley, A.J., H.F. Paterson, C.L. Johnston, D. Diekmann and A. Hall, 1992 - The small GTP-binding protein rac regualtes growth factor-induced membrane ruffling. *Cell* **70**, 401–410.

Rosqvist, R., A. Forsberg and H. Wolf-Watz, 1991 - Intracellular targeting of the *Yersinia* YopE cytotoxin in mammalian cells induces actin microfilament disruption. *Infect. Immun.* **59**, 4562–4569.

Rosqvist, R., K.E. Magnusson and H. Wolf-Watz, 1994 - Target cell contact triggers expression and polarized transfer of Yersinia YopE cytotoxin into mammalian cells. *EMBO J.* **13**, 964–72.

Simonet, M., S. Richard and P. Berche, 1990 - Electron microscopic evidence for in vivo extracellular localization of *Yersinia pseudotuberculosis* harboring the pYV plasmid. *Infect. Immun.* **58**, 841–845.

Skurnik, M. and H. Wolf-Watz, 1989 - Analysis of the yopA gene encoding the Yop1 virulence determinant Yersinia spp. *Mol. Microbiol.* **3**, 517–529.

Straley, S.C., G.V. Plano, E. Skrzypek, P.L. Haddix and K.A. Fields, 1993 - Regulation by Ca^{2+} in the Yersinia low-Ca^{2+} response. *Mol. Microbiol.* **8**, 1005–1010.

Sturgill-Koszycki, S., P.H. Schlesinger, P. Chakraborty, P.L. Haddix, H.L. Collins, A.K. Fok, R.D. Allen, S.L. Gluck, J. Heuser and D.G. Russell, 1994 - Lack of acidification in *Mycobacterium* phagosomes produce by exclusion of the vesicular proton-ATPase. *Science* **263**, 678–681.

Takeuchi, A., 1967 - Electron microscope studies of experimental Salmonella infection. I. Penetration into the intestinal epithelium by *Salmonella typhimurium*. *Amer. J. Path.* **50**, 109–136.

Tartera, C. and E.S. Metcalf, 1993 - Osmolarity and growth phase overlap in regulation of *Salmonella typhi* adherence to and invasion of human intestinal cells. *Infect. Immun.* **61**, 3084–3089.

Yang, Y. and R.R. Isberg, 1993 - Cellular internalization in the absence of invasin expression is promoted by the *Yersinia pseudotuberculosis yadA* product. *Infect. Immun.* **61**, 3907–3913.

Zychlinsky, A., M.C. Prevost and P.J. Sansonetti, 1992 - *Shigella flexneri* induces apoptosis in infected macrophages. *Nature* **358**, 167–169.

Andrew Camilli, Claudette Gardel, John Wm. Tobias, Michael J. Mahan, James M. Slauch, Philip C. Hanna, John R. Collier and John J. Mekalanos

Molecular Cross Talk between Bacteria and their Hosts

Abstract

The investigation of the bacterial-host interaction has been dominated by the study of host immune responses. Little is known about how microbes specifically respond to environments within the host. We have developed new genetic approaches to define the genes bacteria express while in host tissues. Understanding these regulatory responses should provide insights into pathogenesis and the control of infectious agents.

Molecular cross talk between bacteria and their hosts

By nature, pathogenic bacteria must be able to survive and/or multiply on living host tissues and produce virulence factors to enhance this interaction. Classical virulence factors (e.g., adherence factors, toxins, invasins, etc.) are seldom essential components of cell structure and thus are usually not expressed constitutively under laboratory conditions (Mekalanos, 1992). When bacteria cycle between environments outside and inside a host, it must be assumed that they exercise economy by expressing the appropriate genes. While the expression of some virulence factors are probably turned on shortly after introduction into the host (e.g., upon encounter of the epithelial cell mucosal surface), others may only be induced after the organism enters specific host sub-compartments (e.g., the endosomal or lysosomal lumenal space). This hierarchy in the temporal order and spatial location of gene expression has probably evolved to maximize the chance of establishing a successful infection and then resisting the specific and nonspecific host immune responses to the incipient microbial invasion.

We must assume that the expression of virulence factors within the host is presumably accomplished via the same regulatory systems that have been defined under laboratory growth conditions. Unfortunately, these regulatory systems may recognize different signals in the laboratory than they do during the interaction of a pathogen with the host. Accordingly, we have been studying the virulence regulatory responses of bacteria within the context of infection by applying a family of molecular techniques that aim to define genes expressed by bacteria during their interaction with host tissues. While several different model systems have been employed in this analysis, the two that have been most successful to date involve the organisms *Salmonella typhimurium* and *Vibrio cholerae*.

In vivo expression technology utilizing *purA* as a reporter

In 1993, we reported our initial results with a new experimental strategy to identify bacterial genes that are specifically induced in host tissues. This new approach has been termed *in vivo* expression technology (or 'IVET') and was first utilized with the *Salmonella typhimurium*-BalbC mouse pathogen-host system (Mahan, 1993b).

This IVET selection system involved complementation of a bacterial strain carrying an auxotrophic mutation (*purA*) that highly attenuated its virulence at the level of growth or survival *in vivo*. Gene fusions between random promoters and a promoterless copy of the same biosynthetic gene (*purA*) were constructed and introduced into the auxotrophic strain. The resultant fusion pool was then introduced into a host animal. The environment inside the animal then selected for active promoters which allowed expression of the essential biosynthetic gene thus providing a positive enrichment for the bacterial gene fusions that were specifically expressed in animal tissues. The original pIVET1 vector also fused the random promoters to the *lacZY* genes of *E. coli* and thus provided a means of assessing the expression of gene fusions *in vitro* on laboratory media. A subset of gene fusions can thereby be identified that correspond to genes which are poorly expressed on laboratory media but which are highly expressed during the mouse infection. The analyzed data to date suggests that as much as 5% of the *S. typhimurium* chromosome (est. 200 genes) is devoted to sequences that are expressed during infection but not on MacConkey lactose agar inculated at 37°C under aerobic conditions (M. Mahan, J. Slauch, J. Tobias, and J. Mekalanos, unpublished results). We refer to these gene sequences as *in vivo* induced or '*ivi*' genes.

Characterization of *ivi* genes involved cloning and sequencing of the fusion junctions. In addition to biosynthetic genes originally reported (Mahan *et al.*, 1993b) a number of interesting genes that may represent possible 'adaptive response' genes were identified as *ivi* candidates. One such *ivi* was the *mutS* gene. MutS encodes a protein that binds to and is involved in the repair of mismatched DNA base pairs (Haber, 1988). The regulation of *mutS* is not understood and under laboratory media conditions only 10–20 molecules of MutS exist per cell. Thus, if *mutS* gene is induced during infection, one might predict that there is a greater need to repair DNA damage at the level of mismatched base pairs within the animal environment than on laboratory media. Perhaps DNA damage caused by highly reactive oxidation products produced within macrophages, is the source of this *in vivo* signal or alternatively another host signal (e.g., low pH) is used to tell the bacterium that it has entered an environment (the phagosome) where elevated DNA repair enzymes will be needed.

Antibiotic-based IVET selection strategy

The first IVET method we developed depended on the fact that an auxotrophic mutation could be defined in a pathogen of interest that resulted in its attenuation in an animal model for infection and disease. In order to extend the IVET approach to pathogens where such auxotrophic mutations have not yet been characterized, we have recently developed a new IVET vector that allows antibiotic resistance to be used to select *in vivo* induced genes (Mahan, 1995). Once again, *S. typhimurium* was used as a test organism to evaluate this new vector.

The antibiotic-IVET approach begins with the construction of a pool of recombinant plasmids that contain random fragments of *S. typhimurium* DNA cloned into a transcriptional vector, pIVET8. This plasmid is a derivative of the suicide vector pGP704 (Miller, 1988). Plasmid pIVET8 contains a promoterless chloramphenicol acetyl transferase (*cat*) gene joined to promoterless *lacZY* genes (the latter to allow transcription levels to be monitored *in vivo* and *in vitro*; (Mahan *et al.*, 1993b). The pool of recombinant plasmid clones is mated into Sm^r *S. typhimurium* strain, MT110, which cannot replicate pGP704 derivatives. Thus, the selected Ap^r Sm^r exconjugates have integrated the plasmid pool into the *S. typhimurium* chromosome by homologous recombination, using the cloned bacterial DNA as the source of homology. The product of the integration event generates a duplication of *S. typhimurium* material (including any potential *ivi* promoters) in which one promoter drives the *cat-lac* fusion, while the other promoter drives the expression of a wild-type copy of a putative *ivi* gene whose expression may be required for infection.

MacConkey Lactose indicator medium can be used to monitor *in vitro* expression levels by scoring the Lac phenotype of the fusion strain. Red colonies are Lac$^+$ and white colonies are Lac$^-$. Monitoring the population of *cat-lac* fusion strains on this medium is very important in optimizing the conditions under which transcriptionally active promoters are selected *in vivo*. When the pool of *cat-lac* fusions are grown in a given host, all constitutively active promoters are expected to answer the IVET selection because the selected gene product (*purA* or *cat*) would be produced all of the time. Because the pool of clones that are recovered from the animal show an increase in percentage of Lac$^+$ clones (red colonies) compared to the pre-selected pool, we have termed this expected shift, the 'red shift' (Mahan, 1994). The optimal conditions required to maximize the red shift is thus important to the success of the antibiotic-IVET selection. The concentration of antibiotic used to treat infected animals and the time table on this treatment is critical in order to select for transcriptionally active promoters *in vivo*. For the *S. typhimurium* model, the optimal red shift occurred under the following condition: 10^5 to 10^6 cells of the *cat-lac* fusion pool were injected i.p. into BALB/c mice followed by 18hr incubation. Infected mice were given 0.2 ml i.p. injections of 0.09 mg/ml chloramphenicol twice daily and 2.5 mg/ml chloramphenicol was also provided in the mouse drinking water. After 2 days, the infected mice were sacrificed and the bacterial cells were recovered from the spleen and the procedure repeated. Reconstruction experiments suggested that only bacterial cells that contain fusions to genes that are transcriptionally active are predicted to survive and propagate in animals so treated with chloramphenicol. Consistent with this prediction, a substantial red shift was observed after the mouse selection. In the pre-selected pool, 21% (37/180) of the *cat-lac* fusions were 'ON' *in vitro* (red or pink) and 79% (143/180) were 'OFF' (white). In contrast, after two rounds of selection with chloramphenicol *in vivo*, 95% (184/193) were 'ON' and 5% (9/193) were 'OFF'. The rare 5% Lac⁻ class of fusions that were recovered from the spleen presumably represent *ivi* gene fusions since they expressed high enough levels of Cat to overcome the antibiotic when the strain was grown in the animal, but expressed LacZ poorly when the strain was grown on laboratory medium.

The *ivi* gene fusions from several strains isolated from mouse *cat-lac* selection were cloned directly from the bacterial chromosome according to methods we have recently described (Mahan, 1993a). The *cat-lac* fusion joint points were then sequenced. One of the *ivi* fusions that answered the mouse *cat-lac* selection was located in *fadB*, a gene involved in the degradation of long and short chain fatty acids (Nunn, 1987). We showed that this *cat-lac* fusion is under the transcriptional control of the *fadB* promoter by demonstrating its induction in the presence of 5mm oleate on solid medium. Thus, the *in vivo* induction of *fadB* may reflect the high concentration of fatty acids in either phagocytic cells or the extracellular inflammatory milieu. It is known that phospholipase A_2 is activated during phagocytosis of bacteria and this enzyme produces arachidonic acid and ultimately other proinflammatory factors such as prostaglandins and leukotrienes (Pace, 1993; Svensson, 1991). We hypothesize that ß-oxidation by salmonellae of fatty acids such as arachidonate might act to suppress the local inflammatory response triggered by these metabolites. Additionally, it is well known that many different saturated and unsaturated fatty acids display toxicity associated with either their detergent action or free radical formation coincident with their peroxidation (Knapp, 1986). Thus, we propose that metabolism of fatty acids *via fadB*-dependent mechanisms might provide a protective mechanism for *S. typhimurium* from these host bacteriocidal mechanisms.

Although most bacterial species are destroyed within the phagocyte, *S. typhimurium* has evolved mechanisms to survive within the phagolysososme. The lysosomal vesicle is a hostile environment containing bactericidal elements such as hydrolytic enzymes (lysozyme, proteases, lipases, etc.), low pH, lactoferrin (iron deprivation), defensins (cationic pore-forming peptides), and highly reactive oxygen species (superoxide anion, hydrogen peroxide, free radical hydroxyl anion, hypochlorate, nitrous oxide etc.) (Spitznagel, 1993). The antibiotic-based IVET approach has turned out to be particularly useful in selecting bacterial genes that are specifically induced in the intracellular environment within macrophages. The protocol we used involved incubation of the *cat-lac* fusion pool with RAW 264.7 cultured macrophages for 2 hrs after which the antibiotic gentamicin was added to kill any extracellular *S. typhimurium*. Chloramphenicol (which enters mammalian cells) was then added to the culture medium and after an overnight incubation in the presence of the antibiotic, the surviving intracellular bacteria were recovered by lysing the macrophages in H_2O. The selection was repeated one more time. Using this protocol, a marked red shift was observed in favor of Lac^+ clones, from 21% (37/180) in the pre-selected pool to 86% (25/29) in the post-selected pool, suggesting that transcriptionally active promoters were selected within the macrophages by antibiotic treatment.

IVET vectors designed to probe transient changes in bacterial gene expression during host infection

The *purA*-based and antibiotic-based IVET vectors both demand continuous expression of *in vivo* induced genes during the infection cycle in order to complement or provide antibiotic resistance, respectively. It is probable that many virulence genes will not be expressed throughout the infection cycle but rather will be expressed only in short 'bursts' coincident with the bacterium's passage through host inducing environments. Accordingly, we have recently reported a new IVET approach based on transcriptional fusions to *tnpR*, encoding the site specific recombinase resolvase (Camilli, 1994). Resolvase acts on a 150 base pair DNA sequence called *res*. In our new system, the induction of the transcriptional *tnpR* gene fusions results in production of resolvase which, in turn, catalyzes excision of a linked tetracycline-resistance reporter gene flanked by direct repeats of *res*. Thus, the loss of tetracycline-resistance in bacterial progeny serves as an heritable marker of prior gene expression. This gene fusion approach allows one to assay the induction of gene expression in as few as one cell and also allows gene expression to be monitored at a different time and place from the inducing environment (a useful property in complex animal infection models). This new IVET system should be adaptable to virtually any pathogenic organism because TnpR requires only Mg^{2+} and negatively supercoiled DNA as substrates.

We used the well characterized, low iron-inducible, *irgA* gene of *V. cholerae* (Goldberg, 1992) to evaluate the use of the TnpR-based IVET system. We constructed a *irgA::tnpR* transcriptional fusion and showed first that it obeyed the previously established *in vitro* conditions for repression and induction of *irgA* by limiting iron in growth media. Growth of the *irgA::tnpR* fusion strain in high-iron medium resulted in few detectable Tc^s progeny while growth in a low-iron medium resulted in essentially complete loss of tetracycline-resistance within the bacterial population (99.5% Tc^s progeny). Moreover, when the fusion strain was shifted from a high-iron medium to a low-iron medium, tetracycline sensitive bacteria appeared within 20 minutes. To test the hypothesis that the intestine represented a low iron environment, animals were intraintestinally infected with the fusion strain and after *in vivo* growth, resolution was monitored by scoring tetracycline resistance among the bacteria recovered from intestinal contents. No detectable resolution occurred even after consecutive passages of the fusion strain in infant mice and adult rabbits suggesting that the small intestine was a non-inducing environment for the *irgA-tnpR* fusion. In contrast, injection of the reported strain into the mouse peritoneal cavity, resulted in extensive resolution demonstrating that the *irgA-tnpR* fusion was capable of being induced *in vivo*.

We were surprised by the apparent lack of high levels of *irgA* expression during intestinal infection but believe that this result indicates that either iron sources are readily available in this host compartment or that regulation of *irgA* in the intestine is more complex than *in vitro* experiments would suggest. The anaerobic environment present in the small intestine might result in significant availability of iron in its reduced (Fe^{2+}) form which is not sequestered by host iron-binding proteins like lactoferrin and transferrin. Within the mouse peritoneal cavity this is apparently not the case and indeed the *irgA-tnpR* fusion induced nicely within this compartment. Thus, the resolvase fusion to *irgA* was capable of recognizing two different host compartments demonstrating clearly the ability of a pathogenic bacterium to sense these different host anatomical locations based on presumably a difference in the availability of iron.

We have recently used the resolvase IVET vector to identify genes of *V. cholerae* that are highly induced *in vivo* within the intestine. This was done by generating a random *tnpR*-gene fusion library, infecting a host, recovering the bacteria after a certain time, and screening for Tc^s recombinants (A. Camilli, and J. Mekalanos, unpublished results). Strains which had resolved and lost the reporter gene *in vivo* contain *tnpR* fusions to genes which were presumably expressed during infection (i.e., *ivi* genes). After cloning and sequencing of the selected *ivi* fusion junctions, the identity of a number of different *V. cholerae ivi* genes could be inferred based on their sequence similarity to genes in the sequence data base. These included genes involved in anaerobic metabolism, permeases, an outer membrane protein, and a lipase. Interestingly, among over twenty gene fusions analyzed by DNA sequencing to date, none were found to be identical to any of the 18 known ToxR-regulated genes. ToxR is the regulator responsible for transcriptional activation of cholera toxin, the toxin co-regulated pilus, and other virulence genes of *V. cholerae* (DiRita, 1992). The lack of ToxR-regulated genes among the *ivi* genes identified with the resolvase vector might be explained in a number of different ways. It is possible, for example, that ToxR-regulated genes are simply expressed at too high a level *in vitro* (i.e., on laboratory media) for them to answer the *ivi* definition. Alternatively, ToxR-regulated genes might be reduced in expression *in vivo* as has been hypothesized earlier in studies that showed that transcription of ToxR is modulated by the heat shock response (Parsot, 1990). Most recently we have obtained results that suggest that the ToxR regulatory system is coupled to the status of the motility-chemotaxis system of *V. cholerae*. Interestingly, at least one *ivi* gene fusion was found to be located in the *flaA-flaC* intragenic region in the opposite orientation to *fla* gene transcription. There are two possible explanations for the *in vivo* expression of this resolvase gene fusion. First, transcription in the *fla* region is down-regulated during *in vivo* growth allowing expression from a cryptic low level promoter located in this region in an opposite orientation. Second, an *ivi*

Molecular cross talk between bacteria and their hosts

promoter in the *fla* region defined by the *tnpR* gene fusion is upregulated *in vivo* and might therefore lead to a decrease in *flaAC* expression through an 'anti-sense' mechanism.

Cross talk between motility and the ToxR regulatory system of *V. cholerae*

We have noted a connection between alterations in the motility phenotype of *V. cholerae* and ToxR regulation that complements the observations noted above in the TnpR fusion studies. Namely, we have found that a number of different virulence phenotypes, including some which are ToxR-regulated, are affected by mutations that either increase or decrease the motility/chemotaxis 'fitness' of *V. cholerae* (C. Gardel and J. Mekalanos, unpublished results). Two different classes of mutants have been isolated termed 'hyperswarmer' and 'nonmotile' which either penetrate soft agar more rapidly than wild type strains or not at all, respectively. Most hypermotile mutants of *V. cholerae*, show a dramatic reduction in the expression of ToxR-regulated gene products such as cholera toxin and toxin coregulated pili (TCP). These same hyperswarmer mutants show elevated expression of protease and a fucose-sensitive hemagglutinin (FSHA). In contrast, nonmotile mutants show elevated expression of ToxR-regulated gene products particularly under growth conditions that are not optimal for production of these factors *in vitro* (e.g., media of alkaline pH). Nonmotile mutants also produce low levels of FSHA and protease. Thus, these two groups of potential virulence factors are expressed in a reciprocal fashion *in vitro* at least in regard to how they respond to mutational alterations in the motility/chemotaxis phenotype. Interestingly, two ToxR-regulated genes called TcpI and AcfB have been recently identified that appear to be a homologs of methyl accepting chemoreceptors (Everiss, 1994). Moreover, one of the genes in the *hly* operon of *V. cholerae* (termed *hlyB*) has also been identified as a homolog of a methyl accepting chemoreceptor (Jeffery, 1993). The TnpR-based resolvase system described above has recently shown that *hlyC*, the gene immediately downstream from *hlyB* and presumably in the same transcriptional unit (Alm, 1990), is in fact an *in vivo* induced gene (C. Camilli and J. Mekalanos, unpublished). Thus, it is apparent that alterations in the expression of motility, chemotaxis, and ToxR-regulated virulence genes are occurring *in vivo* presumably in response to changing signals within intestinal microenvironments.

We propose that the expression of virulence factors by *V. cholerae* occurs in at least three distinct phases. We have previously presented evidence that the heat shock response can down regulate expression of *toxR* transcription and may reflect the initial contact between the vibrios and the harsh environment within the stomach of the infected host (Parsot *et al.*, 1990). A transient 'ToxR⁻ state' results, and may in fact help the transition of the vibrios into the next stage of the colonization process. In the next phase of the colonization process, the vibrios are presummed to be highly motile and chemotatic and thus swim toward the intestinal mucus and down deep into the intestinal crypts (Freter,

1981). It is in this phase that factors such as protease and FSHA are highly expressed and thus are able to aid in the binding to and penetration of the mucus gel. ToxR-regulated gene products such as cholera toxin and TCP are not expressed during this motile phase of the colonization process. Shortly after penetration of the mucus gel and colonization of the intestinal crypts, the vibrios find themselves in yet a new microenvironment. This environment signals significant down-regulation of motility and chemotaxis phenotypes (perhaps through the *flaA* antisense mechanisms noted above) and a commensurate up-regulation of ToxR-regulated gene products. It is during this phase that the vibrios become tightly adherent to absorptive epithelial and crypt cells through the expression of TCP pili and where they first produce significant amounts of cholera toxin. The chemoreceptors (TcpI, AcfB and HlyB) that are expressed via ToxR-mediated or other *in vivo* activated promoters are presumably expressed in this adherent, nonmotile phase. We postulate that these chemoreceptors may actually be involved in sensing subsequent changes in the intestinal environment that occur concomitantly with the fluid secretory response and extensive multiplication of the vibrios on the mucosal epithelium. These late stage environmental changes cause the vibrios to swim away from the mucosa and thus deciminate most efficiently through the massive diarrheal purge that characterizes cholera.

Conclusions

Clearly the interaction between bacteria and their hosts is complex. Most of the time we tend to emphasize disease as the normal consequence of microbial-host interactions that involve pathogenic species of microbes. However, it is important to also remember that subclinical infections are more common than overt disease. Indeed it has been generally appreciated that the progressive evolution of a pathogen can lead to its decreased virulence rather than its increased virulence (Mims, 1987). Pathogens might modulate their virulence in ways that prolong the host interaction and thereby optimize transmission as well as growth yield of the microbe. Presumably, an important way that pathogens achieve this optimal microbial-host interaction is through regulation. Upon entry into the host, appropriate gene expression might lead to increases or decreases in virulence gene expression depending on host conditions (e.g., permissive or nonpermissive growth environments), or microbial conditions (e.g., population density or accumulation of toxic byproducts of metabolism) (Mekalanos, 1992). *Salmonella typhimurium* and *Vibrio cholerae* provide wonderful experimental systems to probe deeper into these complex host-parasite interactions. IVET experiments have surprisingly demonstrated that our preconceptions about certain host environments and the expression of various bacterial virulence factors may be wrong. Clearly, there is still much to learn about the bacterial response to host signals. We are optimistic that this knowledge will provide new insights into microbial pathogenesis and thus better strategies for control of infectious agents.

References

Alm, R.A. and P.A. Manning, 1990 - Characterization of the *hlyB* gene and its role in the production of the El Tor haemolysin of *Vibrio cholerae*. *Mol. Microbiol.* **4**, 413–425.

Camilli, A., D. Beattie and J. Mekalanos, 1994 - Use of genetic recombination as a reporter of gene expression. *Proc. Natl. Acad. Sci. USA* **91**, 2634–2638.

DiRita, V.J., 1992 - Co-ordinate expression of virulence genes by ToxR in *Vibrio cholerae*. *Mol. Microbiol.* **6**, 451–458.

Everiss, K.D., K.J. Hughes, M.E. Kovach and K.M. Peterson, 1994 - The *Vibrio cholerae acfB* colonization determinant encodes an inner membrane protein that is related to a family of signal-transducing proteins. *Infect. Immun.* **62**, 3289–3298.

Freter, R., P.C.M. O'Brien and M.M.S. Macsai, 1981 - Role of chemotaxis in the association of motile bacteria with intestinal mucose *in vivo* studies. *Infect. Immun.* **34**, 234–240.

Goldberg, M.C., S.A. Boyko, J.R. Butterton, J.A. Stoebner, S.M. Payne and S.B. Calderwood, 1992 - Characterization of a *Vibrio cholerae* virulence factor homologous to the family of TonB-dependent proteins. *Mol. Microbiol.* **6**, 2407–2418.

Haber, L.T., P.P. Pang, D.I. Sobell, J.A. Mankovich and G.C. Walker, 1988 - Nucleotide Sequence of the *Salmonella typhimurium mutS* Gene Required for Mismatch Repair: Homology of MutS and HexA of *Streptococcus pneumoniae*. *J. Bacteriol.* **170**, 197–202.

Jeffery, C.J. and J.D.E. Koshland, 1993 - *Vibrio cholerae hlyB* is a member of the chemotaxis receptor gene family. *Protein Sci.* **2**, 1532–1535.

Knapp, H.R. and M.A. Melly, 1986 - Bacteriocidal effects of polyunsaturated fatty acids. *J. Infect. Dis.* **154**, 84–94.

Mahan, M.J., J.M. Slauch, P.C. Hanna, A. Camilli, J.W. Tobias, M.K. Waldor and M. J.J., 1994 - Selection for bacterial genes that are specifically induced in host tissues: the hunt for virulence factors., pp. 263–268. In: S. Falkow (Ed.): *Infectious Agents and Disease*, Raven Press, New York.

Mahan, M.J., J.M. Slauch and J.J. Mekalanos, 1993a - Bacteriophage P22 transduction of integrated plasmids: single-step cloning of *Salmonella typhimurium* gene fusions. *J. Bacteriol.* **175**, 7086–7091.

Mahan, M.J., J.M. Slauch and J.J. Mekalanos, 1993b - Selection of bacterial virulence genes that are specifically induced in host tissues. *Science* **259**, 686–688.

Mahan, M.J., J.W. Tobias, J.M. Slauch, P.C. Hanna, R.J. Collier and J.J. Mekalanos, 1995 - Antibiotic-based IVET selection for bacterial virulence genes that are specifically induced during infection. *Proc. Natl. Acad. Sci. USA in press*.

Mekalanos, J.J., 1992 - Environmental signals controlling expression of virulence determinants in bacteria. *J. Bacteriol.* **174**, 1–7.

Miller, V.L. and J.J. Mekalanos, 1988 - A novel suicide vector and its use in construction of insertion mutations: osmoregulation of outer membrane proteins and virulence determinants in *Vibrio cholerae* requires *toxR. J. Bacteriol.* **170**, 2575–2583.

Mims, C.A., 1987 - The Pathogenesis of Infectious Disease, pp. 1–7. In: C.A. Mims (Ed.): *The Pathogenesis of Infectious Disease*, Academic Press, London.

Nunn, W.D., 1987 - Two-carbon compounds and fatty acids as carbon sources, pp. 285–301. In: F.C. Neidhardt (Ed.): *Escherichia coli and Salmonella typhimurium Cellular and Molecular Biology*, American Society for Microbiology, Washington, DC

Pace, J., M.J. Hayman and J.E. Galan, 1993 - Signal transduction and invasion of epithelial cells by *S. typhimurium. Cell* **72**, 505–514.

Parsot, C. and J.J. Mekalanos, 1990 - Expression of ToxR, the transcriptional activator of the virulence factors in Vibrio cholerae, is modulated by the heat shock response. *Proc. Natl. Acad. Sci. USA* **87**, 9898–902.

Spitznagel, J.K., 1993 - Constitutive Defenses of the Body, pp. 90–113. In: M. Schaechter, G. Medoff, and B. I. Eisenstein (Eds): *Mechanisms of microbial disease*, Williams and Wilkins, Baltimore, Maryland.

Svensson, U., E. Holst and R. Sundler, 1991 - Proteinkinase-C-independent activation of arachidonate release and prostaglandin E2 formation in macrophages interacting with certain bacteria. *Eur. J. Biochem.* **200**, 699–705.

P. Baumann

Biology of Aphid Endosymbionts (Genus *Buchnera*)

Abstract

Most aphids are dependent on an association with an intracellular prokaryotic endosymbiont (*Buchnera*). Evolutionary studies are consistent with an infection of an aphid ancestor with *Buchnera* and subsequent cospeciation of the host and the bacterium. Genetic studies show that *Buchnera* resembles free-living bacteria in having genes coding for proteins involved in DNA replication, transcription, translation and a variety of other functions. Studies of the genetics of the tryptophan biosynthetic pathway indicate that *trpEG* genes of *Buchnera* are on plasmids and are amplified, relative to the remaining chromosomal genes. The *trpEG* genes encode anthranilate synthase, the first enzyme of the pathway, which is feedback-inhibited by tryptophan. Amplification of *trpEG* is consistent with past evidence suggesting that one of the functions of *Buchnera* is the over-production of tryptophan for the aphid host.

Introduction

Aphids (class, Insecta; order, Homoptera; superfamily, Aphidoidea) are insects that feed on plant sap (Buchner, 1965; Douglas, 1989; Hauk and Griffiths, 1980). Aphids penetrate plant tissue by means of flexible stylets which probe until they reach the sieve tubes in the phloem tissue. This mode of feeding is conducive to the transmission of disease. Aphids are important vectors of plant viruses and cause major economic losses in agriculture. The general properties of aphids are shared by whiteflies (Aleyrodoidea) and mealybugs (Pseudococcidae), which are related insects within the order Homoptera. All of these insects have a mutualistic association with intracellular prokaryotes (Douglas, 1989; Houk and Griffiths, 1980). The endosymbionts of aphids have been studied most extensively and have been assigned to the genus *Buchnera*, which currently has one species, *B. aphidicola*. (Recent reviews on endosymbionts are those of Douglas, 1989; Ishikawa, 1989; and Baumann *et al.*, 1995ab. Due to space limitations, many relevant references could not be cited in this discussion and are included in Baumann *et al.*, 1995ab).

Morphology, growth and transmission

Within the body cavity of most aphids is a bilobed structure (bacteriome) consisting of 60 to 90 cells called bacteriocytes. Within these cells are host-derived vesicles (symbiosomes) which contain *Buchnera* (Figure 1). This organism is oval-shaped and has a gram-negative cell wall. *Buchnera* and the aphid are dependent on each other. The endosymbionts have not been cultivated outside the host. Elimination of the endosymbionts by antibiotics or other treatments causes decreased growth of the aphid, sterility and eventual death. Some species of aphids have additional intracellular bacteria designated as secondary endosymbionts, which are absent from bacteriocytes and which do not appear to play an essential role in the life of the aphid.

Aphids vary greatly in their annual life cycles and host plant preferences. During their most active reproductive stage, aphids are parthenogenetic females which contain embryos and give birth to live young. Under laboratory conditions a typical aphid, *Schizaphis graminum*, which is a major pest of cereals, gives birth to young having an average weight of 24 μg and containing 0.2×10^6 endosymbionts. The increase in the number of *Buchnera* cells during aphid growth approximately parallels the increase in the weight and protein and total

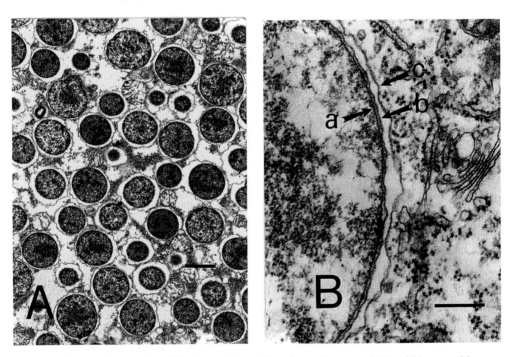

Fig. 1.   Electron micrographs of *Buchnera* (A) within a bacteriocyte and (B) within a symbiosome showing the (a) cell membrane and (b) outer membrane of the endosymbiont and (c) the symbiosome membrane. Bar in (A) and (B), represents 2 μm and 0.5 μm, respectively. Photograph courtesy of D. McLean and M. Kinsey.

DNA content of the aphid, indicating a close integration of growth of the endosymbiont with that of the host. The aphid reaches a maximal weight of 540 ug in 10 to 11 days and contains 5×10^6 endosymbionts, an approximately 28-fold increase in the *Buchnera* population. During this time there is an increase in the bacteriocyte volume, but not bacteriocyte number (Douglas and Dixon, 1987). New aphids are born about 8 days after the birth of the mother, and each aphid can produce 50 to 60 live young. *Buchnera* is transmitted maternally to the offspring by complex mechanisms which have not been extensively studied.

Evolutionary relationships and rRNA gene organization

Sequence comparisons of endosymbiont genes coding for 16S rRNA (rDNA) were used to establish evolutionary relationships. The results for *Buchnera* are presented in Figure 2. The nearest relatives were members of the *Enterobacteriaceae* (which includes *Escherichia coli*) and the newly characterized bacteriocyte endosymbionts of the tsetse fly (Aksoy *et al.*, 1994) (results not included). The latter were more closely related to *E. coli* than to *Buchnera* (Aksoy, 1994; Aksoy *et al.*, 1994). All of these organisms are in the gamma-3

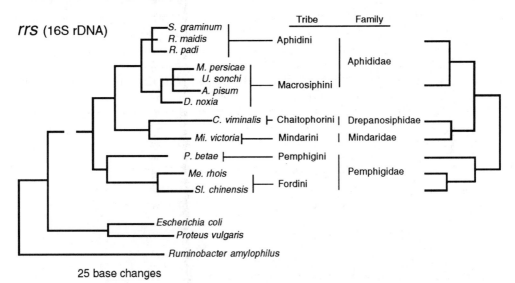

Fig. 2. *Buchnera* phylogeny based on 16S rDNA sequences and comparison with a proposed phylogeny of the aphid hosts. Names designate the aphid host. The following abbreviations designate aphid genera: *S, Schizaphis*; *R, Rhopalosiphum*; *M, Myzus*; *U, Uroleucon*; *A, Acyrthosiphon*; *D, Diuraphis*; *C. Chaitophorus*; *Mi, Mindarus*; *P, Pemphigus*; *Me, Melaphis*; *Sl, Schlechtendalia*. Redrawn from Baumann *et al.* (1995a) and Moran *et al.* (1993).

subdivision of the *Proteobacteria*. An inspection of Figure 2 indicates that the groupings of *Buchnera* agree with those of classical aphid taxonomy based on morphology and that the branching order within the *Buchnera* phylogenetic tree is identical to the proposed phylogeny of aphids (Moran and Baumann, 1993; Moran *et al.*, 1993). On the basis of the fossil record for aphids, dates could be assigned to the branch points of the *Buchnera* phylogenetic tree, allowing an estimation of the rate of change of 16S rRNA sequences (Moran *et al.*, 1993). The totality of these results is consistent with the following interpretation. Approximately 200 to 250 million years ago an ancestor of present-day aphids was infected with a free-living bacterium and an endosymbiotic association became established. Subsequent parallel divergence led to cospeciation of *Buchnera* and host, resulting in the present species of aphids and strains of *Buchnera*. A more limited analysis of the endosymbionts of whiteflies and mealybugs indicated that they constitute two different lineages distinct from *Buchnera*.

In most bacteria the genes for rRNA are arranged as a single transcription unit consisting of *16S-23S-5S*. *Buchnera* differs from these organisms in having the rRNA genes on two transcription units containing (i) *16S* and (ii) *23S-5S* (Figure 3) (Munson *et al.*, 1993; Rouhbakhsh and Baumann, 1995). Based on the linkage arrangements illustrated in Figure 3, pairs of oligonucleotide primers (*argS-16S*) and (*aroE-23S*) were designed and used in conjunction with the polymerase chain reaction to allow the identification of *Buchnera* (Rouhbakhsh *et al.*, 1995). Both *16S* and *23S* were preceded by conserved DNA sequences corresponding to putative -35 (TTGAC^A/T) and -10 (TGTA^A/T^T) promoter regions. A DNA fragment upstream of *16S* (Fig. 3) functioned as a promoter in *E. coli* and a DNA fragment downstream of *16S* functioned as a terminator (Munson *et al.*, 1993). As is characteristic of other slow-growing bacteria, *Buchnera* contains only one copy of the rRNA genes in its genome (Baumann and Baumann, 1994; Wolfe and Haygood, 1993).

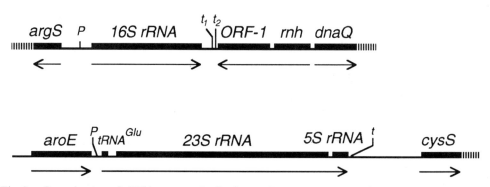

Fig. 3. Organization of rRNA operons in *Buchnera*. *P*, promoter; *t*, terminator; *ORF*, open reading frame; striped line, partial sequence of gene; arrow, direction of transcription. For explanation of gene designations see Tables 1. Redrawn from Munson *et al.* (1993) and Rouhbakhsh and Baumann (1995).

Genetics and physiology

The DNA of *Buchnera* has a guanine + cytosine content of 28 to 30 mol %, a value similar to that of the aphid host. Its genome size (1.4×10^{10} daltons) is approximately five times that of *E. coli* (Ishikawa, 1989). Over 60 kilobase pairs (kbp) of *Buchnera* DNA have been cloned and sequenced. Genes coding for proteins involved in DNA synthesis, transcription and translation, enzymes of the common portion of the aromatic amino acid biosynthetic pathways, enzymes of the tryptophan biosynthetic pathway, chaperonins, as well as genes for other functions have been detected in the endosymbiont (Table 1, Figure 4). Consistent with these results, it has been shown that isolated *Buchnera* are able to synthesize DNA, rRNA, and over 210 different proteins (Ishikawa, 1989). As in the case of other intracellular bacteria, *Buchnera* has elevated levels of GroEL (Aksoy, 1994; Ohtaka *et al.*, 1992). The totality of these observations indicates that *Buchnera* has many of the genetic and physiological properties of free-living bacteria.

In *E. coli*, many of the genes homologous to those of *Buchnera* have upstream and downstream DNA sequences involved in regulation of gene expression. In *Buchnera* such sequences have for the most part not been detected. There are a few differences which may be of interest in that they could represent modifications which are an adaptation to the endosymbiotic association. DnaA is a protein which initiates chromosome replication by binding to a DNA segment known as the origin of replication (Yoshikawa and Ogasawara, 1991). The characteristic features of the origin of replication are several nine-nucleotide

Table 1.   Genes detected in *Buchnera* and the designations of the deduced products.[a]

Proteins involved in DNA synthesis: DnaA (*dnaA*), primase (*dnaG*), β- and ε-subunit of DNA polymerase III (*dnaN*, *dnaQ*), subunit B of gyrase (*gyrB*), RNase H (*rnh*).

RNA polymerase: α-(*rpoA*), β-(*rpoB*), β′-(*rpoC*), σ-(*rpoD*) subunits.

Ribosomal RNAs: 16S-(*rrs*), 23S-(*rrl*), 5S-(*rrf*) rRNA.

Ribosomal proteins: S4 (*rpsD*), S11 (*rpsK*), L7/L12 (*rplL*), L20 (*rplT*), L34 (*rpmH*), L35 (*rpmI*).

tRNA synthases: argS, cysS, thrS.

Chaperonins: SecB (*secB*), GroEL (*groEL*), GroES (*groES*).

Amino acid biosynthesis: Tryptophan biosynthetic pathway, serine acetyltransferase (*cysE*), 3-deoxy-D-*arabino*-heptulosonate 7-phosphate synthase (*aroH*), shikimate dehydrogenase (*aroE*).

Miscellaneous: Initiation factor-3 (*infC*), RNase P (*rnpA*), β-subunit of ATP synthase (*atpD*), β-subunit of integration host factor (*himD*), glyceraldehyde-3-phosphate dehydrogenase (*gapA*), triose phosphate isomerase (*tpiA*).

---

[a]Protein designation followed by gene designation in parentheses. Data from Lai and Baumann (1992ab), Lai *et al.* (1994), Munson and Baumann (1993), Munson *et al.* (1993) Ohtaka *et al.* (1992), Rouhbakhsh and Baumann (1995), and additional references given in Baumann *et al.* (1995a).

sequences known as DnaA boxes and adenine- and thymine-rich direct repeats. The linkage relationship of genes around *dnaA* is highly conserved in bacteria: the order in most cases is *rnpA-rpmH-dnaA-dnaN-recF-gyrB* (Ogasawara and Yoshikawa, 1992). In most organisms the origin of replication is between *rpmH* and *dnaA*, but in *E. coli* it is approximately 40 kilobases away. In this species, a DnaA box is present upstream of *dnaA* and is involved in the autoregulation of DnaA protein. The *dnaA* region of *Buchnera* differs from that of most other organisms in two features (Baumann *et al.*, 1995a; Lai and Baumann, 1992a). The first is the absence of DnaA boxes and other properties characteristic of an origin of replication between *rpmH* and *dnaA*, suggesting that, as in *E. coli*, the origin of replication lies elsewhere. The absence of a DnaA box upstream of *Buchnera dnaA* may be an indication of a different mechanism of regulation of DnaA synthesis and, hence, initiation of chromosome replication. This regulation could be under the control of host signals. A second difference in the *Buchnera dnaA* region is the absence of *recF* between *dnaN* and *gyrB*. This gene could be located elsewhere or, alternatively, since RecF is involved in the repair of UV-damaged DNA, it is possible that due to the intracellular location of *Buchnera*, this function is no longer necessary. The same absence of *recF* was also recently noted in *Spiroplasma citri*, another organism which leads a sheltered existence within plant tissue (Ye *et al.*, 1994). In *E. coli* and a variety of other organisms, *rpoD* (σ^{70}) is followed by one or two inverted repeats characteristic of *rho*-independent terminators; inverted repeats are not found downstream of *Buchnera rpoD* (Lai and Baumann, 1992b).

Tryptophan biosynthesis

Plant sap, the diet of aphids, is rich in carbohydrates but deficient in amino acids and other nitrogenous compounds. Insects are thought to require ten essential amino acids and one of the proposed functions of the endosymbionts is the synthesis of these amino acids for the aphid host. Some aphids are able to grow and reproduce on a synthetic diet. There is an extensive literature on the amino acid requirements of aphids. In principle, the demonstration of a requirement in the presence but not in the absence of an antibiotic is strong evidence that the biosynthetic activities of the endosymbionts are the source of the amino acid. In practice, such clear-cut results have rarely been obtained and the results are often difficult to interpret. Nevertheless, the consensus of opinion derived from such experiments is that endosymbionts produce essential amino acids for the aphid host (Baumann *et al.*, 1995ab; Douglas, 1989; Ishikawa, 1989). Using nutritional methods as well as radioactive tracers evidence has been obtained indicating that *Buchnera* is able to reduce sulfate to sulfide and synthesize methionine and cysteine (Douglas, 1990). By far, the best evidence has been obtained for the synthesis of tryptophan by the endosymbionts. Douglas and Prosser (1992) have found that most aphids survive to adulthood on a synthetic diet containing tryptophan and chlortetracycline, while the omission of tryptophan leads to death of the aphids. In addition, these investigators have detected in *Buchnera*, tryptophan synthase, the last enzyme of the tryptophan biosynthetic pathway. The inclusion of chlortetracycline in the diet led to the elimination of tryptophan synthase activity. While this work was in progress we independently initiated studies on the genetics of the *Buchnera* tryptophan biosynthetic pathway (Lai *et al.*, 1994; Munson and Baumann, 1993).

The modifications which *Buchnera* potentially must undergo in order to overproduce tryptophan or any other biosynthetic endproduct involve a major change in the regulation of the biosynthetic pathway (Baumann *et al.*, 1995ab; Lai *et al.*, 1994). The ancestor of *Buchnera* probably resembled other free-living bacteria in that it had mechanisms which integrated the rate of tryptophan synthesis to the intracellular and extracellular availability of this amino acid. In almost all bacteria, the immediate effect of tryptophan accumulation is feedback inhibition of anthranilate synthase (AS, encoded by *trpEG*), the first enzyme of the pathway. The long-term effect of tryptophan accumulation is repression of synthesis of the enzymes of this pathway. The first step of endosymbiont adaptation could be a mutation to constitutivity, so that the enzymes of the pathway would be produced in the presence of tryptophan. Such mutations are common in studies of directed evolution. Even if tryptophan is exported from the cell, its overproduction could result in some accumulation which would be expected to reduce activity of AS by feedback inhibition. As in the case of many other allosteric enzymes, considerable activity of AS is present even at high levels of tryptophan. In order to augment AS activity, *Buchnera* could have a mutation in sites which would desensitize the enzyme to allosteric feedback inhibition. An alternative modification is gene amplification resulting in the production of more AS protein, which, even in the presence of tryptophan, would provide sufficient AS activity for the synthesis of this amino acid. Gene amplification is a common mechanism for the overproduction of enzyme protein under conditions where the growth rate is limited by a particular enzyme activity (Anderson and Roth, 1977). Its frequency can be as high as 10^{-4} to 10^{-5}, which is considerably higher then the frequency of mutations leading to changes in structural genes resulting in desensitization of feedback inhibition. Our studies indicate that gene amplification of *trpEG* is the alternative favored by several rapidly growing species of aphids.

Studies of *Buchnera* from the aphid *S. graminum* have indicated the presence of all of the genes of the tryptophan biosynthetic pathway (Fig. 4). The arrangement *trpDC(F)BA* suggests a single transcription unit and restriction enzyme analysis is consistent with a single copy of these genes on the endosymbiont chromosome. On the other hand, *trpEG* is amplified 14- to 15-fold, relative to the chromosomal genes and is found on plasmids consisting of four tandem repeats of a 3.6-kbp unit (Figure 4). Since *Buchnera* AS has all of the amino acid residues which are required for allosteric feedback inhibition of activity (Lai *et al.*, 1994), gene amplification would result in an increase in AS protein which could still provide sufficient activity for the overproduction of tryptophan, even in the presence of this end product.

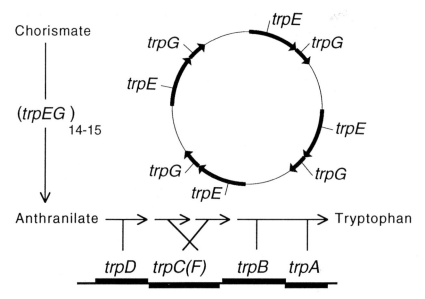

Fig. 4. Genetics of tryptophan biosynthesis in *Buchnera* from the aphid *S. graminum*. *trpEG* is on a plasmid (four tandem repeats) and is amplified 14 to 15-fold relative to the remaining genes of the pathway which are present as one copy on the chromosome. Redrawn from Lai *et al.* (1994) and Munson and Baumann (1993).

Gene amplification of plasmid-borne 3.6-kbp units containing *trpEG* has also been found in *Buchnera* from the aphids *R. maidis* and *A. pisum* (Figure 5). In *R. maidis* the 3.6-kbp unit constitutes a single plasmid, while in *A. pisum* plasmids containing 5, 6, and 10 tandem repeats of this unit have been found. In the latter aphid it is not known whether *Buchnera* from a single aphid has one or several different-sized plasmids. All of these aphids as well as *S. graminum* have a short development time and are in the family Aphididae (Lai *et al.*, 1995). In contrast, the aphid *Schlechtendalia chinensis*, which is in the family

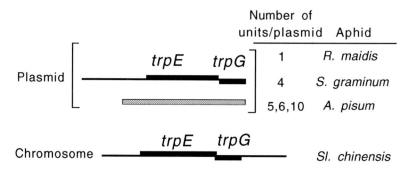

Fig. 5. Arrangements of *trpEG* in *Buchnera* from different aphid hosts. Brackets designate a *trpEG*-containing 3.6-kbp unit which, singly or as tandem repeats, constitutes a plasmid. Stippled line indicates conserved DNA sequences in the plasmid units. Redrawn from Baumann *et al.* (1995b).

Pemphigidae, has a long development time (Lai *et al.*, 1995). We have cloned and sequenced the *Buchnera* genes for the tryptophan biosynthetic pathway from this aphid. The results indicate that the genes are organized into two single chromosomal transcription units consisting of *trpEG* and *trpDC(F)BA*. The absence of amplification of *trpEG* in the endosymbiont of *Sl. chinensis* may be due to the fact that its development time is long and consequently the demand for tryptrophan is reduced.

Comparisons of the sequences of the 3.6-kbp units from *Buchnera* of three aphid species have indicated that the nucleotide sequence of the genes and the amino acid sequences of the proteins are highly conserved (Figure 5). A phylogenetic tree based on these sequences gives a branching order identical to that observed in the tree derived from 16S rDNA (Figure 2) which is consistent with the vertical evolution of the endosymbionts and the *trpEG* plasmids. A sequence approximately 600 base pairs upstream of *trpEG* is also highly conserved (Fig. 5). The conserved sequence proximal to *trpEG* is the putative ribosome binding site and the promoter. The more distal conserved upstream sequence has a number of properties, such as DnaA boxes and in some cases tandem high AT-containing repeats, which suggest that it functions as the plasmid origin of replication. There is no conservation of the remaining upstream sequence of approximately 900 base pairs. In the case of *Buchnera* from *S. graminum*, graminum, two different 3.6-kbp units have been sequenced and the intergenic region between *trpG* and *trpE* has been found to be virtually identical. The major difference in the intergenic sequence of plasmids from *Buchnera* of the three closely related aphid species and the virtual identity of the intergenic sequence in the units from the plasmid of *Buchnera* from the same aphid suggest that the number of tandem repeats is subject to relatively rapid variation. One possible mechanism of gene amplification is an increase in the number of tandem repeats which constitute a plasmid. Another is an increase in the copy number of a plasmid. These mechanisms may be a response to the nutritional status of the aphid: aphids provided with a good source of food and growing rapidly would have a greater *trpEG* amplification than aphids growing slowly on a poor nutrient source.

As in the case of the obligate intracellular pathogens, *Rickettsia* and *Chlamydia*, application of recombinant DNA methodology to aphid endosymbionts has resulted in considerable new information on the genetics, physiology and evolutionary relationships of these organisms. Much, however, remains to be learned concerning the nutritional contributions which *Buchnera* makes to the aphid host and nothing is known about the mechanisms which are involved in the transmission of *Buchnera* to aphid progeny.

References

Aksoy, S., 1995 - Molecular analysis of the endosymbionts of tsetse flie: 16S rDNA locus and over-expression of a chaperonin. *Insect Mol. Biol.* **4**, 23–29.

Aksoy, S., A.A. Pourhosseini and A. Chow, 1995 - Mycetome endosymbionts of tsetse flies constitute a distinct lineage related to *Enterobacteriaceae. Insect Mol. Biol.* **4**, 15–22.

Anderson, R.P. and J.R. Roth, 1977 - Tandem genetic duplications in phage and bacteria. *Annu. Rev. Microbiol.* **31**, 473–505.

Baumann, L. and P. Baumann, 1994 - Growth kinetics of the endosymbiont *Buchnera aphidicola* in the aphid *Schizaphis graminum. Appl. Environ. Microbiol.* **60**, 3440–3443.

Baumann, P., L. Baumann, C.Y. Lai, D. Rouhbakhsh, N.A. Moran and M.A. Clark, 1995a - Genetics, physiology and evolutionary relationships of the genus *Buchnera*: intracellular symbionts of aphids. *Annu. Rev. Microbiol.* **49**, 55–94.

Baumann, P., C.-Y. Lai, L. Baumann, D. Rouhbakhsh, N.A. Moran and M.A. Clark, 1995b - Mutualsitic associations of aphids and prokaryotes: biology of the genus *Buchnera. Appl. Environ. Microbiol.* **61**, 1–7.

Buchner, P., 1965 - Endosymbiosis of Animals with Plant Microorganisms, p. 210–338. Interscience Publishers, Inc., New York.

Douglas, A.E., 1989 - Mycetocyte symbiosis in insects. *Biol. Rev. Camb. Phil. Soc.* **64**, 409–434.

Douglas, A.E., 1990 - Nutritional interactions between *Myzus persicae* and its symbionts, p. 319–327. Aphid-plant genotype interactions, R.K. Campbell and R.D. Eikenbary (ed.). Elsevier Biomedical Press, Amsterdam.

Douglas, A.E. and A.F.G. Dixon, 1987 - The mycetocyte symbiosis of aphids: variation with age and morph in virginoparae of *Megoura viciae* and *Acyrthosiphon pisum. J. Insect Physiol.* **33**, 109–113.

Douglas, A.E. and W.A. Prosser, 1992 - Synthesis of the essential amino acid tryptophan in the pea aphid (*Acyrthosiphon pisum*) symbiosis. *J. Insect Physiol.* **38**, 565–568.

Houk, E.J. and G.W. Griffiths, 1980 - Intracellular symbiotes of the Homoptera. *Annu. Rev. Entomol* **25**, 161–187.

Ishikawa, H., 1989 - Biochemical and molecular aspects of endosymbiosis in insects. *Int. Rev. Cytol.* **116**, 1–45.

Lai, C.-Y. and P. Baumann, 1992a - Genetic analysis of an aphid endosymbiont DNA fragment homologous to the *rnpA-rpmH-dnaA-dnaN-gyrB* region of eubacteria. *Gene* **113**, 175–181.

Lai, C.-Y. and P. Baumann, 1992b - Sequence analysis of a DNA fragment from *Buchnera aphidicola* (an endosymbiont of aphids) containing genes homologous to *dnaG, rpoD, cysE,* and *secB. Gene* **119**, 113–118.

Lai, C.-Y., L. Baumann and P. Baumann, 1994 - Amplification of *trpEG*; adaptation of *Buchnera aphidicola* to an endosymbiotic association with aphids. *Proc. Natl. Acad. Sci. USA* **91**, 3819–3823.

Lai, C.-Y., P. Baumann and N.A. Moran, 1995 - Genetics of the tryptophan biosynthetic pathway of the prokaryotic endosymbiont (*Buchnera*) of the aphid *Schlechtendalia chinensis. Insect Mol. Biol.* **4**, 47–59.

Moran, N.A. and P. Baumann, 1993 - Phylogenetics of cytoplasmically inherited microorganisms of arthropods. *Trends Ecol. Evol.* **9**, 15–20.

Moran, N.A., M.A. Munson, P. Baumann and H. Ishikawa, 1993 - A molecular clock in endosymbiotic bacteria is calibrated using the insect hosts. *Proc. R. Soc. Lond. B* **253**, 167–171.

Munson, M.A. and P. Baumann, 1993 - Molecular cloning and nucleotide sequence of a putative *trpDC(F)BA* operon in *Buchnera aphidicola* (endosymbiont of the aphid *Schizaphis graminum*). *J. Bacteriol.* **175**, 6426–6432.

Munson, M.A., L. Baumann and P. Baumann, 1993 - *Buchnera aphidicola* (a prokaryotic endosymbiont of aphids) contains a putative 16S rRNA operon unlinked to the 23S rRNA-encoding gene: sequence determination, and promoter and terminator analysis. *Gene* **137**, 171–178.

Ogasawara, N. and Y. Yoshikawa, 1992 - Genes and their organization in the replication origin region of the bacterial chromosome. *Mol. Microbiol.* **6**, 629–634.

Ohtaka, C., H. Nakamura and H. Ishikawa, 1992 - Structures of chaperonins from an intracellular symbiont and their functional expression in *Escherichia coli groE* mutants. *J. Bacteriol.* **174**, 1869–1874.

Rouhbakhsh, D. and P. Baumann, 1995 - Characterization of a putative 23S-5S rRNA operon of *Buchnera aphidicola* (endosymbiont of aphids) unlinked to the 16S rRNA-encoding gene. *Gene* **155**, 107–112.

Rouhbakhsh, D., N.A. Moran, L. Baumann, D.J. Voegtlin and P. Baumann, 1994 - Detection of *Buchnera*, the primary prokaryotic endosymbiont of aphids, using the polymerase chain reaction. *Insect Mol. Biol.* **3**, 213–217.

Wolfe, C.J. and M.G. Haygood, 1993 - Bioluminescent symbionts of the Caribbean flashlight fish (*Kryptophanaron alfredi*) have a single rRNA operon. *Mol. Mar. Microbiol.* **2**, 189–197.

Ye, F., J. Renaudin, J.-M. Bové and F. Laigret, 1994 - Cloning and sequencing of the replication origin (*oriC*) of the *Spiroplasma citri* chromosome and construction of autonomously replicating artificial plasmids. *Curr. Microbiol.* **29**, 23–29.

Yoshikawa, H. and N. Ogasawara, 1991 - Structure and function of DnaA and the DnaA-box in eubacteria: evolutionary relationships of bacterial replication origins. *Mol. Microbiol.* **5**, 2589–2597.

Acknowledgments

Work from the author's laboratory was supported by the National Science Foundation IBN-9201285, MCB-9402813, DEB-9306495 (to Nancy A. Moran), Entotech Inc. (Novo Nordisk), and the University of California Experiment Station.

Microbiology Section, University of California, Davis, CA, USA 95616-8665

J. Heesemann, S. Schubert, A. Roggenkamp, A. Rakin and I. Autenrieth

Pathogenicity of Yersinia: A Strategy for Extracellular Survival and Multiplication

Abstract

Yersinia enterocolitica and *Y. pseudotuberculosis* are enteropathogenic for humans and rodents. After oral uptake, yersiniae invade the Peyer's patches followed by rapid extracellular multiplication and dissemination presumably via blood and lymphatic vessels into spleen, liver, lung and mesenteric lymph nodes.

Plasmid- and chromosomally-encoded factors have been identified enabling yersiniae to resist the primary unspecific host response. The plasmid-encoded yersinia adhesin YadA mediates binding to extracellular matrix proteins, inhibition of serum complement activation and cell adherence. The protein-tyrosine phosphatase YopH suppresses the generation of oxygen radicals by professional phagocytes. To compete with the high-affinity iron binding proteins of the host, *Yersinia* has evolved diverse pathways for ferric iron uptake. The most efficient of those is the yersiniabactin system. For eradication of the pathogen the host has to activate a specific cellular and humoral immune response including IFN-producing specific T-cells and YadA-specific antibodies.

Introduction

The impact of foodborne intestinal infectious diseases all over the world is well established. Improvement of the hygiene standards and efficient vaccination strategies are required to eradicate enteric pathogens in the environment and to protect humans, children in particular. However such measures demand exact knowledge of the pathogenicity, epidemiology and ecology of these pathogens. Up to now there are only few bacterial microorganisms of which infectious strategies have been at least partially dissected on a molecular level. Amongst these are the three pathogenic species of the genus *Yersinia*, namely *Y. pestis*, *Y. pseudotuberculosis* and *Y. enterocolitica*. These species are gramnegative rods and belong to the family of *Enterobacteriaceae*.

In 1980 it was recognized that the pathogenicity of yersiniae is controlled by a 70-kilobase (kb) plasmid which is now called pYV (*p*lasmid of *Yersinia* *v*irulence) (Zink *et al.*, 1980). This virulence plasmid is present in all three pathogenic *Yersinia spp.* and encodes diverse pathogenic factors which will be discussed later. The sequence similarities between pYV plasmids of the three species are very high (70–90%) (Heesemann *et al.*, 1983; Cornelis, 1994). Interestingly, the agent of bubonic plague, *Y. pestis*, harbours two further plasmids in addition to pYV: pPCP is a 10 kb plasmid encoding pesticin (a bacteriocin) as well as a plasminogen activator which enhances bacterial dissemination after transmission by a flea bite; and pTOX , a 100 kb plasmid encoding a mouse toxin and fraction 1 protein (capsule-forming protein) which is believed to protect *Y. pestis* against phagocytosis.

Chromosomal determinants with proven or putative virulence functions have also been identified in yersiniae. Two proteins with cell adherence and invasion functions have been characterized (Isberg, 1989; Miller *et al.*, 1988). The first one named Invasin (Inv) is an outer membrane protein of about 100 kilodalton (kDa) which is well expressed below 30°C by pathogenic *Y. pseudotuberculosis* and *Y. enterocolitica* strains. Inv triggers the internalization of the attached pathogen after interaction with β1 integrins on the surface of mammalian cells. The second invasin called Ail, (encoded by the *a*ttachment *i*nvasin *l*ocus) is restricted to enteropathogenic *Y. enterocolitica* strains (Miller *et al.*, 1988). This 20 kDa outer membrane protein has cell adherence functions and enables yersiniae to survive in liquid medium supplemented with 5%–10% human serum. However, there are presently only weak evidences that these two adhesin factors are absolutely required for entry, survival and multiplication in the hosts such as mice.

It is commonly established that enterotoxins produced by enterics are directly involved in the pathogenesis of diarrhea. Accordingly, *Y. enterocolitica* produces a heat-stable enterotoxin (Yst) which is closely related to the known heat-stable enterotoxin of *E. coli* (ST). Yst-negative mutants of *Y. enterocolitica* generated by insertional mutagenesis of the chromosomally located gene *yst* turned out to be attenuated in causing diarrhea in the young rabbit oral infection model (Delor and Cornelis, 1992). Strikingly, the invasiveness of *yst* mutant was hardly affected in this model indicating that other virulence genes control this phenotype. In contrast to *Y. enterocolitica*, *Y. pseudotuberculosis* lacks the *yst* gene. This may explain why *Y. pseudotuberculosis* infections are rarely associated with watery of bloody diarrhea. Instead, the typical clinical manifestation of *Y. pseudotuberculosis* infection is known as mesenteric lymphadenitis.

The pathogenicity of *Y. enterocolitica* was in question for many years because of inconsistencies in mouse virulence. First, it was observed that *Y. enterocolitica* strains of biotype IB (so-called American serotypes 08, 013, 020, 021) lost their mouse virulence potential after repeated subcultivation in the laboratory (Carter, 1975). This phenomenon is ascribed to the selective growth advantage of plasmid-cured derivatives at 37°C. Second, *Y. enterocolitica* strains of European origin, which are of biotype 2 (serotype 09) or of biotype 4 (serotype 03) are not mouse virulent in spite of the presence of pYV (Heesemann *et al.*, 1984). However, if mice were pretreated with ferric iron or the iron chelator desferrioxamine, European serotypes of *Y. enterocolitica* likewise turned out to be mouse virulent (Robins-Browne and Prpic, 1985; Autenrieth *et al.*, 1994;

Boelaert *et al.*, 1987). Obviously, non-biotype 1 B strains of *Y. enterocolitica* lack a sufficient iron-utilization system required for multiplication in host tissue and therefore are of moderate pathogenicity for mice. (This issue will be discussed in the section on iron uptake and virulence of yersiniae).

Orogastric infection of mice

The mouse virulent *Y. enterocolitica* strains of serotype 08 have been used by several research groups to study the infection process after orogastric challenge of mice (Carter, 1975; Grutzkau *et al.*, 1990; Hanski *et al.*, 1991; Hanski *et al.*, 1989). Within hours after challenge yersiniae preferentially enter the Peyer's patches (PPs) of the small bowel. There are evidences that M-cells are involved in translocation of yersiniae. Carefully performed kinetic studies by Hanski *et al.* revealed that the efficiency of the initial translocation process was similar for both, plasmid-harbouring strains and their plasmidless derivatives (Hanski *et al.*, 1991). However, survival, multiplication and dissemination of translocated yersiniae were controlled by the virulence plasmid pYV. While plasmid-positive strains survived and disseminated into mesenteric lymph nodes, spleen, liver and lung (probably via blood and lymphatic vessels), resulting in the formation of granuloma-like lesions and abscesses, plasmidless yersiniae were rapidly eradicated within the PPs. Carefully performed eletronmicroscopical and immunohistological investigations of infected tissues revealed that yersiniae are located exclusively in the extracellular matrix, surrounded by polymorphonuclear leukocytes, macrophages and lymphocytes (Hanski *et al.*, 1989; Heesemann *et al.*, 1993; Simonet *et al.*, 1990). From these results we conclude that enteropathogenic yersiniae must be well equipped for extracellular survival and multiplication in host tissue.

Plasmid-encoded virulence functions

The virulence plasmid pYV encodes for outer membrane proteins (e.g. *y*ersinia *a*dhesin, YadA), secreted proteins (*y*ersinia *o*uter *p*roteins: YopE, YopD, YopH, YopM and others), gene regulator proteins (e.g. VirF), proteins involved in the Yop-secretion (lcrD and Ysc-proteins) and a translocation machinery (e.g. YopD). For further details concerning Yop secretion and Yop-gene regulation the reader is referred to the recent review of G. Cornelis, 1994).

Recently it was demonstrated that YopE is translocated into epithelial cells after attachment of yersiniae to the host cell membrane (Rosqvist *et al.*, 1990; Rosqvist *et al.*, 1994). Moreover, there is accumulating evidence that YopD functions as Yop-protein translocator at the bacterial host cell contact point. Presumably, also YopH, YopO and YopM are processed via this polarized translocation pathway. After YopE is translocated into the cytoplasm of the target cell, cell-rounding and detachment is observed and accompanied by aggregation of actin fibrillae and destruction of the cytoskeleton (cytotoxic effect).

One of the best characterized Yops is YopH. By amino acid sequence comparisonYopH was identified as protein-tyrosine phosphatase (PTPase) (Guan and Dixon, 1990). The PTPase activity of YopH was found to be optimal at about pH 5.0. After infection of the murine macrophage-like cell line J774A.1 with plasmid-positive yersiniae two tyrosine-dephosphorylated proteins of 55 kDa and 120 kDa could be identified (Bliska *et al.*, 1992). We compared the chemiluminescence signal of PMNLs induced by in vitro infection with plasmidless (strain WA-C), plasmid-positive (strain WA-314) and YopH-mutant (strain WA-C (pYV *yopH*)) *Y. enterocolitica* strains, respectively (Ruckdeschel *et al.*, in preparation). Within the first 60 min. after infection WA-C generated a high and WA-314 a low chemiluminescence signal, whereas the signal of YopH mutant was moderate. After two hours of infection the PMNLs were restimulated with opsonized zymosan. A high oxidative burst was observed in case of WA-C- and WA-C (pYV *yopH*), whereas WA-314 infected PMNLs did not respond. These results demonstrate that YopH has the capacity to turn down or to block the generation of superoxide anion radicals. Moreover, the PTPase activity of YopH may also be responsible for blocking the phagocytic capacity of PMNLs and macrophages (Bliska *et al.*, 1992; Rosqvist *et al.*, 1988). There is strong evidence that besides YopH YadA also favours the extracellular location of yersiniae (Heesemann and Laufs, 1985; Heesemann J. and Grüter L. 1987). First, YadA prevents activation of complement by binding of the C3-convertase-inhibitor factor H. Second, YadA covers the surface of the bacterial cell and thus blocks the interaction between Inv and cellular β1-integrins. Whether YopO (also called YpkA), which has protein-kinase activity,

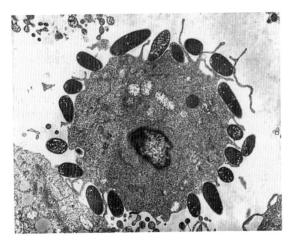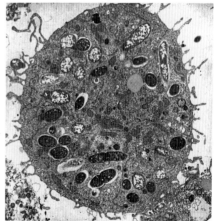

Fig. 1. Transmission electronmicrograph of mouse peritoneal macrophages infected with plasmid-positive *Y. enterocolitica* strain WA-314 (left) and plasmid-negative derivative WA-C (right), respectively.

does also contribute to inhibition of phagocytosis is not yet known (Galyov *et al.*, 1993). Probably, several plasmid-encoded proteins are involved in suppression of phagocytosis (Lian *et al.*, 1987). In Fig. 1 mouse macrophages infected with plasmid-positive and plasmid-negative *Y. enterocolitica*, respectively, are shown to demonstrate the different properties of an isogenic pair.

Finally YopM which seems to be involved in blood coagulation process should be mentioned. Short stretches of YopM exhibit amino acid sequence identity to the platelet receptor GP1bα. Therefore, it is not surprising that YopM binds thrombin and inhibits thrombin-induced platelet aggregation (Leung *et al.*, 1990; Reisner and Straley, 1992). Although the *in vivo* function of YopM is not known, testing of YopM mutant of *Y. pestis* in the mouse model turned out that YopM is required for full virulence expression.

Yersinia adhesin YadA - a multifunctional protein

The first gene of the virulence plasmid pYV which has been cloned and sequenced was *yadA* (Skurnik and Wolf Watz, 1989). *yadA* encodes a protein (formerly called as P1 or Yop-1) which forms multimeric fibrillae on the surface of enteropathogenic yersiniae (Kapperud *et al.*, 1987). The apparent molecular weight as determined by SDS-PAGE depends on the solublization conditions: extraction of YadA from outer membranes at 30°C results in a single broad band of 120 kDa (presumably the native form); extraction at 100°C leads to two bands one oligomeric form of about 200 kDa and one monomeric form of about 50 kDa (as predicted from yadA sequence); treatment of outer membranes with 6 M urea results in the exclusive appearance of the monomeric form (Skurnik and Wolf Watz, 1989; Mack *et al.*, 1994; Tamm *et al.*, 1993). Expression of YadA depends on temperature (37°C) and VirF (Cornelis, 1994).

yadA genes of enteropathogenic *Yersinia species* comprise a gene family with common structural elements, conserved domains and strain-specific domains which can be distinguished by polyclonal and monoclonal antibodies (Skurnik and Wolf Watz, 1989; Sory *et al.*, 1990). YadA knock-out mutants of *Y. enterocolitica* are of reduced virulence for mice (increase of the 50% mouse lethal dose, LD_{50}) and YadA can thus be considered as a pathogenic factor of *Y. enterocolitica* (Kapperud *et al.*, 1987; Tamm *et al.*, 1993; Roggenkamp *et al.*, 1995). Diverse functions have been ascribed to YadA: (i) YadA mediates autoagglutination of yersiniae at 37°C (Skurnik and Wolf Watz, 1989). This feature may favour formation of microcolonies in the host. (ii) YadA competes with Inv for cell adherence. According to the inverse temperature regulation of *yadA* (37°C) and *inv* (<30°C), and the surface properties of YadA (masking of Inv), YadA appears to be the dominant cell adhesin *in vivo* (Kapperud *et al.*, 1987; Cornelis, 1994; Heesemann J. and Grüter L. 1987). (iii) YadA turned out to have extroordinary capacities to bind various extracellular matrix (ECM) proteins such as collagen type I, II, III, IV, V, IX, XI, cellular fibronectin, and laminin-1 (Emody *et al.*, 1989; Flügel *et al.*, 1994; Schulze Koops *et al.*, 1992;

Site-directed Mutagenesis of *yad A*

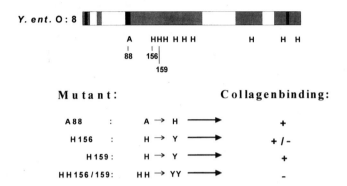

Fig. 2. Schematic drawing of YadA domains and histidyl residues (H); black: hydrophobic domains; halftone: conserved domains; white: variable domains.

Schulze Koops *et al.*, 1993). (iv) Plasmid-positive *Y. enterocolitica* strains are able to survive in 50% human serum (Heesemann *et al.*, 1983; Pilz *et al.*, 1992). It could be demonstrated that YadA inhibits formation of the complement attack complex on the bacterial surface, presumably by binding of the C3-convertase inhibitor factor H (Cornelis, 1994). (V) There are evidences that interaction of YadA with the surface of epithelial cells bypasses the phagocytosis trigger which is mediated by Inv- 1 integrin interaction (Ruckdeschel *et al.*, in preparation).

These multifunctional features of YadA prompted us to dissect functional domains. Using site-directed mutagenesis we succeeded in abolishing the binding activity of YadA for diverse ECM proteins by substitution in YadA of two histidyl residues (His 156/His 159) by tyrosine (Fig. 2). This *yadA* mutant was also unable to adhere to Hep-2 or Hela cells and turned out to be attenuated in mouse virulence, whereas resistance to human serum (complement) and autoagglutination were not affected (Roggenkamp *et al.*, 1995). These results are in contrast to those of Tamm *et al.* who constructed a *yadA* mutant by complete deletion of a hydrophobic domain of 20 amino acids of YadA (Tamm *et al.*, 1993): in this mutant loss of collagen-binding was associated with loss of autoagglutination.

Iron-uptake and virulence of yersiniae

Transfer of the pYV plasmid from mouse-virulent 08 strain WA-314 (biotype 1 B) to non-mouse virulent 03 or 09 strains (biotype 4 and 3, respectively) did not result in concomitant transfer of the mouse virulent phenotype (Heesemann *et al.*, 1984). This result prompted us to look for chromosomal virulence determinants. Using the siderophore indicator agar (chrome azurol S agar, CAS) we were able to demonstrate that biotype 1 B *Y. enterocolitica* strains produce siderophores (CAS-positive) in contrast to biotyp 1 A, 2 and 4 strains which were CAS-negative (Heesemann, 1987). Moreover, CAS-positive strains turned out to be highly susceptible to pesticin, a bacteriocin which is produced by *Y. pestis* harbouring pPCP (Heesemann *et al.*, 1993). Previously, it had been described that *Y. enterocolitica* serotype 08 and *Y. pseudotuberculosis* serotype 1 lost their mouse virulence phenotype after selection for pesticin resistance (Une and Brubaker, 1984). From these observations we concluded a link between the pesticin receptor and a putative mouse virulence factor, presumably a siderophor receptor. To verify this hypothesis we introduced a cosmid library of *Y. enterocolitica* serotype 08 into a pesticin-resistant mutant of *Y. enterocolitica 08* and selected the obtained transconjugants for mouse virulence by intraperitoneal infection of mice. By this procedure we obtained transconjugants from mouse tissues which harboured a unique cosmid and regained the pesticin-sensitive phenotype (Rakin *et al.*, 1994). Subcloning and sequencing revealed a Fur-regulated (iron-repressible) open reading frame of 2022 bp which encodes an outer membrane protein of 71 kDa with high homologies to other iron regulated Ton B-dependent outer membrane proteins with siderophore receptor functions. Moreover, we were able to demonstrate that the 71 kDa protein functioned as a receptor both for pesticin and Yersiniabactin and was required for full mouse virulence. Because of this *f*erric *y*ersiniabactin *u*ptake function the 71 kDa protein was called FyuA. Moreover we could demonstrate that pesticin-susceptible bacteria such as *Y. enterocolitica* of serotypes 013, 020 and 021, *Y. pseudotuberculosis* serotype 1 and *Y. pestis* express FyuA. Sequence comparison of *fyuA* genes of diverse *Yersinia spp.* revealed more than 99% sequence homology and two evolutionary lineages of highly pathogenic yersiniae: (i) *Y. enterocolitica* biotype 1 B and (ii) *Y. pseudotuberculosis* serotype 1 and *Y. pestis* (including pesticin-sensitive *E. coli*) (Rakin *et al.*, 1995). Functional FyuA could not be detected in *Y. enterocolitica* of biotype 1 A, 2 and 4 and *Y. pseudotuberculosis* of serotypes 2 and 3 which is consistent with their pesticin-resistant phenotype but not with the mouse-virulence phenotpye of *Y. pseudotuberculosis*. However, we have evidences that certain strains of *Y. pseudotuberculosis*, serotype 3 produce a siderophore distinct from yersiniabactin which mediates mouse virulence (unpublished results).

Presently, there are only few data concerning the structure of yersiniabactin and the determinants for synthesis (Haag *et al.*, 1993; Heesemann *et al.*, 1993). Since mutations in *aroA* and *irp2* (*irp2* is homologous to *entF* of *E. coli*) result in abrogation of yersiniabactin synthesis, we assume a enterochelin-like structure of yersiniabactin (Heesemann *et al.*, 1993; Guilvout *et al.*, 1993).

In conclusion, mouse virulence of *Y. enterocolitica* is closely associated with efficient ferric iron provision mediated by the yersiniabactin determinant *fyu*. However, yersiniae are able to express also other iron uptake systems which may be important for iron provision in diverse ecological niches (Fig. 3). Human

Yersinia enterocolitica
biotype 1 B strains

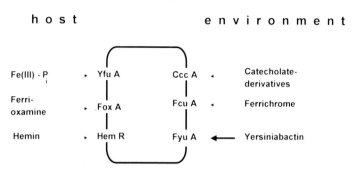

host   environment

Fig. 3. Iron-uptake systems identified in *Y. enterocolitica* of serotype 08, biotype 1B (mouse-virulent strain). Non-biotype 1B strains are lacking yersiniabactin uptake determinant (fyu).

pathogenic *Y. enterocolitica* express TonB-dependent specific receptors for uptake of ferrichrome (FcuA), ferrioxamines (FoxA) and hemin (HemR) (Bäumler and Hantke, 1992; Bäumler *et al.*, 1993; Stojiljkovic and Hantke, 1992). Moreover, ferric iron bound to polyphosphates can be utilized by the TonB-independent transport system *yfu* (Saken *et al.*, in prepraration). The impact of these transport systems for virulence depends on the ability of *Y. enterocolitica* to use the yersiniabactin uptake system. In case of *fyu*-negative strains (biotype 2 and 4) disruption of *hemR* or *yfuB* results in virulence attenuation whereas corresponding mutants of *fyu*-positive strains (e.g. *Y. enterocolitica 08*) are not affected in virulence.

The host response against *Y. enterocolitica*

Mice and rats are suitable animal models to analyze the host defence mechanisms against *Yersinia enterocolitica* (Heesemann *et al.*, 1993). During the early phase of infection (up to three to five days after challenge) the unspecific host defence (e.g. complement attack, polymorphonuclear leukocytes) fail to eliminate the invading yersiniae (Autenrieth *et al.*, 1993; Autenrieth *et al.*, 1993). C57Bl/6 mice which are able to recruit sufficiently IFN-g-producing *Yersinia*-specific T-cells are able to eradicate yersiniae efficiently from spleen and liver (*Yersinia*-resistant mice). In contrast, the *Yersinia*-specific T-cell response in BALB/c mice is delayed, weak and IFN-g-production could not be detected before three weeks after infection (*Yersinia*-susceptible mice) (Autenrieth *et al.*, 1994; Autenrieth and Heesemann, 1992; Autenrieth *et al.*, 1993). Recently, the heat shock protein HSP60 could be identified as protective T-cell specific antigen of *Y. enterocolitica 08* (Noll *et al.*, 1994). Besides T-cells, a specific humoral antibody response can be protective as has been demonstrated by pretreatment of mice with YadA-specific rabbit antiserum (Vogel *et al.*, 1993). Interestingly, YadA-specific antiserum was not protective for strains expressing heterologous YadA (no cross-protection against *Y. enterocolitica* of different serotypes). In summary, *Y. enterocolitica* appears to be well equipped for extracellular survival in host lymphatic tissue and able to resist the unspecific primary host defence reaction. Whether yersiniae can be totally eradicated by an efficient cell-mediated immune response of the host or are still able to evade into protected niches (causing latent persisting infection) has to be elucidated.

References

Autenrieth, I.B., M. Beer, E. Bohn, S.H.E. Kaufmann and J. Heesemann, 1994 - Immune responses to *Yersinia enterocolitica* in susceptible BALB/c and resistant C57BL/6 mice: an essential role for gamma interferon, *Infect. Immun.* **62**, 2590.

Autenrieth, I.B., P. Hantschmann, B. Heymer and J. Heesemann, 1993 - Immunohistological characterization of the cellular immune response against *Yersinia enterocolitica* in mice: evidence for the involvement of T lymphocytes, *Immunobiology* **187**, 1.

Autenrieth, I.B. and J. Heesemann, 1992 - In vivo neutralization of tumor necrosis factor alpha and interferon-gamma abrogates resistance to *Yersinia enterocolitica* in mice, *Med. Microbiol. Immunol.* **181**, 333.

Autenrieth, I.B., R. Reisbrodt, E. Saken, R. Berner, U. Vogel, W. Rabsch and J. Heesemann, 1994 - Desferrioxamine-promoted virulence of *Yersinia enterocolitica* for mice depends on both Desferrioxamine species and mouse strains, *J. Infect. Dis.* **169**, 562.

Autenrieth, I.B., U. Vogel, S. Preger, B. Heymer and J. Heesemann, 1993 - Experimental *Yersinia enterocolitica* infection in euthymic and T-cell-deficient athymic nude C57BL/6 mice: Comparison of time course, histomorphology, and immune response, *Infect. Immun.* **61**, 2585.

Bäumler, A.J. and K. Hantke, 1992 - Ferrioxamine uptake in *Yersinia enterocolitica*: characterization of the receptor protein FoxA, *Mol. Microbiol.* **6**, 1309.

Bäumler, A.J., R. Koebnik, I. Stojiljkovic, J. Heesemann, V. Braun and K. Hantke, 1993 - Survey on newly characterized iron uptake systems of *Yersinia enterocolitica*, *Zbl. Bact.* **278**, 416.

Bliska, J.B., J.C. Clemens, J.E. Dixon and S. Falkow, 1992 - The Yersinia tyrosine phosphatase: specificity of a bacterial virulence determinant for phosphoproteins in the J774A.1 macrophage, *J. Exp. Med.* **176**, 1625.

Boelaert, J.R., H.W. van Landuyt, Y.J. Valcke, B. Cantinieaux, W.F. Lornoy, J.L. Vanherweghem, P. Moreillon and J.M. Vandepitte, 1987 - The role of iron overload in *Yersinia enterocolitica* and *Yersinia pseudotuberculosis* bacteremia in hemodialysis patients, *J. Infect. Dis.* **156**, 384.

Carter, P.B., 1975 - Pathogenecity of *Yersinia enterocolitica* for mice, *Infect. Immun.* **11**, 164.

Cornelis, G.R., 1994 - *Yersinia* pathogenicity factors, *Curr. Top. Microbiol. Immunol.* **192**, 243.

Delor, I. and G.R. Cornelis, 1992 - Role of *Yersinia enterocolitica* Yst toxin in experimental infection of young rabbits, *Infect. Immun.* **60**, 4269.

Emody, L., J. Heesemann, H. Wolf Watz, M. Skurnik, G. Kapperud, P. O'Toole and T. Wadstrom, 1989 - Binding to collagen by *Yersinia enterocolitica* and *Yersinia pseudotuberculosis*: evidence for yopA-mediated and chromosomally encoded mechanisms, *J. Bacteriol.* **171**, 6674.

Flügel, A., H. Schulze-Koops, J. Heesemann, K. Kühn, H. Sorokin, K. Burkhardt, A. von der Mark and F. Emmrich, 1994 - Interaction of enteropathogenic *Yersinia enterocolitica* with complex basement membranes and the extracellular matrix proteins collagen type IV, Laminin-1 and -2, and Nidogen/Entactin, *J. Biol. Chem.* **269**, 29732.

Galyov, E.E., S. Hakansson, A. Forsberg and H. Wolf-Watz, 1993 - A secreted protein kinase of *Yersinia pseudotuberculosis* is an indispensible virulence determinant, *Nature* **361**, 730.

Grutzkau, A., C. Hanski, H. Hahn E.O. and E.O. Riecken, 1990 - Involvement of M cells in the bacterial invasion of Peyer's patches: a common mechanism shared by *Yersinia enterocolitica* and other enteroinvasive bacteria, *Gut* **31**, 1011.

Guan, K.L. and J.E. Dixon, 1990 - Protein tyrosine phosphatase activity of an essential virulence determinant in *Yersinia*, *Science* **249**, 553.

Guilvout, I., O. Mercereau Puijalon, S. Bonnefoy, A.P. Pugsley and E. Carniel, 1993 - High-molecular-weight protein 2 of *Yersinia enterocolitica* is homologous to AngR of *Vibrio anguillarum* and belongs to a family of proteins involved in nonribosomal peptide synthesis, *J. Bacteriol.* **175**, 5488.

Haag, H., K. Hantke, H. Drechsel, I. Stojiljkovic, G. Jung and H. Zähner, 1993 - Purification of Yersiniabactin: a siderophore and a possible virulence factor of *Yersinia enterocolitica*, *J. Genet. Microbiol.* **139**, 2159.

Hanski, C., U. Kutschka, H.P. Schmoranzer, M. Naumann, A. Stallmach, H. Hahn, H. Menge and E.O. Riecken, 1989 - Immunohistochemical and electron microscopic study of interaction of *Yersinia enterocolitica* serotype O8 with intestinal mucosa during experimental enteritis, *Infect. Immun.* **57**, 673.

Hanski, C., M. Naumann, A. Grutzkau, G. Pluschke, B. Friedrich, H. Hahn and E.O. Riecken, 1991 - Humoral and cellular defense against intestinal murine infection with *Yersinia enterocolitica*, *Infect. Immun.* **59**, 1106.

Heesemann J. and L. Grüter, 1987 - Genetic evidence that the outer membrane protein Yop1 of *Yersinia enterocolitica* mediates adherence and phagocytosis resistance to human epithelial cells, *FEMS Microbiol. Lett.* **40**, 37.

Heesemann, J., 1987 - Chromosomal-encoded siderophores are required for mouse virulence of enteropathogenic Yersinia species, *FEMS Microbiol. Lett.* **48**, 229.

Heesemann, J., B. Algermissen and R. Laufs, 1984 - Genetically manipulated virulence of *Yersinia enterocolitica*, *Infect. Immun.* **46**, 105.

Heesemann, J., K. Gaede and I.B. Autenrieth, 1993 - Experimental *Yersinia enterocolitica* infection in rodents: a model for human yersiniosis, *APMIS* **101**, 417.

Heesemann, J., K. Hantke, T. Vocke, E. Saken, A. Rakin, I. Stojiljkovic and R. Berner, 1993 - Virulence of *Yersinia enterocolitica* is closely associated with siderophore production, expression of an iron-repressible outer membrane protein of 65000 Da and pesticin sensitivity, *Mol. Microbiol.* **8**, 397.

Heesemann, J., C. Keller, R. Morawa, N. Schmidt, H.J. Siemens and R. Laufs, 1983 - Plasmids of human strains of *Yersinia enterocolitica*: molecular relatedness and possible importance for pathogenesis, *J. Infect. Dis.* **147**, 107.

Heesemann, J. and R. Laufs, 1985 - Double immunofluorescence microscopic technique for accurate differentiation of extracellularly and intracellularly located bacteria in cell culture, *J. Clin. Microbiol.* **22**, 168.

Isberg, R.R., 1989 - Mammalian cell adhesion functions and cellular penetration of enteropathogenic *Yersinia* species, *Mol. Microbiol.* **3**, 1449.

Kapperud, G., E. Namork, M. Skurnik and T. Nesbakken, 1987 - Plasmid-mediated surface fibrillae of *Yersinia pseudotuberculosis* and *Yersinia enterocolitica*: relationship to the outer membrane protein YOP1 and possible importance for pathogenesis, *Infect. Immun.* **55**, 2247.

Leung, K.Y., B.S. Reisner and S.C. Straley, 1990 - YopM inhibits platelet aggregation and is necessary for virulence of *Yersinia pestis* in mice, *Infect. Immun.* **58**, 3262.

Lian, C.J., W.S. Hwang and C.H. Pai, 1987 - Plasmid-mediated resistance to phagocytosis in *Yersinia enterocolitica*, *Infect. Immun.* **55**, 1176.

Mack, D., J. Heesemann and R. Laufs, 1994 - Characterization of different oligomeric species of the *Yersinia enterocolitica* outer membrane protein YadA, *Med. Microbiol. Immunol.* **183**, 217.

Miller, V.L., B.B. Finlad and S. Falkow, 1988 - Factors essential for the penetration of mammalian cells by *Yersinia*, *Curr. Top. Microbiol. Immunol.* **138**, 15.

Noll, A., A. Roggenkamp, J. Heesemann and I.B. Autenrieth, 1994 - Protective Role for Heat Shock Protein-Reactive alpha/beta T Cells in Murine Yersiniosis, *Infect. Immun.* **62**, 2784.

Pilz, D., T. Vocke, J. Heesemann and V. Brade, 1992 - Mechanism of YadA-mediated serum resistance of *Yersinia enterocolitica* serotype O3, *Infect. Immun.* **60**, 189.

Rakin, A., E. Saken, D. Harmsen and J. Heesemann, 1994 - The pesticin receptor of *Yersinia enterocolitica*: a novel virulence factor with dual function, *Mol. Microbiol.* **13**, 253.

Rakin, A., P. Urbitsch and J. Heesemann, 1995 - Evidence for two evolutionary lineages of highly pathogenic *Yersinia, J. Bacteriol.*, in press.

Reisner, B.S. and S.C. Straley, 1992 - *Yersinia pestis* YopM: thrombin binding and overexpression, *Infect. Immun.* **60**, 5242.

Robins-Browne, R.M. and J.K. Prpic, 1985 - Effects of iron and desferrioxamine on infections with *Yersinia enterocolitica, Infect. Immun.* **47**, 774.

Roggenkamp, A., H.-R. Neuberger, A. Flügel, T. Schmoll and J. Heesemann, 1995 - Substitution of two histidine residues in YadA protein of *Yersinia enterocolitica* abrogates collagen-binding, cell-adherence and mouse virulence, *Mol. Microbiol.* **16**, 1207–1219.

Rosqvist, R., I. Bolin and H. Wolf Watz, 1988 - Inhibition of phagocytosis in *Yersinia pseudotuberculosis*: a virulence plasmid-encoded ability involving the Yop2b protein, *Infect. Immun.* **56**, 2139.

Rosqvist, R., A. Forsberg, M. Rimpilainen, T. Bergman and H. Wolf Watz, 1990 - The cytotoxic protein YopE of Yersinia obstructs the primary host defence, *Mol. Microbiol.* **4**, 657.

Rosqvist, R., K.E. Magnusson and H. Wolf Watz, 1994 - Target cell contact triggers expression and polarized transfer of Yersinia YopE cytotoxin into mammalian cells, *EMBO J.* **13**, 964.

Schulze Koops, H., H. Burkhardt, J. Heesemann, T. Kirsch, B. Swoboda, C. Bull, S. Goodman and F. Emmrich, 1993 - Outer membrane protein YadA of enteropathogenic yersiniae mediates specific binding to cellular but not plasma fibronectin, *Infect. Immun.* **61**, 2513.

Schulze Koops, H., H. Burkhardt, J. Heesemann, K. von der Mark and F. Emmrich, 1992 - Plasmid-encoded outer membrane protein YadA mediates specific binding of enteropathogenic yersiniae to various types of collagen, *Infect. Immun.* **60**, 2153.

Simonet, M., S. Richard and P. Berche, 1990 - Electron microscopic evidence for in vivo extracellular localization of *Yersinia pseudotuberculosis* harboring the pYV plasmid, *Infect. Immun.* **58**, 841.

Skurnik, M. and H. Wolf Watz, 1989 - Analysis of the yopA gene encoding the Yop1 virulence determinants of Yersinia spp., *Mol. Microbiol.* **3**, 517.

Sory, M.P., J. Tollenaere, C. Laszlo, T. Biot, G.R. Cornelis and G. Wauters, 1990 - Detection of pYV+ *Yersinia enterocolitica* isolates by P1 slide agglutination, *J. Clin. Microbiol.* **28**, 2403.

Stojiljkovic, I. and K. Hantke, 1992 - Hemin uptake system of *Yersinia enterocolitica*: similarities with other TonB-dependent systems in gram-negative bacteria, *EMBO J.* **11**, 4359.

Tamm, A., A. Tarkkanen, P.K. Korhonen, P. Toivanen and M. Skurnik, 1993 - Hydrophobic domains affect the collagen-binding specificity and surface polymerization as well as the virulence potential of the YadA protein of *Yersinia enterocolitica, Mol. Microbiol.* **10**, 995.

Une, T. and R.R. Brubaker, 1984 - In vivo comparison of avirulent Vwa- and Pgm- or Pstr phenotypes of yersiniae, *Infect. Immun.* **43**, 895.

Vogel, U., I.B. Autenrieth, R. Berner and J. Heesemann, 1993 - Role of plasmid-encoded antigens of *Yersinia enterocolitica* in humoral immunity against secondary *Y. enterocolitica* infection in mice, *Microb. Pathogen.* **15**, 23.

Zink, D.L., J.C. Feeley, J.G. Wells, C. Vanderzant, J.C. Vickery, W.D. Roof and G.A. O'Donovan, 1980 - Plasmid-mediated tissue invasiveness in *Yersinia enterocolitica*, *Nature* **283**, 224.

Molecular and Cellular Bases of Invasion of the Intestinal Mucosa by *Shigella flexneri*

Abstract

Shigella flexneri, a gram-negative bacillus, is a member of the family enterobacteriaceae. It causes bacillary dysentery by invading the human colonic mucosa and inducing an inflammatory reaction. Recent data suggest a model of the infectious process. *In vivo*, bacteria enter into the mucosa *via* M-cells, specialized cells present in the epithelial dome covering the lymphoid follicular structures of the intestinal mucosa. Once inside the submucosa, shigellae encounter resident tissue macrophages, which are infected and programmed cell death (i.e. apoptosis) is rapidly induced in these phagocytic cells. During programmed cell death, the inflammatory cytokine Interleukin-1 (IL-1) is released. It triggers an inflammatory reaction characterized by extravasation of polymorphonuclear (PMN) cells. Inflammation is probably potentiated by the production of other cytokines by epithelial, endothelial and PMN cells. PMN cells migrate through the epithelium into the lumen of the colon, thus destabilizing the integrity of the epithelial barrier. The damaged epithelium allows massive entry of bacteria into subepithelial tissues. Further colonization of the epithelium aggravates inflammation which in turn causes extensive tissue destruction. This colonization process encompasses entry into epithelial cells, escape into the host cell cytoplasm and cell to cell spread. Both the *in vitro* and *in vivo* results that support this model are discussed here.

Introduction

Diarrhea is a major public health issue. About five millions children die annually worldwide of diarrheal diseases (Barua, 1981). *Shigella*e are among the important etiologic agents of these diseases (Sanyal, 1981), causing a bloody diarrhea called bacillary dysentery. In developing countries, *Shigella flexneri* is the major etiological agent of the endemic form of the disease. *Shigella dysenteriae* 1 is less common but causes devastating epidemics. Development of vaccines allowing prevention of bacillary dysentery is a priority (Maurelli & Sansonetti, 1988; Lindberg & Pal, 1993).

The major characteristic of the disease is bacterial invasion of the rectal and colonic mucosa. Histopathological analysis of the recto-colon of patients with shigellosis shows severe destruction of the epithelium characterized by mucosal erosion and inflammation dominated by an infiltration and a major exudation of polymorphonuclear leukocytes (PMN) (Anand *et al.*, 1986; LaBrec *et al.*, 1964; Mathan & Mathan, 1991).

A major property of *S. flexneri* is its capacity to invade eukaryotic cells (LaBrec *et al.*, 1964). After phagocytosis, *Shigella* lyses the phagocytic vacuole and escapes into the cytoplasm (Sansonetti *et al.*, 1986; Maurelli & Sansonetti, 1988). In shigellosis, although very few bacteria can cause dysentery, this microorganism is non-pathogenic in experimental animals (Lindberg & Pal, 1993; Maurelli & Sansonetti, 1988) except macaque monkeys. Paradoxically, *in vitro*, *S. flexneri* can efficiently invade all vertebrate cells tested so far. *Shigella* pathogenicity can be analyzed using cell culture of both explanted cells and established cell lines, as well as *in vivo* models like the rabbit ligated loop assay and the Serény test (Serény, 1955; LaBrec *et al.*, 1964). Rabbits are not naturally sensitive to *Shigella*, but injection of the bacterial pathogen into the lumen of ligated intestinal loops mimics the physiopathology observed in experimental human and monkey infections. The Serény test is based on the capacity of invasive shigellae to induce a purulent keratoconjunctivitis in guinea pigs when inoculated directly onto the conjunctiva.

S. flexneri invasiveness is encoded by a 220-kilobase plasmid. Through transposon mutagenesis and cosmid vector cloning, the invasion capability of *S. flexneri* has been localized to 31 kilobases in the pathogenicity-plasmid (Maurelli *et al.*, 1985). This 31-kilobase contains essentially the *ipa* genes (*inva*sion *p*lasmid *a*ntigens) and the *mxi/spa* genes (*m*embrane *ex*pression of *I*pas, *s*urface *p*resentation of Ipas). The *ipa* genes encode the IpaA, IpaB, IpaC and IpaD polypeptides which are the dominant antigens in the humoral response to shigellosis. Using transposon insertion and deletion mutagenesis it has been demonstrated that the *ipa*B, *ipa*C and *ipa*D genes, which belong to the same transcriptional unit, are essential for entry and vacuolar escape (Sasakawa *et al.*, 1988; High *et al.*, 1992; Ménard *et al.*, 1993). IpaB (62 kDa) and IpaC (42 kDa) are chaperoned and partitioned in the bacterial cytoplasm by IpgC, a 17 kDa protein encoded by a gene located upstream *ipa*B. Once released into the bacterial supernatant via the Mxi/Spa apparatus, the IpaB and IpaC proteins form a molecular complex which interacts with the host cell surface, thus triggering major cytoskeletal rearrangements which cause entry of the pathogen (Ménard *et al.*, 1994a). These invasion-associated proteins are maintained as a cytoplasmic pool in the bacterial cytoplasm, IpaB and IpaD forming a 'cap' which blocks their release via the Mxi/Spa apparatus. Upon contact with the host cell surface, the cap is released and the invasion-associated proteins, particularly IpaB and IpaC appear massively in the bacterial surpernatant (Ménard *et al.*, 1994b). This is an example of cross talk between a bacterium and its cellular target. Both the *mxi* and *spa* genes code for the secretion apparatus to release other plasmid-encoded proteins (Andrews *et al.*, 1991; Allaoui *et al.*,

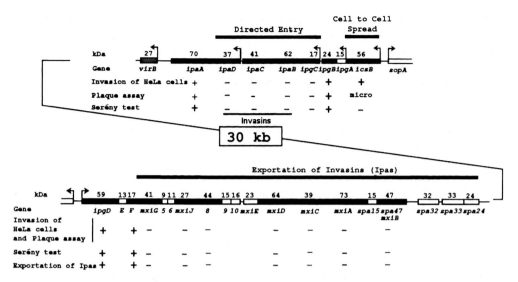

Fig. 1.   Genetic map of the 30-kb entry region of *Shigella flexneri* virulence plasmid.

1992; Allaoui *et al.*, 1993). These two divergently transcribed operons are shown on Figure 1. The plasmid also contains *ics*A (*vir*G), a gene essential for intracellular and intercellular movement (Bernardini *et al.*, 1989).

Intracellular movement and epithelial colonization

*Shigella*e do not have flagella and therefore are non-motile. *S. flexneri* uses the host-cell cytoskeleton to move around the cytoplasm and from cell to cell (Goldberg & Sansonetti, 1993). In infected cells, short filaments of actin form tight bundles at one pole of intracellular bacteria. The actin filaments subsequently form a tail that can be several micrometers long and contains actin-binding proteins such as plastin (Prévost *et al.*, 1992). This actin tail forms on one pole of the bacterium and makes it move as a probable consequence of filaments elongation and aggregation.

Mutants of the *ics*A gene are invasive, but once in the cytoplasm, they do not form an actin tail, do not move and cannot spread to adjacent cells (Bernardini *et al.*, 1989). IcsA is a surface protein with ATPase activity which either directly or indirectly induces actin nucleation and is localized to only one pole of the bacterium (Goldberg *et al.*, 1993). This polarity of IcsA localization provides the system with an asymmetry of actin localization which is likely to allow the motor's efficiency. This protein can be phosphorylated by a cAMP-dependent protein kinase (d'Hauteville & Sansonetti, 1992), it is cleaved into a 95 kDa molecular species which is released into the bactierial supernatant.

Pathogenicity of an *ics*A mutant was tested on macaque monkeys and evaluated by endoscopy and histopathology (Sansonetti *et al.*, 1991). In contrast to monkeys infected with the wild type parental strain, the *ics*A mutant caused only mild clinical symptoms. This mutant caused a few scattered abscesses with nodular morphology and small bloody ulcerations. In biopsies, these infectious foci showed superficial alterations of the mucosa overlaying lymphoid nodules, or in the case of ulcerations there was destruction of the mucosal surface, over lymphoid nodules, that became exposed to the colonic lumen.

The mild symptoms seen in monkeys infected with the *ics*A mutant indicate that intracellular movement, as well as cell to cell spread, play a crucial role in the development of full blown shigellosis. The fact that the few abscesses caused by this mutant localized to lymphoid nodules strongly suggests that *Shigella* penetrates the submucosa *via* M-cells.

The importance of intercellular spread in shigellosis is also examplified by the function of another pathogenicity plasmid gene: *ics*B (Allaoui *et al.*, 1992) (Figure 1). This gene is essential for promoting passage from one infected epithelial cell to the cytoplasm of the next cell. A mutant in *ics*B does not cause keratoconjunctivitis in guinea pigs, suggesting that cell to cell spread by itself is essential for pathogenicity.

Based on the reported observations, passage from cell to cell turns out to be an essential component of the epithelial colonization process by *Shigellae*. This passage causes the formation of protrusions, expansions of the membrane of the infected cell by the moving microorganism which enters the next cell. We have recently demonstrated that in the context of the colonization of an epithelial layer, protrusions are actively endocytosed by neighbouring cells and that this process involves cadherins (Sansonetti *et al.*, 1994), a family of cell adhesion molecules that are expressed essentially in the area of cells' intermediate junctions. These data allow to describe a cycle of epithelial infection and allowing extensive epithelial colonization without an extracellular phase for the bacterium. The potential efficiency of this system that protects intracellular bacteria against effector components of immune defenses is certainly reflected in the dramatic effect that the *ics*A mutation has on reducing the severity of intestinal lesions and intensity of clinical symptoms.

Bacterial effraction into the colonic mucosa

S. flexneri is only capable of invading epithelial cells through their basolateral membrane. This paradoxical observation was made in a study investigating invasion by *Shigella* of the human colonic epithelial cell line Caco-2 which establishes a confluent epithelial monolayer where cells are polarized and form an apical brush border. Therefore, the apical face of a Caco-2 monolayer mimicks the epithelial surface that a bacterium should encounter in the *in vivo* situation. When Caco-2 cells are infected with *S. flexneri*, only a few bacteria interact with the apical surface of cells, and are incapable of entering them. When the epithelial monolayer is pretreated with EGTA that disrupts the intercellular junctions by chelating Ca^{2+}, the cells become efficiently infected (Mounier *et al.*, 1992). These data suggest that *S. flexneri* cannot directly infect epithelial cells in intact epithelia and that during a natural infection, the bacteria may have to reach the subepithelial tissues in order to enter the epithelial lining. These results are consistent with observations in electron microscopy of infected ileal loops made in rabbits. When epithelia were observed shortly after infection, there were no bacteria detectable inside epithelial cells (Perdomo *et al.*, 1994). *Shigella*e appear to be rather unique in their selectivity for the basolateral membrane. Other enteric pathogens, like *Salmonellae*, can invade cells through the apical pole (Falkow *et al.*, 1992).

M-cells are specialized cells which develop only in the epithelial dome covering the lymphoid follicles associated with the mucosa (Kraehenbühl & Neutra, 1992). These cells have the function of non-selectively transporting intact antigens from the lumen into the gut-associated lymphoid tissues (GALT) to ensure a mucosal immune response. M-cells can be differentiated from enterocytes by their characteristic morphology: shorter villi (microfolds), intense activity of endocytosis, invagination by lymphocytes and macrophages. Several enteric pathogens appear to use M-cells as a pathway to cross the epithelium. These include reovirus, poliovirus, retroviruses, bacterial pathogens such as *Salmonellae* and *Yersiniae*. M-cells also transport *Shigella*e into the lymphoid tissue (Wassef *et al.*, 1989). Observations, both in the rabbit ligated ileal loop model and in biopsies of experimentally infected monkeys indicate that the initial entry of *S. flexneri* into the mucosa is *via* M-cells (Wassef *et al.*, 1989; Perdomo *et al.*, 1994).

After translocation through M-cells, the microorganisms are delivered into the follicular structures which represents the inducive site that generates mucosal immune response (Kraehenbühl & Neutra, 1992; Liu & MacPherson, 1993; Pavli *et al.*, 1993) and also the first line of natural immune defense, essentially due to the presence of resident tissue macrophages (Soestayo *et al.*, 1990; Jarry *et al.*, 1989). Most microorganisms that encounter this cell are killed, due to the numerous antibacterial components that they produce. Pathogenic bacteria have evolved different mechanisms to survive this hostile environment. *Legionella pneumophila* and *Mycobacterium tuberculosis* inhibit fusion of lysosomes to the phagocytic vacuole. Other microorganisms, like *Coxiella burnetti*, resist the phagolysosomal environment (Falkow *et al.*, 1992). As an alternative strategy, *Shigella* avoids being killed by the macrophage by triggering the phagocyte's suicide program (Zychlinsky *et al.*, 1992).

S. flexneri induces apoptosis of macrophages

Necrosis and apoptosis are the two major forms of cell death. Necrosis is a passive process, which occurs when a cell dies because of physical alteration. Apoptosis, or programmed cell death, needs active participation of the cell. Apoptotic cell death has been described during normal embryonic development and differentiation, in tumor regression and during growth factor deprivation (Arends & Wyllie, 1991; Ellis *et al.*, 1991).

We have reported that the mechanism of cytotoxicity by which *S. flexneri* kills macrophages (Clerc *et al.*, 1987) is induction of programmed cell death (Zychlinsky *et al.*, 1992). Apoptosis is induced when either a membrane or a cytoplasmic receptor binds an appropriate ligand which induces expression of a second messenger (Arends & Wyllie, 1991; Ellis *et al.*, 1991). An increase in the concentration of intracellular calcium (Caron-Leslie & Cidlowski, 1991; Ojcius *et al.*, 1991) and cAMP (McConkey *et al.*, 1993; Vintermyr *et al.*, 1993) have been implicated, thus inducing expression of the genes necessary for cell death. There are few eukaryotic genes known to be involved in apoptosis. Expression of the tumor suppressor gene *p53* is apparently sufficient to commit a cell to undergo apoptosis. Expression of the oncogenes *c-myc* and *c-fos* is also required, but is not sufficient for the induction of apoptosis. On the other hand, the oncogene *bcl-2* can block the process of programmed cell death (Freeman *et al.*, 1993). *Shigella* only kills its host-cell if it escapes from the phagolysosome into its cytoplasm. Further investigations will hopefully allow complete understanding of the molecular bases of *Shigella*'s relationship to the macrophage (Zychlinsky *et al.*, 1993). IpaB, one of the *Shigella* invasins, accounts for macrophage death (Zychlinsky *et al.*, 1994a).

In addition to their microbicidal activity, macrophages have a crucial role in signalling to other cells the presence of an invasive agent and the generation of inflammation (Dinarello, 1992). In response to a variety of stimuli, macrophages can express three of the most important inflammatory cytokines: Interleukin-1 (IL1), IL-6 and TNFα. IL-6 and TNFα are transcribed, translated and secreted as soon as the cell is stimulated, while IL-1 is in part accumulated in the cytosol. The two forms of IL-1, IL-1α and IL-1β, bind to the same receptors and have similar biological activities. Both forms are synthesized as precursors of 35 kDa which are subsequently proteolytically cleaved by specific proteases to yield mature forms of 17.5 kDa. Both the precursors and the mature form of IL1α and only the mature form of IL-1β are biologically active. The precursor forms of IL-1 are synthesized and accumulated in the cytosol of macrophages. The mature forms are found exclusively in tissue culture supernatants. In the absence of a secretion signal sequence, IL-1 molecules are not released *via* a classic secretory pathway (Dinarello, 1992). It has been shown that one of the possible mechanisms for this cytokine release is apoptosis (Hogquist *et al.*, 1991).

In order to confirm that macrophage apoptosis may play a significant role in the initiation of inflammation, we studied the release of inflammaroty cytokines by infected macrophages *in vitro*. We tested cytokine release by LPS-stimulated murine peritoneal macrophages infected with *S. flexneri*. These cells contain pools of IL-1 and may reflect the activation state of colonic macrophages (Youngman *et al.*, 1993; Mahida *et al.*, 1989; Mahida *et al.*, 1989; Soestayo *et al.*, 1990; Jarry *et al.*, 1989) which are likely to be permanently exposed to bacterial products originating from the intestinal flora. Large amounts of IL-1, but not IL-6 or TNFα, are released by stimulated peritoneal macrophages infected with wild types *S. flexneri*, but not with a non-invasive derivative. Time course experiments of cytokine release demonstrate that IL-1 is present in the supernant of infected cells as early as 15 minutes after infection. IL-1 release asssayed either by its biological activity or antigenically in an ELISA assay, happens before macrophage integrity is compromised. The supernants of LPS-stimulated macrophages infected with *Shigella* contain IL-1α in its active precursor form and IL-1β both in its precursor and mature forms. These results suggest that release of IL-1 happens early in apoptosis and that the release is an active process and not the result of leakage of intracellular stores of cytokines when the integrity of the plasma membrane is compromised (Zychlinsky *et al.*, 1994b).

Bacterial-induced apoptosis of macrophages might play an active role *in vivo* by eliciting an early inflammatory response in epithelial tissues. Release of IL-1 would be a primary, if not the first signal to initiate the inflammatory process. This signal will subsequently be amplified by the induction of the production of other inflammatory cytokines such as IL-6, IL-8 and TNFα by other cells: non-infected macrophages, lymphocytes, endothelial and epithelial cells (Agace *et al.*, 1993; Nakamura *et al.*, 1991).

PMN leukocytes facilitate *S. flexneri* invasion

A major characteristic of shigellosis is the extensive inflammatory reaction and tissue destruction found far beyond Peyer's patches in the rabbit ligated ileal loop model and lymphoid follicles in biopsies of humans and monkeys (Anand *et al.*, 1986; Sansonetti *et al.*, 1991). In these late stages numerous bacteria are found inside epithelial cells. These data suggest that other secondary sites of bacterial entry may exist besides M-cells or that lymphoid follicles and associated dome epithelium are the center of a centrifugal inflammation that extends progressively away from the initial site of bacterial entry.

We hypothesized that the early inflammatory reaction induced by the release of IL-1 by apoptotic macrophages may provoke edema and extravasation of PMN cells. PMN cells (Dinarello, 1992) have a strong chemotactic activity toward gram-negative bacteria and migrate to the lumen of the colon. The transmigration of PMN cells would destabilize and eventually destroy the epithelial barrier, allowing access to the basolateral membrane of colonocytes and their subsequent invasion. Data *in vitro* strongly support this model (Perdomo *et al.*, 1994). The migration of PMN leukocytes was tested using the cell line T-84. This human colonic cell line is grown on permeable supports, the cells become polarized, they present microvilli on their apical side and develop junctions (McRoberts & Barrett, 1989). PMN leukocytes migrate through the epithelium in response to the presence of *Shigella* on the apical side of colonocytes. This migration disrupts intercellular junctions and opens the paracellular pathway for bacteria to reach the basolateral side of epithelial cells and to invade. The structure of the T-84 epithelial lining is reminiscent of intestinal crypts. This system has been used to study chemotactic substances that induce the transmigration of neutrophils across epithelia (Colgan *et al.*, 1993).

When PMN leukocytes are placed on the basolateral side of the epithelium and bacteria on the apical side, both the wild-type strain of *S. flexneri* and a plasmid-cured, non-pathogenic derivative provoke efficient transmigration of neutrophils across a 3-day old T-84 monolayer. However, only the wild-type strains efficiently invade the epithelial cells. In control experiments, where only bacteria were added to the apical side without PMN cells in the system, there was no significant invasion of T-84 cells as previously mentioned in this review. These results indicate that *S. flexneri*, like other enterobacteriaceae, can induce the transmigration of PMN cells and that destruction of the epithelial barrier provides bacteria an access to the basolateral membrane cells. Release of oxygen radicals as well as proteolytic enzymes, like elastase, metallo-proteases and serine proteases, by PMN cells could destroy the epithelium through an 'innocent by-stander' effect, providing even greater access for bacteria to infect the basolateral membrane of epithelial cells (Weiss, 1989).

Transmigration requires specific adhesion of PMNs to epithelial cells. The interaction between these two cells is essentially mediated by the integrin CD11b/CD18 (Mac 1) (Parkos *et al.*, 1991). Monoclonal antibodies against CD18 can neutralize PMN cell transmigration, as well as consequent epithelial cell invasion. The importance of PMN leukocytes in the invasion of *Shigella* has recently been confirmed in experiments carried out in the rabbit ligated ileal loop assay. In these experiments (Perdomo *et al.*, 1994) rabbits have been preloaded with a monoclonal antibody against CD18, before ligating the ileal loops and infecting them with wild-type *Shigella*. Under these conditions a very strong inhibition of tissue inflammation was observed, and almost no bacterial invasion could be detected. These results confirm that bacterial passage through the epithelial barrier depends very much on transmigration of PMN cells and consequent destruction of epithelial cell junctions.

Conclusion

Taking together information from tissue cultured cells, animal models and histopathology from experimentally infected monkeys and patients, we propose here a model for the initiation of shigellosis. Figure 2 shows the proposed sequence of events. First, *S. flexneri* makes contact with M-cells in the colon and is transcytosed from the lumen into the mucosa. M-cells deliver bacteria directly into the dome of lymphoid follicles. These areas are densely populated by resident tissue macrophages, which are infected by *Shigella*. Infection induces macrophage apoptosis, with the concomitant release of IL-1. *Shigella* then starts disseminating through the epithelium and the *lamina propria*. IL-1 released by macrophages starts an inflammatory response. Consecutive extravasation of PMN leukocytes from the circulation into the submucosa, followed by chemoattraction into the lumen of the colon, disrupts the integrity of the epithelial barrier. *S. flexneri* massively infects epithelial cells through their basolateral membrane. Bacterial products induce the production of more cytokines which potentiate inflammation. In the final stage, major destruction of the epithelium is observed. This process resembles certain aspects of acute inflammatory bowel

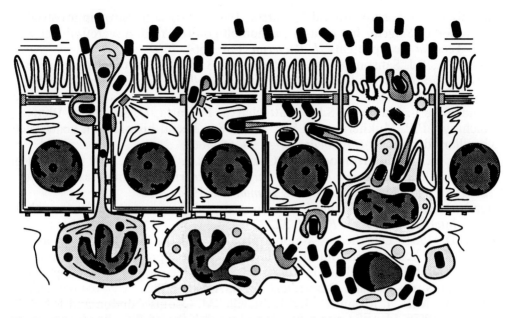

Fig. 2. Scheme of the global process of invasion of the epithelial barrier by *Shigella flexneri.*
Initial event involving entry into M-cells, phagocytosis by local macrophages in the vicinity of lymphoid follicles, induction of macrophages apoptotic death with release of inflammatory cytokines. Subsequent events involving invasion of the *lamina propria* by polymorphonuclear cells (PMN), destabilization of epithelial layer by PMN transmigrating through, under chemoattractant potential of luminal bacteria, entry through basolateral side of epithelial cell and development of the colonization process by cell to cell spread.

diseases such as ulcerative colitis. It must be considered, especially for future vaccine development.

Acknowledgments

I wish to acknowledge the participation of A. Allaoui, J.-M. Cavaillon, M. Huerre, R. Ménard, C. Parsot, J.J. Perdomo, M.-C. Prévost and A. Zychlinsky to the work that has been presented here.

References

Agace, W., S. Hedges, U. Andersson, J. Andersson, M. Ceska and C. Svanborg, 1993 - Selective production by epithelial cells following exposure to *Escherichia coli. Infect. Immun.* **61**, 602–609.
Allaoui, A., J. Mounier, M.C. Prévost, P.J. Sansonetti and C. Parsot, 1992 - *ics*B: a virulence gene necessary for the lysis of protrusions during intercellular spread. *Mol. Microbiol.* **6**, 1605–1616.

Allaoui, A., P.J. Sansonetti and C. Parsot, 1992 - MxiJ, a lipoprotein involved in secretion of *Shigella* Ipa invasins, is homologous to YscJ, a secretion factor of the *Yersinia* Yop proteins. *J. Bacteriol.* **174**, 7661–7669.

Allaoui, A., P.J. Sansonetti and C. Parsot, 1993 - MxiD: an outer membrane protein necessary for the secretion of the *Shigella flexneri* Ipa invasins. *Mol. Microbiol.* **7**, 59–68.

Anand, B.S., V. Malhorta, S.K. Bhattacharya, P. Datta, D. Sen, M.K. Bhattacharya, P.P. Mukherjee and S.C. Pal, 1986 - Rectal histology in acute bacillary dysentery. *Gastroenterology* **90**, 654–660.

Andrews, G.P., A.E. Hromockyj, C. Coker and A.T. Maurelli, 1991 - Two novel virulence loci, *mxi*A and *mxi*B, in *Shigella flexneri* 2A facilitate excretion of invasion plasmid antigens. *Infect. Immun.* **59**, 1997–2005.

Arends, M.J. and A.H. Wyllie, 1991 - Apoptsis: mechanisms and roles in pathology. *Internat. Rev. Exp. Pathol.* **32**, 223–254.

Barua, D., 1981 - Diarrhea as a global problem and the WHO program for its control *In* Acute enteric infections in children. New prospects for treatment and prevention. T. Holme, J. Holmgren, M.H. Merson and R. Möllby. 1–6 Elsevier/North Holland Biomedical Press, Amsterdam.

Bernardini, M.L., J. Mounier, H. d'Hauteville, M. Coquis-Rondon and P.J. Sansonetti, 1989 - Identification of *ics*A a plasmid locus of *Shigella flexneri* that governs bacterial intra and intercellular spread through interaction with F-actin. *Proc. Natl. Acad. Sci. USA* **86**, 3867–3871.

Caron-Leslie, L.-M.M. and J.A. Cidlowski, 1991 - Similar actions of glucocorticoids and calcium on the regulation of apoptosis in S49 cells. *Mol. Endocrinol.* **5**, 1169–1179.

Clerc, P., A. Ryter, J. Mounier and P.J. Sansonetti, 1987 - Plasmid-mediated early killing of eukaryotic cells by *Shigella flexneri* as studied by infection of J774 macrophages. *Infect. Immun.* **55**, 521–527.

Colgan, S.P., C.A. Parkos, C. Delp, M.A. Arnaout and J.L. Madara, 1993 - Neutrophil migration across cultured intestinal epithelium monolayers is modulated by epithelial exposure to IFN-γ in a highly polarized fashion. *J. Cell Biol.* **120**, 785–798.

d'Hauteville, H. and P.J. Sansonetti, 1992 - Phosphorylation of IcsA by cAMP-dependent protein kinase and its effects on intercellular spread of *Shigella flexneri*. *Mol. Microbiol.* **6**, 833–841.

Dinarello, C.A., 1992 - Role of interleukin-1 and tumor necrosis factor in systemic response to infection and inflammation *In* Inflammation, basic principles and clinical correlates. J.I. Gallin, I.M. Goldstein and R. Snyderman. 211–232. Raven Press, New York.

Ellis, R.E., J. Yuan and H.R. Horvitz, 1991 - Mechanisms and functions of cell death. *Annu. Rev. Cell Biol.* **7**, 663–698.

Falkow, S., R.R. Isberg and D.A. Portnoy, 1992 - The interaction of bacteria with mammalian cell. *Ann. Rev. Cell Biol.* **8**, 333–363.

Freeman, R.S., S. Estus, K. Horigome and E.M.J. Johnson, 1993 - Cell death genes in invertebrates and (maybe) vertebrates. *Curr. Opin. Neurobiol.* **3**, 25–31.

Goldberg, M. and P.J. Sansonetti, 1993 - *Shigella* subversion of the cellular cytoskeleton: a strategy for epithelial colonization. *Infect. Immun.* **61**, 4941–4946.

Goldberg, M., O. Bârzu, C. Parsot and P.J. Sansonetti, 1993 - Unipolar localization and ATPase activity of IcsA, a *Shigella flexneri* protein involved in intracellular movement. *J. Bacteriol.* **175**, 2189–2196.

High, N., J. Mounier, M.C. Prévost and P.J. Sansonetti, 1992 - IpaB of *Shigella flexneri* causes entry into epithelial cells and escape from the phagocytic vacuole. *EMBO J.* **11**, 1991–1999.

Hogquist, K.A., M.A. Nett, E.R. Unanue and D.D. Chaplin, 1991 - Interleukin-1 is processed and released during apoptosis. *Proc. Natl. Acad. Sci. USA* **88**, 8485–8489.

Jarry, A., M. Robaszkiewicz, N. Brousse and GF. Potet, 1989 - Immune cells associated with M-cells in the follicle-associated epithelium of Peyer's patches in the rat. *Cell Tissue Res.* **255**, 293–298.

Kraehenbühl, J.P. and M.R. Neutra, 1992 - Molecular and cellular basis of immune protection of mucosal surfaces. *Physiol. Rev.* **72**, 853–849.

LaBrec, E.H., H. Schneider, T.J. Magnani and S.B. Formal, 1964 - Epithelial cell penetration as an essential step in the pathogenesis of bacillary dysentery. *J. Bacteriol.* **88**, 1503–1518.

Lindberg, A.A. and T. Pal, 1993 - Strategies for development of potential candidate *Shigella* vaccines. *Vaccine* **11**, 168–179.

Liu, L.M. and G.G. MacPherson, 1993 - Antigen acquisition by dendritic cells: intestinal dendritic cell acquire antigen administered orally and can prime naive T cells *in vivo*. *J. Exp. Med.* **177**, 1299–1307.

Mahida, Y.R., K. Wu and D.P. Jewell, 1989 - Enhanced production of interleukin-1β by mononuclear cells isolated from mucosa with active ulcerative colitis of Crohn's disease. *Gut* **30**, 835–838.

Mahida, Y.R., S. Patel, P. Gionchetti, D. Vaux and D.P. Jewell, 1989 - Macrophages subpopulation in *lamina propria* of normal and inflamed colon and terminal ileum. *Gut* **30**, 826–834.

Mathan, M.M. and V.I. Mathan, 1991 - Morphology of rectal mucosa of patients with shigellosis. *Rev. Infect. Dis.* **13**(S4), S314–318.

Maurelli, A.T. and P.J. Sansonetti, 1988 - Genetic determinants of *Shigella* pathogenicity. *Ann. Rev. Microbiol.* **42**, 127–150.

Maurelli, A.T., B. Baudry, H. d'Hauteville, T.L. Hale and P.J. Sansonetti, 1985 - Cloning of plasmid DNA sequences involved in invasion of HeLa cells by *Shigella flexneri*. *Infect. Immun.* **49**, 164–171.

McConkey, D.J., S. Orrenius, S. Okret and M. Jondal, 1993 - Cyclic AMP potentiates glucocorticoid-induced endogenous endonuclease activation in thymocytes. *FASEB J.* **7**, 580–585.

McRoberts, J.A. and K.E. Barrett, 1989 - Hormone-regulated ion transport in T84 colonic cells *In* Functional epithelial cells in culture. 235–265. Alan R. Lyss. Inc. New York.

Ménard, R., P.J. Sansonetti and C. Parsot, 1993 - Non polar mutagenesis of the *ipa* genes defines IpaB, IpaC and IpaD as effectors of *Shigella flexneri* entry into epithelial cells. *J. Bacteriol.* **175**, 5899–5906.

Ménard R., P.J. Sansonetti, C. Parsot and T. Vasselon. Extracellular association and cytoplasmic partitioning of the IpaB and IpaC invasins of *Shigella flexneri*. 1994 - *Cell* **79**, 515–525.

Ménard R., P.J. Sansonetti and C. Parsot, 1994 - The secretion of the *Shigella flexneri* Ipa invasins is induced by the epithelial cell and controlled by IpaB and IpaD. *EMBO J.* **13**, 5293–5302.

Mounier, J., T. Vasselon, R. Hellio, M. Lesourd and P.J. Sansonetti, 1992 - *Shigella flexneri* enters human colonic Caco-2 epithelial cells through the basolateral pole. *Infect. Immun.* **60**, 237–248.

Nakamura, H., R. Yoshimura, H.A. Jaffe and R.G. Crystal, 1991 - Interleukin-8 gene expression in human bronchial epithelial cells. *J. Biol. Chem.* **266**, 19611–19617.

Ojcius, D.M., A. Zychlinsky, L.M. Zheng and J.D.-E. Young, 1991 - Ionophore-induced apoptosis. Role of DNA fragmentation and calcium fluxes. *Exp. Cell Res.* **197**, 43–49.

Parkos, C.A., C. Delp, M.A. Arnaout and J.L. Madara, 1991 - Neutrophil migration across a cultured intestinal epithelium. Dependence on a CD11b/CD18-mediated event and enhanced efficiency in physiological direction. *J. Clin. Invest.* **88**, 1605–1612.

Pavli, P., D.A. Hume, E. van den Pol and W.F. Doe, 1993 - Dendritic cells, the major antigen-presenting cells of the human colonic *lamina propria. Immunology* **78**, 132–141.

Perdomo, J.J., P. Gounon and P.J. Sansonetti, 1994 - Polymorphonuclear leukocyte transmigration promotes invasion of colonic epithelial monolayer by *Shigella flexneri. J. Clin. Invest.* **93**, 633–643.

Perdomo J.J., J.M. Cavaillon, M. Huerre, M. Ohayon, P. Gounon and P.J. Sansonetti, 1994 - Acute inflammation causes epithelial invasion and mucosal destruction in experimental shigellosis. *J. Exp. Med.* **180**, 1307–1319.

Prévost, M.C., M. Lesourd, M. Arpin, F. Vernel, J. Mounier, R. Hellio and P.J. Sansonetti, 1992 - Unipolar reorganization of F-actin layer at bacterial division and bundling of actin filaments by plastin correlate with movement of *Shigella flexneri* within HeLa cells. *Infect. Immun.* **60**, 4088–4099.

Sansonetti, P.J., A. Ryter, P. Clerc, A.T. Maurelli and J. Mounier, 1986 - Multiplication of *Shigella flexneri* within HeLa cells: lysis of the phagocytic vacuole and plasmid-mediated contact hemolysis. *Infect. Immun.* **51**, 461–469.

Sansonetti, P.J., J. Arondel, A. Fontaine, H. d'Hauteville and M.L. Bernardini, 1991 - Ompb (osmo-regulation) and *ics*A (cell to cell spread) mutant of *Shigella flexneri*: vaccine candidates and probes to study the pathogenesis of shigellosis. *Vaccine* **9**, 416–422.

Sansonetti, P.J., J. Mounier, M.C. Prévost and R.M. Mège, 1994 - Cadherin expression is required for the spread of *Shigella flexneri* between epithelial cells. *Cell* **76**, 1–20.

Sanyal, S.C., 1981 - Epidemiological importance of diarrheal agents in India *In* Acute enteric infections in children. New prospects for treatment and prevention. T. Holme, J. Holmgren, M.H. Merson and R. Möllby. 149–157 Elsevier/ North Holland Biomedical Press. Amsterdam.

Sasakawa, C., K. Kamata, T. Sakai, S. Makino, M. Yamada, N. Okada and M. Yoshikawa, 1988 - Virulence-associated genetic regions comprising 31 kb of the 230-kb plasmid in *Shigella flexneri* 2A. *J. Bacteriol.* **170**, 2480–2484.

Serény, B., 1955 - Experimental *Shigella* keratocunjunctivitis. *Acta Microbiol. Acad. Sci. Hung* **2**, 293–296.

Soestayo, M., J. Biewenga, G. Kraal and T. Sminia, 1990 - The localization of macrophages subsets and dendritic cells in the gastrointestinal tract of the mouse with special reference to the presence of high endothelial venules. An immuno- and enzyme-histochemical study. *Cell Tissue Res.* **259**, 587–593.

Vintermyr, O.K., B.J. Gjertsen, M. Lanotte and S.O. Doskeland, 1993 - Microinjected catalytic subunit of cAMP-dependent protein kinase induces apoptosis in myeloid leukemia (IPC-81) cells. *Exp. Cell Res.* **206**, 157–161.

Wassef, J.S., D.F. Keren and J.L. Mailloux, 1989 - Role of M-cells in initial antigen uptake and in ulcer formation in rabbit intestinal loop model of shigellosis. *Infect. Immun.* **57**, 858–863.

Weiss, S.J., 1989 - Tissue destruction by neutrophils. *New Engl. J. Med.* **320**, 365–376.

Youngman, K.R., P.L. Simon, G.A. West, F. Cominelli, D. Rachmilewitz, J.S. Klein and C. Fiocchi, 1993 - Localization of intestinal interleukin-1 activity and protein and genes expression to *lamina propria* cells. *Gastroenterology* **104**, 749–758.

Zychlinsky, A., 1993 - Programmed cell death in infectious diseases. *Trends Microbiol.* **1**, 114–117.

Zychlinsky, A., C. Fitting, J.M. Cavaillon and P.J. Sansonetti, 1994 - Interleukin-1 is released by macrophages during *Shigella flexneri* induced apoptosis. *J. Clin. Invest.* **94**, 1328–1332.

Zychlinsky, A., M.C. Prévost and P.J. Sansonetti, 1992 - *Shigella flexneri* induces apoptosis in infected macrophages. *Nature* **358**, 167–169.

Zychlinsky, A., B. Kenny, R. Ménard, M.C. Prévost, I.B. Holland and P.J. Sansonetti, 1994 - IpaB mediates macrophage apoptosis induced by *Shigella flexneri*. *Mol. Microbiol.* **11**, 619–927.

Jan D.A. van Embden[1], Petra de Haas[2], Herre Heersma[1], Leo Schouls[1], Jim Douglas[3], Lishi Qiang[3], Peter W.M. Hermans[4], Feriele Messadi[5], Francoise Portaels[6] and Dick van Soolingen[2]

Repetitive DNA as a Tool to Study the Genetic Variation and Epidemiology of *Mycobacterium tuberculosis*

Abstract

The species *Mycobacterium tuberculosis* constitutes a very homogenous genetic group of bacteria. Repetitive DNA elements are presently the only cellular targets that can be used to discriminate clinical isolates for epidemiological purposes. The insertion sequence IS*6110* is usually present in multiple copies in *M. tuberculosis* and due to the IS*6110*-associated DNA polymorphism, it is the most widely used marker to establish the genetic relatedness between clinical isolates of this pathogen. This study will discuss how large scale DNA fingerprinting can be exploited for epidemiological studies and the hypothesis is brought forward that BCG vaccination has influenced the population structure in countries where vaccination is common practice.

Introduction

Tuberculosis is the world's leading infectious disease in terms of mortality. The World Health Organization estimates yearly 7 million new cases and a death toll of 2.5 million (Raviglione *et al.*, 1995). The incidence is on the increase in most countries and the recent emergence of multidrug resistant *Mycobacterium tuberculosis* strains can set treatment back to the preantibiotic days of tuberculosis (Bloom, 1992; Edlin, 1992). One of the key factors in the control of tuberculosis is contact tracing to arrest further transmission. Recent studies on repetitive DNA elements in *Mycobacterium tuberculosis* have shown that these elements are associated with DNA polymorphism in the chromosome. This polymorphism enables to distinguish different strains of *M. tuberculosis*. Therefore, these elements have been found to be extremely useful for epidemiological studies of tuberculosis like outbreak investigations, transmission studies in the community and the dissemination of multi-drug resistant clones (Beck-Sauge *et al.*; 1992, Daley *et al.*, 1992; Dwyer *et al.*, 1993; Edlin *et al.*, 1992; Fischl et *al.*, 1992; Mazurek *et al.*, 1991; Small *et al.*, 1993).

Two classes of repetitive DNA elements have been used for the molecular epidemiology of tuberculosis: (i) insertion elements, which have the capacity to move within the genome with little or no target specificity and which have a size of about 1300 bp (Mazurek *et al.*, 1991, van Soolingen *et al.*, 1992) and (ii) small repetitive DNAs, varying in size from three to 36 bp (Small and van Embden, 1994). The nature of the genetic rearrangements driven by the small repetitive elements has been investigated only for the Direct Repeat (DR, 36bp) region and homologous recombination between DRs was found to be the predominant kind of rearrangement in the DR cluster (Groenen *et al.*,1993). It is likely that the same mechanism contributes to DNA polymorphism associated with other small repetitive sequences, like the Polymorphic GC-rich Repeat Sequence (PGRS, 9 bp; Ross, 1992), the Major Polymorphic Tandem Repeat (MPTR, 10 bp; Hermans *et al.*, 1992) and the triplet repeat $(GTG)_5$ (Wiid *et al.*, 1994). Except for the DNA polymorphism associated with repetitive DNA very little genetic heterogeneity is found in *M. tuberculosis*. A recent sequence comparison of a number of eight loci in housekeeping genes, comprising about 200,000 nucleotides revealed almost a complete absence of nucleotide variation among strains from diverse geographic origin (Kapur *et al.*, 1994). The average number of synonymous substitutions per site was found to be about 0.0001, which is 10000 times less as found in *Escherichia coli*. As the mutation frequency in *M. tuberculosis* is not different from other bacteria like *Escherichia coli*, the investigators concluded that the present day isolates of *M. tuberculosis* found among humans probably evolved from a common ancester some 8000-10000 years ago, during an episode of periodic selection.

The insertion element IS*6110* is the most widely used marker for epidemiological studies, because of the high degree of differentiation obtained with this element. Furthermore, international consensus exists on a standardized method of IS*6110* fingerprinting, thus enabling to compare DNA types from different laboratories (van Embden *et al.*, 1993). Most studies on the DNA polymorphism in *M. tuberculosis* has been exploited to answer short term epidemiological questions, taking advantage of the knowledge that identical fingerprints from different isolates is usually evidence for recent person to person transmission or endogenous reactivation. However, little is known about the significance of non-identical, but related patterns of IS*6110*-associated RFLPs of *M. tuberculosis* in different human populations and the degree of geographic isolation of *M. tuberculosis* in different parts of the world. As the transposition of IS*6110* is a time-dependent process, the degree of IS*6110* polymorphism among the descendents of a particular clone in a population is a reflection of the time, which elapsed scince its dissemination. Thus analysis of the *M. tuberculosis* population structure by IS*6110*-associated Restriction Fragment Length Polymorphism (RFLP) may provide information about the history and the pathways of global dissemination of tuberculosis and the factors favouring the (re)emergence of this infectious disease. Here we describe preliminary results on differences in the population structure of *M. tuberculosis* in four different countries.

Analysis of the population structure of *M. tuberculosis* in Ethiopia, Tunisia and the Netherlands

IS*6110* DNA fingerprints were analyzed from about 500 isolates from Ethiopia, Tunisia and the Netherlands. The IS*6110* banding patterns of the strains from each country were analysed for similarity by computer analysis and all patterns were ordered by similarity according to a previously described algorithm (van Soolingen *et al.*, 1991). To visualize the relatedness between the banding patterns between all isolates, a similarity matrix was generated for the IS*6110* fingerprints from strains of each country. In these matrices the degree of relatedness of each IS*6110* banding pattern with any other in the collection are visualized. All clustered strains (with identical fingerprints) constitute black triangles just below the diagonal, and all families of related strains are visualized by triangular groupings in varying grey values.

About two third of the Ethiopian isolates belonged to clusters of identical strains or to related families (figure 1a). A substantial number of these isolates carried only a single or a few IS*6110* copies. It is known that *M. tuberculosis* strains carrying one or a few IS*6110* copies are often difficult to differentiate by IS*6110* RFLP, due to a site-specific preference of insertion of the IS element (Hermans *et al.*, 1991, van Soolingen *et al.*, 1993). Using the genetic markers PGRS and DR about half of these strains could be further distinguished. Taking this heterogeneity into account, about 36% of the Ethiopian strains were grouped in families of closely related strains. The population structure of *M. tuberculosis* in Tunisia differed considerably in that a larger proportion, 62%, of the Tunisian isolates grouped into three large families with closely related IS*6110* DNA banding patterns (see figure 1b). The strains of each family contain more than 10 IS*6110* copies and the members of any of these 3 families differed only in one or a few bands. This suggests that the majority of the Tunisian strains descended from 3 recently expanded clones. The degree of IS*6110* DNA polymorphism among the strains isolated in the Netherlands was found to be much greater than that among the *M. tuberculosis* strains originating from Ethiopia and Tunisia. Only two families of distantly related strains could be distinguished, and these accounted for 24% of all strains (see figure 1c).

Surprisingly, none of the Ethiopian strains shared a fingerprint with any of the Tunisian isolates. Two of the Ethiopian fingerprints matched with Dutch ones and one Tunisian isolate was identical to a Dutch one. Because a previous study suggested an association between fingerprint type and geographic origin, we investigated the patient data of the 3 Dutch patients from whom *M. tuberculosis* was isolated that shared fingerprints with those of Ethiopia and Tunisia. The single patient with a Tunisian type was a Dutch truck driver. He frequently delivered cattle from the Netherlands to Marocco and Tunisia. The patients with an Ethiopian *M. tuberculosis* type were born in Ethiopia and Somalia, respectively and living since a few years since in the Netherlands. These data indicate an association between *M. tuberculosis* DNA type and geographical origin. Analysis of patient data from Dutch *M. tuberculosis* strains having fingerprints

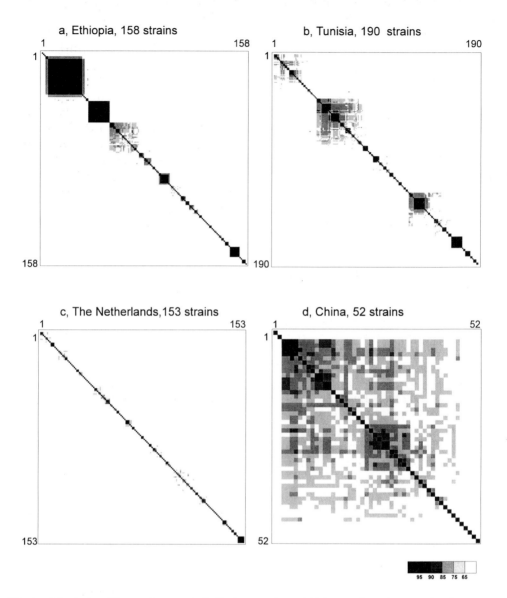

Fig. 1. IS*6110* banding patterns and similarity matrices of 158 *M. tuberculosis* strains from Ethiopia (a), 190 strains from Tunisia (b), 153 strains from the Netherlands (c) and 52 strains from China (d). The banding patterns (not shown) were ordered by similarity and the similarities are depicted between any strain (ordered horizontally) with any other strain (ordered vertically in the same order as the horizontal ones). The scale depicts similarity coefficients as defined previously (van Soolingen *et al.*, 1991). The value of the similarity coefficient only between values of 65% and 100% is depicted by the 5 different grey tones in the matrices. These values roughly correspond to the percentage of bands shared between two strains. The diagonal is formed by the 100% similarity coefficient values of the corresponding strains.

Repetitive DNA as a tool to study

that are related, but not identical to Ethiopian ones, indicated that the majority of these patients originated from Ethiopia or Somalia, again strengthening the idea of the existance of families of genetically closely related *M. tuberculosis* strains, which have been geographically isolated for long periods of time.

The population structure of *M. tuberculosis* in China and some other Asian countries

Fifty two *M. tuberculosis* strains isolated from patients in China were fingerprinted using IS*6110*. The relatedness of all 52 strains is shown in the similarity matrix of figure 1d. Fourty five of the 52 fingerprints shared at least two thirds of the IS-containing *Pvu*II fragments, indicating that these strains belong to a closely related grouping, which we will refer to as the 'Beijing family', because the vast majority of the Chinese strains originated from patients in Beijing. Only 17 strains, seven from China and 10 from Mongolia, did not belong to this family.

We analyzed the DNA polymorphism in strains from China also with the repetitive DNA elements DR, PGRS, and the insertion element IS*1081*. The strains of the Beijing family were found to be identical or almost identical using these genetic markers, indicating that *M. tuberculosis* isolates of the Beijing family constitute a remarkably distinct group of closely related bacteria. The fingerprint database in Bilthoven was searched for the presence of strains having characteristics of the Beijing banding pattern. About 40% of the strains originating from Mongolia, South Korea, Thailand and Vietnam were of the Beijing type, whereas only a few percent of the strains isolated in several European, African and South American countries were of the Beijing type. Many of the Dutch patients harbouring *M. tuberculosis* of the Beijing type originated from the South East Asia.

These data suggest that in the recent past a single clone of *M. tuberculosis* disseminated rapidly in the Beijing region of China and radiated to other countries and continents. Although no exact data are available about the pace of the molecular clock of IS*6110*, we guess that less than a century elapsed since the clonal expansion from the hypothetical common ancestor.

Factors determining the population structure of *M. tuberculosis*

Presently virtually nothing is known about the forces that influence the population dynamics of *M. tuberculosis*. During the first studies on IS*6110*-associated DNA polymorphism van Soolingen *et al.* (1992) observed that *M. tuberculosis* strains from African countries are genetically much less diverse compared to those originating from the Netherlands. In the latter country the incidence of tuberculosis is low, about 10 cases per year per 100,000 inhabitants and until recently it was assumed that the majority of the tuberculosis cases are due to reactivation of infections that have been contracted many years, often many decades before the onset of disease. Therefore, the spectrum of DNA polymorphism in *M. tuberculosis* strains from this country is likely a reflection of frozen diversity. This diversity from the past is partly explained by the high migration rate in the Netherlands, resulting in the acquisition of strains from diverse geographic areas.

Furthermore, a long period of time between infection and reactivation may allow *M. tuberculosis* to undergo genetic rearrangements and thus contribute to RFLP. In countries with a high incidence of tuberculosis, the rate of transmission is much higher than in low incidence countries like the Netherlands. Therefore, *M. tuberculosis* variants that have some selective advantage will expand more rapidly in countries with a high tuberculosis incidence. This is consistent with the observation that in highly endemic countries like Ethiopia, a high proportion of isolates belong to a limited number of genetically closely related strains. However, although the incidence of tuberculosis in Ethiopia (170 per 100,000) is much higher than that in Tunisia (30 per 100,000) or the Beijing region in China (30 per 100,000), we found more diversity among *M. tuberculosis* in Ethiopia than in Tunesia and China. A factor common to Tunesia and China is BCG vaccination, which has been used for the past decades. This is in contrast to Ethiopia where BCG vaccination is not a common practice. Less than 10% of the population is presently being vaccinated in Ethiopia. Thus this raises the question whether vaccination may have been one of the important selective forces that favoured the selection of particular families of *M. tuberculosis* strains, like the Beijing family.

Although the efficacy of the BCG vaccine has been found to vary considerably in the various vaccine trials (Fine, 1989), it is unlikely that BCG immunity would have no effect at all and that all strains of *M. tuberculosis* would resist BCG- induced immunity to the same degree. Therefore, one may expect that mass BCG vaccination during extended periods of time will have a significant effect on the population structure of *M. tuberculosis*. Clones that resist BCG immunity better than other ones are expected to expand and to radiate to other countries, where BCG vaccination is practised as well. If true, one may expect that the efficacy of BCG vaccination will decrease with time, due the gradual predomination of strains which are resistant or partially resistant to the BCG-induced immune response.

Prospects.

In Bilthoven a project has been undertaken to establish a large IS*6110* DNA fingerprint database, which will contain also patient-related data. Presently the database contains about 4000 fingerprints of *M. tuberculosis* isolates from 30 countries. In 1993 international consensus was reached on a standardized method of *M. tuberculosis* fingerprinting (van Embden, 1993), thus enabling to compare *M. tuberculosis* fingerprints obtained in different laboratories. The fingerprints used in the study described above were prepared in three different laboratories, showing that a concerted international effort on tuberculosis epidemiology is within reach. The database will be used to study the population structure and the global epidemiology of *M. tuberculosis*. It is hoped that this molecular epidemiologic approach will provide clues about issues such as the impact of HIV, migration, drug use and resistance and BCG vaccination on the transmission of tuberculosis within countries and across country borders and lead to more effective methods to control tuberculosis. Furthermore, correlation of fingerprint data with patient-associated data may reveal strain-specific differences in pathogenicity, such as tissue tropism or immune modulation.

Acknowledgments

This study was financially supported by the World Health Organization Programme for Vaccine Development, the European Community Program for Science Technology and Development and the European Community Programme for Biomedical Research.

References

Beck-Sagué, C., S.W. Dooley, M.D. Hutton, J. Otten, A. Breeden, J.T. Crawford, A.E. Pitchenik, C. Woodley, G. Cauthen and W.R. Jarvis, 1992 - Hospital outbreak of multidrug-resistant *Mycobacterium tuberculosis* infections. *JAMA* **268**, 1280–1286.

Bloom, B.R. and C.J.L. Murray, 1992 - Tuberculosis: Commentary on a recent killer. *Science* **257**, 1055–1064.

Daley, C.L., P.M. Small, G.F. Schecter, G.K. Schoolnik, R.A. McAdam, W.R. Jacobs, Jr. and P.C. Hopewell, 1992 - An outbreak of tuberculosis with accelerated progression among persons infected with the human immunodeficiency virus: an analysis using restriction fragment length polymorphisms. *N. Engl. J. Med.* **326**, 231–235.

Dwyer, B., K. Jackson, K. Raios, A. Sievers, E. Wilshire and B. Ross, 1993 - DNA Restriction fragment analysis to define an extended cluster of tuberculosis in homeless men and their associates. *J. Infect. Dis.* **167**, 490–494.

Edlin, B.R., J.I. Tokars, M.H. Grieco, J.T. Crawford, J. Williams, E.M. Sordillo, K.R. Ong, J.O. Kilburn, S.W. Dooley, K.G. Castro, W.R. Jarvis and S.D. Holmberg, 1992 - An Outbreak of multidrug-resistent tuberculosis among hospitalized patients with the acquired immunodeficiency syndrome. *N. Engl. J. Med.* **326**, 1514–1521.

Fischl, M.A., R.B. Uttamchandani, G.L. Daikos *et al.*, 1992 - An outbreak of tuberculosis caused by multiple-drug resistant tubercle bacilli among patients with HIV infection. *Ann. Intern. Med.* **117**, 177–183.

Fine, P.E.M., 1989 - The BCG story: Lessons from the past and imlications for the fututre. *Rev. Infect. Dis.* **11** (Suppl. 2), S353.

Groenen, P.M.A., A.E. van Bunschoten, D. van Soolingen and J.D.A. van Embden, 1993 - Nature of DNA polymorphism in the direct repeat cluster of *Mycobacterium tuberculosis*; Application for strain differentiation by a novel method. *Mol. Microbiol.* **105**, 1057–1065.

Hermans, P.W.M., D. van Soolingen, E.M. Bik, P.E.W. de Haas, J.W. Dale and J.D.A. van Embden, 1991 - The insertion element IS*987* from *M. bovis* BCG is located in a hot spot integration region for insertion elements in *M. tuberculosis* complex strains. *Infect. Immun.* **59**, 2695–2705.

Hermans, P.W.M., D. van Soolingen and J.D.A. van Embden, 1992 - Characterization of a major polymorphic tandem repeat in *Mycobacterium tuberculosis* and its potential use in the epidemiology of *Mycobacterium kansasii* ansasii and *Mucobacterium gordonae*. *J. Bacteriol.* **174**, 4157–4165.

Hermans, P.W.M., F. Messadi, H. Guebrexabher, D. van Soolingen, P.E.W. de Haas, H. Heersma, H. de Neeling, A. Ayoub, F. Portaels, D. Frommel, M. Zribi and Jan D.A. van Embden, 1995 - Usefulness of DNA typing for global tuberculosis epidemiology. *J. Infect. Dis.* **171**, 1504–1513.

Kapur, V., T.S. Whittam and J.M. Musser, 1994 - Is *Mycobacterium tuberculosis* 15,000 years old? *J. Infect. Dis.* **170**, 1348–1349.

Mazurek, G.H., M.D. Cave, K.D. Eisenach, R.J. Wallace, Jr., J.H. Bates and J.T. Crawford, 1991 - Chromosomal DNA fingerprint patterns produced with IS as strain specific markers for epidemiologic study of tuberculosis. *J. Clin. Microbiol.* **29**, 2030–2033.

Raviglione, M.C., D.E. Snider and A. Kochi, 1995 - Global epidemiology of tuberculosis; morbidity and mortality of a worldwide epidemic. *JAMA* **273**, 2207–2276.

Ross, C., K. Raios, K. Jackson and B. Dwyer, 1992 - Molecular cloning of a highly repeated element from *Mycobacterium Tuberculosis* and its use as an epidemiological tool. *J. Clin. Microbiol.* **30**, 942–946.

Small, P.M., R.W. Schafer, P.C. Hopewell, S.P. Singh, M.J. Murphy, E. Desmond, M.F. Sierra and G.K. Schoolnik, 1993 - Exogenous reinfection with multidrug-resistant *M. tuberculosis* in patients with advanced HIV infection. *N. Engl. J. Med.* **328**, 1137–1144.

Small, Peter M. and J.D.A. van Embden, 1994 - Molecular epidemiology of tuberculosis. In Tuberculosis: Pathogenesis, Protection and Control, pp. 569–582. In 'Tuberculosis, pathogenesis, protection, and control'. Ed. B.R. Bloom. ASM Press, Washington DC.

Van Embden, J.D.A., M.D. Cave, J.T. Crawford, J.W. Dale, K.D. Eisenach, B. Gicquel, P.W.M. Hermans, C. Martin, R. Mcadam, T.M. Shinnick and P.M. Small, 1993 - Strain identification of *Mycobacterium tuberculosis* by DNA fingerprinting: Recommendations for a standardized Methodology. *J. Clin. Microbiol.* **31**, 406–409.

Van Soolingen, D., P.W.M. Hermans, P.E.W. de Haas, D.R. Soll and J.D.A. van Embden, 1991 - The occurrence and stability of insertion sequences in

Mycobacterium tuberculosis complex strains; evaluation of IS-dependent DNA polymorphism as a tool in the epidemiology of tuberculosis. *J. Clin. Microbiol.* **29**, 2578–2586.

Van Soolingen, D., P.W.M. Hermans, P.E.W. de Haas and J.D.A. van Embden, 1992 - Insertion element IS*1081*-associated Restriction Fragment Length Polymorphism in *Mycobacterium tuberculosis* Complex spacies: a reliable tool for recognizing *Mycobacterium bovis* BCG. *J. Clin. Microbiol.* **30**, 1772–1777.

Van Soolingen, D., P.E.W. de Haas, P.W.M. Hermans, P.M.A. Groenen and J.D.A. van Embden, 1993 - Comparison of various repetitive Dna elements as genetic markers for strain differentation and epidemiology of *Mycobacterium tuberculosis*. *J. Clin. Microbiol.* **31**, 1987–1995.

Wiid, I.J.F., C. Werely, N. Beyers, P. Donald and P.D. van Helden, 1994 - Oligonucleotide (GTG)$_5$ as amarker for strain identification in *Mycobacterium tuberculosis*. *J. Clin. Microbiol.* **32**, 1318–1321.

Affiliation

Unit Molecular Microbiology[1] and Laboratory of Bacteriology[2], National Institute of Public Health and Environmental Protection, Bilthoven, the Netherlands; Department of Microbiology[2], University of Hawaii at Monoa, Honolulu, USA; Armauer Hansen Research Institute[4], Addis Ababa, Ethiopia; Regional Hygiene Laboratory[5], University Hospital Center Hedi Chakar, Sfax, Tunisia; Institute of Tropical Medicine Prince Leopold[6], Antwerp.

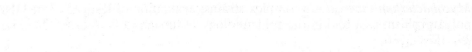

Johannes G. Kusters*[1], Michiel F.J. Blankenvoorde[1], Brian M.M. Ahmer[2], Craig J. Lipps[2], Dan Black[2], Frances Bowe[2], Bernard A.M. van der Zeijst[1] and Fred Heffron[2]

Macrophage-Induced Genes of *Salmonella Typhimurium*

Abstract

We developed an effective strategy for the systematic identification of macrophage-induced genes of *S. typhimurium*. MudJ transposon-insertion mutagenesis was used to create a library of random *lacZ* fusions in *S. typhimurium* strain ATCC 14028. Insertions in macrophage-induced genes were identified by comparing the ability of individual MudJ mutants to ferment X-gal in either the presence or the absence of the murine macrophage cell-line J774. Screening of 940 mutants resulted in the identification of ten MudJ mutants with insertions in macrophage-induced genes. When tested for virulence, 6 out of these 10 mutants were macrophage-sensitive and 3 were avirulent in mice. Southern blot- and sequence analysis of the cloned macrophage-induced genes indicated that all ten MudJ insertions were in different genes. Some genes were found to be specific for *Salmonella* while others are conserved in most pathogenic bacteria. One mutant had a MudJ insertion in the enterotoxin gene *stn*, a known *S. typhimurium* virulence factor, the others are in new virulence genes.

Introduction

When *Salmonella typhimurium* infects a host it is exposed to various environmental changes, such as changes in temperature, nutrient supply, osmolarity and pH (Groisman *et al.*, 1990; Finlay and Falkow, 1988; Fields *et al.*, 1986; Miller *et al.*, 1989; Mekalanos, 1992). In addition the pathogen is exposed to oxygen radicals and defensins produced by the hosts macrophages (Buchmeier and Heffron, 1990). To successfully adapt to this new hostile environment within the

[1] Department of Bacteriology, University of Utrecht, P.O. Box 80.165, 3508 TD, Utrecht, The Netherlands.
[2] Department of Molecular Microbiology and Immunology, Oregon Health Sciences University, Portland, Oregon 97201-3098.
* Present address and correspondence: Department of Medical Microbiology, Vrije Universiteit, Van der Boechorststraat 7, 1081 BT Amsterdam, the Netherlands. E-mail: jg.kusters.mm@med.vu.nl

host, differential expression of bacterial genes must occur. We here describe the development of an effective strategy (Macrophage-Induced Promoter Assay; MIPA) for the systematic identification of *S. typhimurium* genes that are highly expressed when the bacteria are in contact with macrophages but not when they are absent. Use of this MIPA resulted in the identification of 10 macrophage-induced loci of *S. typhimurium*.

Screening for mutants with MudJ insertions in genes of which the expression is altered upon contact with macrophages

MudJ transposon-insertion mutagenesis was used to create a library of random *lacZ* fusions in *S. typhimurium* strain ATCC 14028. From this library we selected 940 individual mutants and screened them for their ability to express β-galactosidase in the presence and absence of J774 macrophages. Only MudJ transposon insertions in actively transcribed genes will result in the production of β-galactosidase. The production of this enzyme can easily be established by its potential to ferment the colourless sugar X-gal (5-bromo-4-chloro-3-indolyl-β-galactose) into an intense blue product. MudJ mutants in macrophage-induced genes can therefore be identified as those mutants that ferment X-gal (i.e. turn blue) in the presence of J774 cells but not in their absence.

Of the 940 individual MudJ mutants tested with the above method, ten showed significant *lacZ* production when in contact with J774 cells while no detectable *lacZ* production was observed when these mutants were grown in tissue culture medium alone. Of the remaining 930 mutants, 718 were white both in the absence and presence of J774 cells, 212 mutants were blue under both conditions. None of the MudJ mutants were blue in the absence of cells while white in their presence.

Analysis of the MudJ mutants that showed macrophage-induced β-galactosidase expression

Although screening of the MudJ libraries did not result in the identification of mutants with MudJ insertions in macrophage repressed genes, 10 MudJ mutants with insertions in genes that are specifically induced upon invasion of macrophages were found. To exclude the possibility that the macrophage-induced phenotype of these mutants was the result of a MudJ insertion in a gene required for the uptake or synthesis of a nutrient lacking inside macrophages all ten MudJ mutants were tested for growth on M9 minimal agar containing X-gal. All mutants grew and none turned blue on these plates. Niether did anaerobic growth, growth at 42°C, or low pH, result in the production of β-galactosidase.

Southernblot analysis was used to 1) exclude that the MudJ insertions were all in the exact same location of the genome, and to 2) confirm that these mutants contained only a single copy of the MudJ transposon. The DNA from all 10 MudJ mutants was analysed with three different restriction endonucleases (*Alu* I, *Hae* III, and *Taq* I). Upon digestion the DNA was separated on a 1.5% agarose gel, blotted to Hybond-N and probed with the left-hand end of the MudJ transposon. All mutants contained only a single copy of the MudJ transposon and each mutant showed a unique hybridisation pattern (data not shown). This indicates that these 10 macrophage-induced mutants are in different genes and therefore probably define 10 different macrophage-induced loci on the salmonella genome. Data on the genomic map position of the MudJ insertions confirms this assumption.

To further characterize these mutants, inverse PCR was used to clone the genomic DNA flanking the MudJ transposon. Southern blot analysis was used to determine the species specificity of the cloned flanking DNA. The cloned DNA was labelled and tested against *Eco* RI digested DNA from *S. typhimurium* (5 independent isolates tested), *Salmonella enteritidis*, *Salmonella dublin*, *Salmonella typhi*, *Salmonella arizona*, *Salmonella heidelberg*, *Salmonella infantis*, *Shigella flexneri*, *Shigella dysenteriae*, *Shigella boydii*, *Shigella sonnei*, *Yersinia enterocolitica*, *Yersinia pseudotuberculosis*, enterohemolytic *Escherichia coli*, enteropathogenic *Escherichia coli*, enterotoxigenic *Escherichia coli*, enteroinvasive *Escherichia coli*, *Proteus mirabilis*, *Vibrio cholerae*, *Erwinia carotovora*, *Klebsiella pneumoniae*, and *Pasteurella haemolytica*. Three basic patterns were observed (Table 1): 1) the gene is exclusively present in *Salmonella typhimurium*, 2) a homologous gene was present in all Salmonella serotypes, but not in any of the other bacteria, and 3) homologue hybridisation signals were detected in (almost) all species.

The nucleotide sequence of the cloned DNA was determined and the obtained sequence was compared to the sequences in the databases using the BLAST programs as provided by NCBI (Altschul *et al.*, 1990). The BLAST-search data are summarized in Table 1.

Table 1.   Sumary of data on macrophage-induced genes.

Mutant	Species specificity	Sequence homology	Virulent in
1	Non-specific	None	mice only
2	Salmonella specific	*E. coli rbsR**	mice only
3	Salmonella specific	None	mice only
4	Salmonella specific	*E. coli poxB*	mice only
5	Salmonella specific	*S. typhimurium stn*	mice only
6	*S. typhimurium* specific	None	mice only
7	Salmonella specific	None	macrophages & mice
8	Salmonella specific	*araD**	macrophages only
9	Non-specific	None	macrophages only
10	Salmonella specific	None	macrophages only

*See text for explanation.

To estabish if these macrophage-induced genes represent virulence factors, we tested the virulence of these mutants both *in vitro* (proteose-peptone elicited peritoneal macrophages) and *in vivo* (oral inoculation in mice). With the exeption of mutant #7 all mutants revealed significant reduction of virulence (Table 1).

Discussion

Several studies demonstrated that adherence to and invasion of host cells results in the *de novo* synthesis of *S. typhimurium* proteins (Finlay *et al.*, 1989; Buchmeier and Heffron, 1990; Aranda *et al.*, 1992; Fierer *et al.*, 1993). It was demonstrated that the contact between *Salmonella* and the host-cell results in the increased synthesis of at least 30 bacterial proteins (Abshire and Neidhardt, 1993; Buchmeier and Heffron, 1990). This *de novo* bacterial protein synthesis seems essential for successful invasion of host cells (Finlay *et al.*, 1989; MacBeth and Lee, 1993; Kusters *et al.*, 1993; Ernst *et al.*, 1990; Schiemann and Shope, 1991). Almost no data exist on the specific host-cell related triggers that cause the induction of *S. typhimurium* virulence-genes. The best studied stimulus known to induce the production of invasion related proteins in the absence of cells is growth under low-oxygen conditions but many other stimuli are probably involved as well (Lee and Falkow, 1990; Ernst *et al.*, 1990; Schieman and Shope, 1991, Jones and Falkow, 1994). Carbon starvation and growth state are some of the factors known to indirectly induce virulence genes by the action of the alternative sigma-factor *katF* (Coynault *et al.*, 1992; Kowarz *et al.*, 1994).

In spite of their importance, only a few of the *Salmonella typhimurium* proteins that are induced upon contact with eukaryotic cells have been identified. They include common stress response proteins like RecA, RecBC, GroEL and DnaK, as well as the virulence related proteins SpvR SpvABCD, PagC and InvE (Buchmeier and Heffron, 1990; Abshire and Neidhardt, 1993; Buchmeier *et al.*, 1993; Miller *et al.*, 1992). Identification and characterization of additional host-induced genes might provide clues on how this bacterium senses its host. Mahan *et al.* have designed an elegant method (IVET) for the identification of host-induced genes *in vivo* (Mahan *et al.*, 1993, 1994). Their method is based on the complementation of a *purA⁻ Salmonella* with a promoterless *purA-lac* construct fused to chromosomal fragments of *Salmonella typhimurium*. However, this method will only identify genes that are induced during all stages of the infection. Repressed genes and genes that are induced only during a brief stage of the infection process can not be identified with this method.

In an attempt to identify the genes missed by the IVET we designed the MIPA (Macrophage-Induced Promoter Assay) as a simple *in vitro* assay for the detection of genes that are induced or repressed during (one particular stage of) the infection. In the MIPA individual mutants, with transposon generated transcriptional *lacZ* fusions, are used to infect macrophages. Following the infection, cells and bacteria are overlaid with X-gal containing agar and screened for blue staining. Comparison of the blue staining of bacteria that are in contact with macrophages with the staining of mutants grown in the absence of cells will identify mutants in which *lacZ* is fused with host-cell regulated genes.

Macrophage induction was demonstrated with 10 mutants from a total of 940 randomly selected MudJ mutants. Since all mutants map at distinct locations in the genome, show distinct hybridization patterns with all three restriction enzymes used, and none of the sequences indicates that two or more insertions are in the same gene or operon, they must represent MudJ instertions in 10 different macrophage-induced loci. None of the MudJ insertions resulted in an auxotrophic phenotype, nor did anaerobic growth or growth at 42°C, low pH, or on minimal agar result in the production of β-galactosidase. This indicates that the observed induction is macrophage specific.

Testing of the MudJ mutants did not result in the identification of mutants that showed macrophage-induced repression of *lacZ*. Maybe such mutants were not present in our library, alternatively, the stability of the β-galactosidase may require infections at a lower MOI and more rigorous washes to remove background staining. Since the MIPA does not require expensive equipment, or the availability of an animal model-system, and since a wide variety of transposons exist for the creation of transcriptional-fusion mutants in pathogenic bacteria, the MIPA is a simple, but powerfull method for the identification of host-induced genes in various bacterial pathogens.

Interestingly all but one mutant show some sort of attenuation. This is indicative of host-induced genes being virulence factors. Sequence analysis of the macrophage-induced genes reveals that the majority of the MudJ insertions is in new virulence genes for which no known homologues exist in any of the databases. Only the the MudJ insertion of mutant #5 was found to be in a known virulence factor; the *S. typhimurium* enterotoxin *stn* (Chopra *et al.*, 1994). Chopra and coworkers were puzzeled by their observation that the *stn* gene is not expressed under normal laboratory conditions. Our finding that this gene is macrophage-induced accounts for their finding.

Although not a known virulence factor, a second gene that was unambiguously identified by its homology to sequences in the databases was the MudJ inactivated gene from mutant #4. The sequence derived from this gene was almost identical to the pyruvate oxidase gene (*poxB*) of *E. coli*. Identity was confirmed by the genomic map position of the MudJ insertion which corresponds with the published location of *poxB*. We can only guess why this gene is induced by macrophages, maybe it serves some function in the elimination of oxidative membrane damage caused by the macrophage.

The sequence of mutant #8 was found to be homologous to the *araD* gene. The macrophage-induced gene disrupted by the MudJ insertion is a homologue of the *araD* gene and not *araD* itself. The MudJ disrupted gene is located at 80' on the genomic map, while the *araD* gene is located at 2' on the *S. typhimurium* genome. A similar gene duplication of the *araD* gene is known to exist in the genome of *E. coli*. In both bacteria the function of the protein encoded by this *araD* homologue is unknown.

The sequence of mutant #2 shows strong homology to the repressor of the ribose operon (*rbsR*) of *E. coli*. In addition some weaker homologies to other repressor genes were found. As with mutant #5 this gene does probably not correspond to the *rbsR* gene but more likely it is a homologous *rbsR*-like gene.

We are currently characterizing the MIPA positive mutants in a quantitative assay to establish the expression levels at different time points upon infection of eukaryotic cells and mice. This will eventually provide insight into the host-related factors that cause the specific host related induction of bacterial virulence genes.

Acknowledgements

We thank Sara Knijff for technical assistance. J.G.K. was supported by a fellowship of the Royal Netherlands Academy of Arts and Sciences, The Netherlands. This work was supported by NIH RO1 grant AI122933 to F.H.

References

Abshire, K. and F.C. Neidhardt, 1993 - Analysis of proteins synthesized by Salmonella typhimurium during growth within a host macrophage. *J. Bacteriol.* **175**, 3734–3743.

Altschul, Stephen F., Warren Gish, Webb Miller, Eugene W. Myers and David J. Lipman, 1990 - Basic local alignment search tool. *J. Mol. Biol.* **215**, 403–10.

Aranda, C.M., J.A. Swanson, W.E. Loomis and S.I. Miller, 1992 - Salmonella typhimurium activates virulence gene transcription within acidified macrophage phagosomes. *Proc. Natl. Acad. Sci. USA* **89**, 10079–10083.

Buchmeier, N.A. and F. Heffron, 1990 - Induction of Salmonella stress proteins upon infection of macrophages. *Science* **248**, 730–732.

Buchmeier, N.A., C.J. Lipps, Y. Magdalene, H. So and F. Heffron, 1993 - Recombination-deficient mutants of Salmonella typhimurium are avirulent and sensitive to the oxidative burst of macrophages. *Mol. Microbiol.* **7**, 933–936.

Chopra, A.K., J.W. Peterson, P. Chary and R. Prasad, 1994 - Molecular characterization of an enterotoxin from Salmonella typhimurium. *Microb. Pathog.* **16**, 85–98.

Coynault, C., V. Robbesaule, M.Y. Popoff, F. Norel, 1992 - Growth Phase and SpvR Regulation of Transcription of Salmonella-Typhimurium spvABC Virulence Genes. *Microb. Pathog.* **13**, 133–143.

Ernst, R.K., D.M. Dombroski and J.M. Merrick, 1990 - Anaerobiosis, type 1 fimbriae, and growth phase are factors that affect invasion of HEP-2 cells by Salmonella typhimurium. *Infect. Immun.* **58**, 2014–2016.

Fields, P.I., R.V. Swanson, C.G. Haidaris and F. Heffron, 1986 - Mutants of Salmonella typhimurium that cannot survive within the macrophage are avirulent. *Proc. Natl. Acad. Sci. USA* **83**, 5189–5193.

Fields, P.I., E.A. Groisman and F. Heffron, 1989 - A Salmonella locus that controls resistance to microbicidal proteins from phagocytic cells. *Science* **243**, 1059–1062.

Finlay, B.B., F. Heffron and S. Falkow, 1989 - Epithelial cell surfaces induce Salmonella proteins required for bacterial adherence and invasion. *Science* **243**, 940–943.

Finlay, B.B. and S. Falkow, 1988 - Virulence factors associated with Salmonella species. *Microbiol. Sci.* **5**, 324–328.

Gahring, L.C., F. Heffron, B.B. Finlay and S. Falkow, 1990 - Invasion and Replication of Salmonella-Typhimurium in Animal Cells. *Infect. Immun.* **58**, 443–448.

Groisman, E.A., E. Chiao, C.J. Lipps and F. Heffron, 1989 - Salmonella typhimurium phoP virulence gene is a transcriptional regulator. *Proc. Natl. Acad. Sci. USA* **86**, 7077–7081.

Groisman, E.A., P.I. Fields and F. Heffron, 1990 - Molecular biology of Salmonella pathogenesis. In: *The Bacteria, a treatise on structure and function, Volume XI, Molecular basis of Bacterial Pathogenesis*, I.C. Gunsalus, J.R. Sokatch and L.N. Ornston (eds), New York, NY: Academic Press, pp. 251–272.

Jones, B.D. and S. Falkow, 1994 - Identification and Characterization of a Salmonella typhimurium Oxygen-Regulated Gene Required for Bacterial Internalization. *Infect. Immun.* **62**, 3745–3752.

Kowarz, L., C. Coynault, V. Robbe-Saule and F. Norel, 1994 - The Salmonella typhimurium katF (rpoS) gene: Cloning, nucleotide sequence, and Regulation of spvR and spvABC virulence genes. *J. Bacteriol.* **176**, 6852–6860.

Kusters, J.G., G.A.W.M. Mulders-Kremers, C.E.M. Van Doornik and B.A.M. Van der Zeijst, 1993 - Effects of multiplicity of infection, bacterial protein synthesis, and growth phase on adhesion to and invasion of human cell lines by Salmonella typhimurium. *Infect. Immun.* **61**, 5013–5020.

Lee, C.A. and S. Falkow, 1990 - The ability of Salmonella to enter mammalian cells is affected by bacterial growth state. *Proc. Natl. Acad. Sci. USA* **87**, 4304–4308.

MacBeth, K.J. and C.A. Lee, 1993 - Prolonged inhibition of bacterial protein synthesis abolishes Salmonella invasion. *Infect. Immun.* **61**, 1544–1546.

Mahan, M.J., J.M. Slauch and J.J Mekalanos, 1993 - Selection of bacterial virulence genes that are specifically induced in host tissues. *Science* **259**, 686–688.

Mahan, M.J., J.M. Slauch, P.C. Hanna, A. Camilli, J.W. Tobias, M.K. Waldor and J.J. Mekalanos, 1994 - Selection for bacterial genes that are specifically induced in host tissues: the hunt for virulence factors. *Infect. Ag. Dis.* **2**, 263–268.

Mekalanos, J.J., 1992 - Environmental signals controlling expression of virulencedeterminants in bacteria. *J. Bacteriol.* **174**, 1–7.

Miller, V., K.B. Beer, W.P. Loomis, J. Olson and S.I. Miller, 1992 - An unusual pagC::TnphoA Mutation leads to an invasion- and virulence-defective phenotype in salmonella. *Infect. Immun.* **60**, 3763–3770.

Miller, J.F., J.J. Mekalanos and S. Falkow, 1989 - Coordinate regulation and sensory transduction in the control of bacterial virulence. *Science* **243**, 916–922.

Rhen, M., P. Riikonen and S. Taira, 1993 - Transcriptional regulation of Salmonella enterica virulence plasmid genes in cultured macrophages. *Mol. Microbiol.* **10**, 45–56.

Schiemann, D.A. and S.R. Shope, 1991 - Anaerobic growth of Salmonella typhimurium results in increased uptake by Henle 407 epithelial and mouse peritoneal cells in vitro and repression of a major outer membrane protein. *Infect. Immun.* **59**, 437–440.

Population genetics and clonal spread

R. Milkman

Recombination and DNA Sequence Variation in *E. coli*

Abstract

The current form of the periodic (clonal) selection model of the microevolution of *E. coli* includes recombination, which compromises the original genome-wide clonal structure, resulting in *meroclones*. These contain a *clonal frame* (relic of the ancestral chromosome) and *clonal segments* (recombinational replacements with different ancestors). The observed mosaic pattern of DNA sequence variation is evidently due to mutational divergence and recombination. Approaches to the estimation of meroclonal age, rate of clone formation, and related parameter values are discussed, as well as information on the patterns of recombinational replacement.

Introduction

Bacterial evolution, long obscured by the shortage of useful phenotypic detail, has now been illuminated by the analysis of data provided by Multi-Locus Enzyme Electrophoresis (MLEE) (Milkman, 1973; Selander and Levin, 1980; Whittam, 1995), Restriction Analysis (Milkman and Bridges, 1990) and DNA Sequencing (Milkman and Crawford, 1983; Crawford, 1989; Dykhuizen and Green, 1991; Nelson *et al.*, 1991 and 1992). The data obtained from 1980 on left no doubt as to the basic accuracy of the periodic selection model (Atwood, Schneider and Ryan, 1951), according to which clones arise with the appearance of a new favorable mutation, a 'motivating allele' which carries the entire 'hitchhiking' genome to high frequency. Ordinarily, a clone does not reach a frequency of 1, probably due in part to environmental heterogeneity (Reeves, 1992), but also because the motivating allele can be transferred to other clones by recombination. It does not remain the exclusive property of the clone it has sponsored. Also, the entire genome does not retain its descent from the original clonal ancestor, because recombination, while rare, occurs frequently enough to dot the chromosome with extraclonal replacements. Thus, the now-compromised clone is better described as a *meroclone* (Milkman and McKane, 1995). Most of these recombinational replacements are presumed to be neutral. When they are seen to appear in numerous strains, they have presumably hitchhiked with the spread of a new clone, which is nested in the meroclone and which has resulted from the selection of a new favorable mutation.

Recently, the study of the molecular evolution of bacteria has benefited from a new level of synthesis: many of us have acquired a collection of findings and concepts from our colleagues, but these have now cohered into a single picture. This has been due both to the expansion of information with increasingly over-lapping implications, and to the deliberate atttempts at a unified view by Smith (1995), Arber (1993) and others.

The present chapter was written after the publication of a symposium entitled *Population genetics of bacteria*, which includes a chapter with a similar focus (Milkman and McKane, 1995). In it will be found additional fundamental details and illustrations, together with related subjects and references. Recombination and physical map locations can be found in Bachmann (1990) and Rudd (1992), respectively.

The *E. coli* strains under study and their patterns of DNA sequence variation

In addition to the ECOR (*E. coli* Reference) collection (Ochman and Selander 1984), various of pathogenic strains have been studied and are discussed in detail elsewhere in this volume. Clearly, *E. coli* is a gigantic and diverse species, and it is not likely that all its major variants have come to our attention. Nevertheless, the strains have been drawn from a geographically diverse group of sources, and from a moderate variety of mammalian hosts. When detailed similarities appear more than once in the ECOR strains (and others will speak for the pathogens), common ancestry is indicated. This ancestry may pertain to the clonal frame or to a set of coextensive clonal segments. In both cases, a vast number of individuals in nature is implicated.

The comparative sequencing of a 10.4 kb stretch of DNA in the *trp* region from about 40 ECOR strains suggests the utility of defining *sequence types* as differing by at least 1% of their nucleotides. Two observations stand out. First, most of the sequences classify into three major groups, corresponding to the A, B_1 and B_2 MLEE groups (Herzer *et al.*, 1990) and here referred to as the **K**, **70** and **51** meroclones. Second, a mosaic pattern of similarities and differences between sequences is striking. Each meroclone is characterized by a *clonal frame*, the relic of the clonal ancestor's genome, and *clonal segments* transferred from other clones. In the **K** and **51** meroclones, the most extensive clonal frames are respectively the K12 and the ECOR 51 sequence type, and they extend over the entire 10.4 kb region (Figure 1). The **70** meroclone's clonal frame, however, is divided between the K12 and ECOR 70 sequence types. This observation brings us to an explicit discussion of the nesting of clones.

What detailed evidence do we have of clones-within-clones (or meroclones-within-meroclones)? First of all, we should ask how different the respective clonal frame sequences in the **K12** meroclone are from one another. Recalling that sequence types are defined to differ from one another by at least 1%, we understand that any clonal frames nested within the **K12** meroclone must differ by less than 1%. In fact, the pairwise differences average out to much less: only

ECOR Strain	Symbol of Sequence Type	Position, kb (Reference: start of *trp* operon)
K meroclone		
		...4.........!.........5.........!.........6.........!.........7.........!.........8.........!.......
		! ! ! ! ! !
K	K	KKKKKKKKKKKKKKKKKKKKKKKKKKKKKKKKKKKKKKKKKKKKKKKKKKKKKKKKKKKKKKKKKKKKKKKKKKKKKKKKKKKKKKKKKKKKKKKKKKKKKK
1, 8, 12		KKKKKKKKKKKKKKKKKKKKKKKKKKKKKKKKKKKKKKKKKKKKKKKKKKKKKKKKKKKKKKKKKKKKKKKKKKKKKKKKKKKKKKKKKKKKKKKKKKKKKK
70 meroclone		
70, 71	7	KK7777777KKKKKKK7777KKKKKKKK77777KKKKKKKKKKKKKKKKKK7777777777KKKKKKKKKKKKKKKKK777777777KKKKKKKKK77777
72		KK7777777KKKKKKK7777KKKKKKKK77777KKKKKKKKKKKKKKKKKK7777777777KKKKKKKKKKKKKKKKK777777777KKKKKKKKK77777
27		KK7777777KKKKKKK7777KKKKKKKK77777KKKKKKKKKKKKKKKKKK7777777777KKKKKKKKKKKKKKKKK777777777KKKKKKKKK77777
69		KK7777777KKKKKKK7777KKKKKKKK77777KKKKKKKKKKKKKKKKKK7777777777KKKKKKKKKKKKKKKKKKKKKKKKKKKKKKKKKKKKKKKKK
45		KK777777**KKKKKKKKKKKKKKKKKKKKKKKKKKKKKKKKKKKK**KKKKKKK7777777777KKKKKKKKKKKKKKKKK777777777KKKKKKKKK77777
28		KK777777**KKKKKKKKKKKKKKKKKKKKKKKKKKKKKKKKKKKK**KKKKKKKKKKKKKKKKKKKKKKKKKKKKKKKKKKKKKKKKKKKKKKKKKK***KKKK
58	Z	KK777777**KKKKKKKKKKKKKKKKKKKKKKKKKKKKKKKKKKKK**KKKKKKKKKKKKKKKKKKZKKKKKKKKKKKKKKKKKKKKKKKKKK*********KKKK

Note: * = DNA not assignable to a specific sequence type.

Fig. 1. Summary of the DNA sequences of K-12 and 11 ECOR strains. Each symbol stands for 50 bp.

Transductants and Backtransductants

Cross	#	NA	AD	GO	GL	BU	ON	LK	AS	SQ	*	CB	ED	BS	SB	TA	AC	AH	PS
47 → K12*trpA33*	4	–	–	–	–	–	–	/d	D	D	**D**	D	D	D	D	D	D	D	–
	9	–	D	D	D	D	D	D	D	D	**D**	–	–	–	–	–	–	–	–
	15	–	–	D	D	D	D	D	D	D	**D**	D	D	–	–	–	–	–	–
	17	–	–	D	D	D	D	D	D	D	**D**	–	–	–	–	–	–	–	–
	7	–	–	–	–	–	–	–	–	–	**D**	D	D	DΔ	–	–	–	–	–
	13	–	–	–	–	–	–	–	/d	D	**D**	D	D	–	–	–	–	–	–
	3	–	–	–	–	–	–	–	–	D	**D**	d/	–	–	–	–	–	–	–
	11	–	–	–	–	–	–	–	–	D	**D**	d/	–	–	–	–	–	–	–
	16	–	–	–	–	–	–	–	/d	D	**D**	D	–	–	–	–	–	–	–
	18	–	–	–	–	–	–	–	–	D	**D**	–	–	–	–	–	–	–	–
(2)	6	–	D	D	D	d/	–	–	D	D	**D**	D	–	–	–	–	–	–	–
	12	–	–	D	D	D	D	D	D	/d	**D**	–	–	–	–	–	–	–	–
	1	–	–	–	–	–	–	D	D	D	**D**	D	D	–	–	–	d/	–	–
	14	–	–	d/	–	–	–	D	D	D	**D**	D	–	–	–	–	d/	–	–
	5	–	–	–	–	/d	d/	–	–	D	**D**	D	–	–	–	–	–	–	–
(3)	8	–	–	–	–	–	–	–	–	D	**D**	–	d/	D	D	D	–	–	–
	2	–	/d	–	–	D	–	/d	D	D	**D**	D	–	–	–	–	–	–	–
(4)	10	–	–	–	–	–	–	–	–	/d	**D**	/d/	d/	–	–	D	–	–	–
47 → ER2476 (=47 → D)	10	–	–	D	D	D	D	D	D	D	**D**	D	D	D	D	D	D	D	D
	11	–	–	D	D	D	D	D	D	D	**D**	D	D	D	D	D	D	D	D
	12	–	–	D	D	D	D	D	D	D	**D**	D	D	D	D	D	D	D	D
	3	–	–	D	D	D	D	D	D	D	**D**	D	D	D	D	D	D	D	–
	14	–	–	D	D	D	D	D	D	D	**D**	D	D	D	D	D	D	D	D
	1	–	–	–	D	D	D	D	D	D	**D**	D	D	D	D	D	D	D	D
	13	–	–	–	–	–	–	–	D	D	**D**	D	D	D	D	D	D	D	D
	9	–	–	D	D	D	D	D	D	D	**D**	D	D	D	D	D	–	–	–
	5	–	–	–	–	–	–	–	D	D	**D**	D	D	D	D	D	D	–	D
	4	–	–	–	–	–	–	–	–	D	**D**	D	D	D	D	D	D	–	–
	7	–	–	–	–	–	–	D	D	D	**D**	D	D	D	–	–	–	–	–
	2	–	–	–	–	–	–	–	–	–	**D**	D	–	–	–	–	–	–	–
	8	–	–	–	–	–	–	–	–	–	**D**	–	–	–	–	–	–	–	–
(2)	15	–	–	–	–	–	–	–	–	–	**D**	–	–	–	–	–	D	–	–
	6	–	–	d/	–	–	–	–	–	–	**D**	–	–	–	–	–	–	–	–
BACKCROSSES 47D10 → D	8	–	–	D	D	D	D	D	D	D	**D**	D	D	D	D	D	D		
	15	–	–	D	D	D	D	D	D	D	**D**	D	D	D	D	D	D		
	1	–	–	D	D	D	D	D	D	D	**D**	D	D	D	D	D	–		
	5	–	–	D	D	D	D	D	D	D	**D**	D	D	D	D	D	–		
	7	–	–	D	D	D	D	D	D	D	**D**	D	D	D	D	D	–		
	10	–	–	D	D	D	D	D	D	D	**D**	D	D	D	D	D	–		
	3	–	–	D	D	D	D	D	D	D	**D**	D	D	D	D	–	–		
	13	–	–	D	D	D	D	D	D	D	**D**	D	D	D	D	–	–		
	14	–	–	D	D	D	D	D	D	D	**D**	D	D	D	D	D	–		
	4	–	–	D	D	D	D	D	D	D	**D**	D	D	D	D	D	d/		
	2	–	–	D	D	D	D	D	D	D	**D**	D	D	–	–	–	–		
	11	–	–	D	D	D	D	D	D	D	**D**	D	D	D	–	–	–		
	12	–	–	D	D	D	D	D	D	D	**D**	D	D	D	–	–	–		
	6	–	–	D	D	D	D	D	D	D	**D**	D	d/	–	–	–			
	9	–	–	D	D	D	D	D	D	D	**D**	–	–	–	–	–			

47K4 → K12	**13**	Identical to 47K4 (see 47 → K Table)
	#2	K12 at AC, otherwise identical
	#3	K12 at both LK sites and at BS, SB, TA and AC
47K9 → 12	**15**	Identical to 47K9 (see 47 → K Table)

Notes: bold **numbers** represent the number of individuals in an identical set; bold **D** is the selected marker; d. indicates donor DNA at left-hand sites only; .d at right only. Modified K12 W3110 *trpA33* recipients: ER2437 has greatly impaired restriction activity; ER2476 has all known restriction genes deleted.

Fig. 2. Chart of the results of transductions. D = donor DNA; – = recipient DNA. Headings are 1.5-kb PCR fragments subjected to restriction analysis. GO and BS are each about 10 kb from the selected marker (*). Actual distances are given in Milkman & McKane (1995) and McKane & Milkman (1995).

about 6 nucleotide substitutions over 10 kb, and the two most extreme differences are about twice that. This means that although the **K12** and **ECOR 70** clonal frames diverged (as we shall see) perhaps about 4 million years ago, the common ancestor of the entire set of 11 ECOR strains sequenced from the K12 meroclone existed about 130,000 years ago. Thus a new clone, nested in an earlier one, has taken its place: the recloning has eliminated a large amount of variation from the meroclone.

The **ECOR 70** meroclone provides an even more dramatic example. It appears that a clonal frame originally consisting of ECOR 70 sequence type DNA, has evidently received numerous recombinational replacements from the **K12** meroclone (and given few in return). In Figure 1 are illustrated summaries of about 5-kb stretches from 5 ECOR strains, 70, 71, 72, 27 and 69, which share a common similarity from positions 4200 to 6400. The few nucleotide differences in replacement (**K12**) DNA leads to the very rough estimate that their recombinant ancestor lived 12,000 years ago. A more recent single recombinational replacement in strains 28, 45 and 58 appears to have taken place in their most recent common ancestor about 3000 years ago. And finally, strains 70 and 71 appear identical over the entire 10.4 kb region. With neither recombinational nor mutational evidence, one can only wait for much more sequence data in this case. The inferred events are summarized in Figure 2.

Why is no 'all-70-sequence-type' strain known? There are at least two plausible answers. First, for any of a number of reasons, the **K12** meroclone may be in the process of swamping the **ECOR 70** meroclone by recombination. And second, for all we know, there may be a vast number of pure 70-type strains that live in hosts or circumstances that we have never sampled. Indeed, *they* could conceivably be the donors of DNA lodged in a K12 clonal frame in the **ECOR 70** meroclone. One thing is clear, however: both recombination and recloning occur frequently enough so that a new large meroclone may arise with a clonal frame that is a dramatic mosaic of clearly recognizable sequence types. [While it remains a formal possibility that the sequenced region is atypical and that the ECOR 70 sequence type is prevalent elsewhere in the chromosome, restriction analyses do not support this view to date (Milkman and McKane Bridges 1990 and unpublished data).]

Methods of dating ancestors

Time is of obvious importance in the study of evolution. The only dating method available for *E. coli* and for specific strains of bacteria in general is the measurement of divergence, the estimation of divergence rate and the estimation of divergence time from their quotient. DNA sequence divergence is easy to determine, counting only nucleotide differences that are thought to be neutral (and it appears that in most cases, virtually all of them are.) The divergence rate is twice the retained nucleotide substitution rate (since two evolutionary lines are diverging); this is essentially the rate of neutral nucleotide substitution, about $1/3 \times 10^{-10}$ (based on Drake, 1991). [For neutral alternatives, the nucleotide substitution rate in a line of descent or in a population of constant size is numerically equal to the rate of mutational nucleotide substitution. Thus, although most new neutral substitutions are lost at random, the chance of retention is the reciprocal of the size of the population in which the mutations occur, and so they cancel out (Crow, 1986). This is why we can speak correctly of the retained substitution rate in the present context.] Various simple non-linear formulas exist to compensate for reverse- and multiple substitutions (Li and Graur, 1991). Homologous sequences, extensive or short, can thus be traced back to their *most recent common ancestor*, provided of course that they are not spatially heterogeneous in their degree of divergence. If they are heterogeneous, they must be divided into regions with homogeneous degrees of difference before dating is attempted.

A derivative potential method of dating ancestry is the use of recombination rate, rather than the retained (neutral) mutation rate. Presumably all recombinant replacements are retained (i.e., they are not selectively removed), and they contain more detail than individual nucleotide substitutions. Their rate of occurrence has been estimated in *E. coli* in comparison with the mutation rate (Milkman and McKane Bridges, 1990; Guttman and Dykhuizen, 1994), but the generality of the ratio of rates is risky to assume until we know more about variation in recombinational accessibility between strains (in each direction!), as well as the effects of restriction endonucleases, as will be discussed. No less important is our ability to detect or confidently infer all replacements that have occurred within a specific recent time.

The frequency of origin of major clones

In the 72 ECOR strains, there are the three major meroclones and at least two other sets of very similar strains (ECOR 38, 39, 40, and 41; ECOR 49 and 50). Further, there are several cases of very similar strains *within* the major groups, indicating, once again, the nesting of clones. This raises the question of the time it takes for a clone to reach substantial size and spatial distribution. *E. coli* seems to be quite vagile, and the minimum time taken to reach great numbers is calculated by a simple formula:

$$N = (1+s)^t,$$

where t is time and s is the *selection coefficient* ($=fitness - 1$). N is the number of individuals to be reached from a single ancestor (or a multiplier of a group of ancestors). A selection coefficient of 0.00001 per generation can lead to a clone size of 10^{19} in about 4 million generations or, at 200 generations per year, about 22,000 years. Similarly, a selection coefficient of 0.00006 could carry a favorable allele and its hitchhiking genome to a frequency of 10^{18} in about 3500 years. These are short times in comparison with the estimated age of the species

(100–150 million years). The clone sizes should be compared to a rough estimate of 10^{20} for the size of the species. It should be noted once again that all ultimately successful favorable alleles are at the mercy of random genetic drift until they reach a *safe number*, which turns out to be about the reciprocal of *s*. Thus an allele whose *s* is 0.00001 must reach a frequency of 100,000 before its frequency is controlled essentially totally by selection (Crow, 1986). Interestingly, though random genetic drift is a slow process on the average, the rare lucky allele makes it to its safe number far faster than it would due to selection in the (absurd) case where drift did not apply.

Recombination

Recombination has been known since 1986 to proceed at a significant rate in natural populations of *E. coli* (Dykhuizen and Green, 1991). Phylogenies of the ECOR strains differ, often strikingly, from region to region: this, of course, means that the phylogenies are not genome phylogenies but merely the phylogenies of local stretches of DNA. Comparative sequencing and restriction analysis of natural isolates (Dubose *et al.*, 1988; others previously cited) has demonstrated the possibility of observing recombinational replacements on a finer scale than could ordinarily be revealed by classical genetic markers.

The entry of a DNA fragment into a cell must be distinguished from the subsequent incorporation of a DNA fragment into a chromosome. This became clear with the observation of small, frequently multiple discrete incorporations of donor DNA in single transduction events between strains (McKane and Milkman, 1995). The possibility that restriction endonucleases might be important in bacterial recombination (DuBose *et al.*, 1988; Milkman and McKane Bridges, 1993) was supported by the results of crosses to apparently restrictionless recipients, as well as backcrosses (Milkman and McKane, 1995 and unpublished data), which resulted in much larger incorporations and far fewer multiples (Figure 3). Extensive polymorphism of restriction/modification systems in *E. coli* has been demonstrated by Murray's group (Barcus and Murray, 1995 and unpublished results). These findings raise the likelihood of large differences in the frequencies of DNA transfer between various strains of *E. coli* beyond those expected merely on the basis of variations in phage adsorption and in conjugational variables. It is thus time to investigate in natural populations of *E. coli* questions such as these: How important, respectively, are conjugation and transduction in recombination? Can natural transformation be excluded as a significant process? Which phages are important mediators of transduction? Can any general patterns of recombinational accessibility (including directional differences) be discerned between strains or groups of strains? What mechanisms are responsible for such patterns?

Our ultimate interest here is to determine the relationship between recombinational events and the mosaic patterns observed in comparative sequencing, as well as the striking local regions of high variability, such as *gnd*, which was dis-

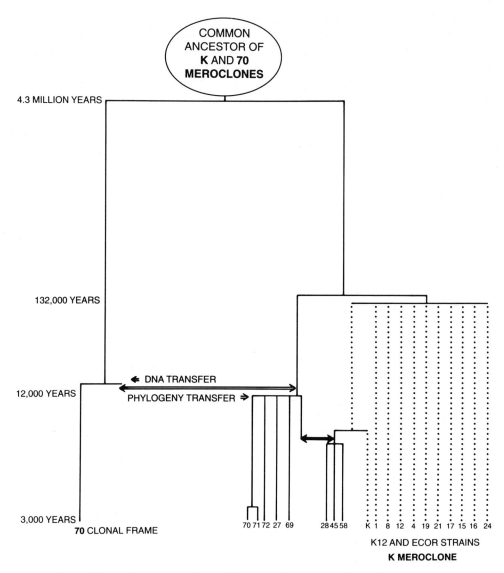

Fig. 3.   Phylogeny of *recombinant replacements* in Fig. 1. See text.

cerned by MLEE (Milkman, 1973, Dykhuizen and Green, 1991). The explanation of this variability lies in strong diversifying selection in the *rfb* gene complex
(Selander, Caugant and Whittam, 1987), which determines the makeup of the O
antigen, a complex polysaccharide (Reeves, 1993; this symposium). The distribution of variants does not follow the MLEE phylogeny in *E. coli* (Stevenson *et
al.*, 1994; Nelson and Selander, 1994; Selander, this symposium).

In such cases, recombinant replacements containing a variant allele (*sensu
lato*), presumably often of ancient origin, add to the fitness of a spreading

genome. Thus, while the sweep of a clonal genome tends to exclude variants, some new neutral replacements appear everywhere and *many* advantageous polymorphs populate a few regions. In these 'bastions of polymorphism,' linked DNA hitchhikes, not with a new favorable mutation that initially carries the entire genome along, but with an established ancient variant. Why are these variants ancient? Because new ones arise very rarely -- *extremely* rarely. Why is that? Presumably because new variants of the O antigen, whose construction requires the activities of an assortment of transferases and mutases, are best assembled from existing components, brought in mainly by horizontal transfer, a rare event indeed (Reeves, 1993; Stevenson *et al.*, 1994). The *hsd* restriction-modification complex appears to behave in a similar way (Barcus and Murray, 1995 and unpublished observations). This process explains why the phylogeny of *gnd* and a sizable region around *rfb* have a phylogeny that requires more than ordinary mutation and ordinary recombination to explain it. The recombinant replacement here is not ordinary for the same reason that a 'motivating allele' is not an ordinary mutation. In each case, the allele is neither neutral nor common. Individual neutral events do not have massive effects on clonal structure. Common favorable events (with a rate of occurrence of 10^{-10} or 10^{-15}) do not either, because they occur frequently in the species.

To see why this is so, consider the region around *tonB*, which by chance is our main region of comparative sequencing. The *tonB* gene product is a protein anchored in the cytoplasmic membrane and connected to (among others) the *fhuA* gene product (Killmann and Braun, 1994), which serves as a receptor for phage T1, phage T5, phage ϕ80 and colicin M. Structural variation in TonB is thought to have an allosteric effect on FhuA, influencing its receptor properties. One would expect to find variation in TonB structure that might make FhuA difficult to recognize, and indeed TonB has an unusually large number of structurally significant amino acid replacements. Yet its region is not a bastion of polymorphism: associated variation is moderate, and the regional phylogeny has a remarkable fit to the genome-wide MLEE phenogram. This implies that variants, not necessarily identical but equivalent in their adaptive significance, are easier to come by. Certainly the rate of nucleotide substitution necessary to cause one of these amino acid replacements, or indeed the rate of insertion and deletion of the type observed is so great that new variants must arise far too frequently to make detectably large clones. Thus the variation has no impact on local phylogeny, each group of strains develops its own variants, as can be seen in Table 1. The distinction between this region and *rfb* seems likeliest to be the difference between a surface-related protein and a complex polysaccharide. Supporting this view, and perhaps of particular interest to this audience, is the recent finding that a newly characterized protein determinant of a virulence phenotype in *E. coli* turns out to be the *yciD* product [John Mahoney, Albany Medical College, personal communication; this protein was formerly called ORF IV: Stoltzfus, Leslie and Milkman, 1988]; *yciD* is 2.2 kb from *tonB* (Rudd *et al.*, 1991; Rudd, 1992). It is also of great interest that Mahoney's *yciD* DNA

Table 1. Amino acid replacements (vs. consensus) in *tonB*.

Meroclone	Strain	Replacement Important Yes	No
K-12	K-12	A	a
	ECOR 1, 8,	A	a
	12, 4, 19	A	a
	21	A, B	a
	17	A	a
	15, 16, 24	A	a
ECOR 70	70, 71	A	
	72, 27, 69	A	
	68, 28	A	b
	29	A	
	45, 58		b
	67	A	
ECOR 51	51, 54	C	
	56, 52	C	
	60	C	c
	61, 62	C	
	65	C, D	d
	64, 66	C	
(Assorted)	40, 35	C	
	50	E	
	46		
	47		e
	48		
	37	F, G	f
	31	H	g

Symbol	Position	Change
A	11942	$p \to 1$
B	11690	$p \to 1$
C	12020-22	Δq
D	11978	$p \to q$
E	>12057	∇_{kp}
F	12011	$p \to q$
G	12312	$p \to s$
H	12132	$e \to k$
a	12189	$a \to t$
b	12000	$v \to i$
c	11814	$v \to i$
d	12333	$1 \to i$
e	12341	$s \to 1$
f	12254	$y \to f$
g	12269	$v \to a$

Strain numbers are listed in the same order as in sequence tables and summaries currently used in our laboratory.

sequence is identical, except for two new amino acid replacements, to the sequences of ECOR 61 and ECOR 62, both of which originated in Swedish schoolgirls with urinary *E. coli* infections (Caugant *et al.*, 1988; Ochman and Selander, 1984).

Clearly, the dynamics of recombination must be quantified before we can develop a quantitative reconstruction of the molecular evolution of the *E. coli* chromosome. Recently, Guttman and Dykhuizen (1994) have made the important point that the effects of recombination and mutation can be expressed in common terms, namely, nucleotide substitutions, which can also be expressed as a rate. They also point out that, while recombination is usually thought of as a homogenizing process, replacements from outside have a diversifying effect on a group. As we have seen, new variation can be brought into a clone from elsewhere in the species, and into a species from other taxa. But while mutation is essentially always diversifying to some extent, recombination is *per se* neither diversifying nor homogenizing. While other caveats expressed earlier also apply here, the classification and quantification of recombination rates and their effects on variation is an important objective, which additional sequence data will help achieve. Finally, it is to be expected that any region whose phylogeny is at substantial variance with the MLEE/clonal frame phylogeny contains a favorable allele whose origin or acquisition is very rare indeed.

Acknowledgements

Melissa McKane criticized the manuscript and organized the transduction experiments, except for the 47D backcrosses, which were made and analyzed by Kerri Pohlmann, who also contributed numerous additional restriction analyses. Elisabeth Raleigh has generously synthesized two restrictionless strains and contributed continuously to our understanding of the phenomenon we are studying. This work has been supported in part by Grants BSR 90-20173 and MCB 94-20613 from the U. S. National Science Foundation.

References

Arber, W., 1993 - Evolution of prokaryotic genomes. *Gene* **135**, 49–56.

Atwood, K.C., L.K. Schneider and F.J. Ryan, 1951 - Selective mechanisms in bacteria. *Cold Spring Harbor Symp. Quant. Biol.* **16**, 345–355.

Bachmann, B.J., 1990 - Linkage map of Escherichia coli K-12, Edition 8. *Microbiol. Rev.* **54**, 130–197.

Barcus, V.A. and N.E. Murray, 1995 - Barriers to recombination: restriction. In: *Population genetics of bacteria, Symposium 52 of the Society for General Microbiology*, pp. 13–30.

Caugant, D.A., Levin, B.R., Lidin-Janson, G., Whittam, T.S., Svanborg Eden, C., and Selander, R.K., 1983 - Genetic diversity and relationships among strains of *Escherichia coli* in the intestine and those causing urinary tract infections, pp. 203–227. In: *Host parasite relationships in gram-negative infections* (Hanson, L.A., Kallos, P. and Westphal, O., eds.), Progress in Allergy, vol. 33. Karger, Basel.

Crow, J.F., 1986 - *Basic Concepts in Population, Quantitative and Evolutionary Genetics*, Freeman, New York.

Drake, J.W., 1991 - A constant rate of spontaneous mutation in DNA-based microbes. *Proc. Natl. Acad. Sci. USA* **88**, 7160–7164.

DuBose, R.F., D.E. Dykhuizen and D.L. Hartl, 1988 - Genetic exchange among natural isolates of bacteria: recombination within the *phoA* gene of *Escherichia coli. Proc. Natl. Acad. Sci. USA* **85**, 7036–7040.

Dykhuizen, D.E. and L. Green, 1991 - Recombination in *Escherichia coli* and the definition of biological species. *J. Bacteriol.* **173**, 7257–7268.

Guttman, D.S. and D.E. Dykhuizen, 1994 - Clonal divergence in *Escherichia coli* as a result of recombination, not mutation. *Science* **266**, 1380–1382.

Herzer, P.J., S. Inouye, M. Inouye and T.S. Whittam, 1990 - Phylogenetic distributon of branched RNA-linked multicopy single-stranded DNA among natural isolates of *Escherichia coli. J. Bacteriol.* **172**, 6175–6181.

Jayaratne, P., D. Bronner, P.R. MacLachlan, C. Dodgson, N. Kido and C. Whitfield, 1994 - Cloning and analysis of duplicated *rfbM* and *rfbK* genes involved in the formation of GDP-mannose in *Escherichia coli* O9:K30 and participation of *rfb* genes in the synthesis of the Group I K30 capsular polysaccharide. *J. Bacteriol.* **176**, 3126–3139.

Kelleher, J.E. and E.A. Raleigh, 1991 - A novel activity in *Escherichia coli* K-12 that directs restriction of DNA modified at CG dinucleotides. *J. Bacteriol.* **173**, 5220–5223.

Killmann, H. and V. Braun, 1994 - Energy-dependent receptor activities of *Escherichia coli* K-12: mutated TonB proteins alter FhuA receptor activities to phages T5, T1, ϕ80 and to colicin M. *FEMS Microbiol. Lett.* **19**, 71–76.

Li, W.-H. and D. Graur, 1991 - *Fundamentals of Molecular Evolution*, Sinauer Associates, Sunderland, MA, USA.

McKane, M. and R. Milkman, 1995 - Transduction, restriction and modification patterns in *Escherichia coli. Genetics* **139**, 35–43.

Milkman, R., 1973 - Electrophoretic variation in *Escherichia coli* from natural sources. *Science* **182**, 1024–1026.

Milkman, R., 1996 - Recombinational Exchange Among Clonal Populations. In: *Escherichia coli and Salmonella Cellular and Molecular Biology, Second Edition*. (Neidhardt, F.C. ed.), American Society for Microbiology, Washington, D. C. 2663–2684.

Milkman, R. and M. McKane, 1995 - DNA sequence variation and recombination in *E. coli*. In: *Population genetics of bacteria, Symposium 52 of the Society for General Microbiology*, pp. 127–142.

Milkman, R. and M. McKane Bridges, 1990 - Molecular evolution of the *E. coli* chromosome. III. Clonal frames. *Genetics* **126**, 505–17. *Corrigendum Genetics* **126**, 1139.

Milkman, R. and M. McKane Bridges, 1993 - Molecular evolution of the *E. coli* chromosome. IV. Sequence comparisons. *Genetics* **133**, 455–468.

Milkman, R. and I.P. Crawford, 1983 - Clustered third-base substitutions among wild strains of *Escherichia coli. Science* **221**, 378–380.

Nelson, K., T.S. Whittam and R.K. Selander, 1991 - Nucleotide polymorphism and evolution in the glyceraldehyde-3-phosphate dehydrogenase gene (*gapA*) in natural populations of *Salmonella* and *Escherichia coli. Proc. Natl. Acad. Sci. USA* **88**, 6667–6671.

Nelson, K., T.S. Whittam and R.K. Selander, 1992 - Evolutionary genetics of the proline permease gene (*putP*) and the control of the proline utilization operon in populations of *Salmonella* and *Escherichia coli. J. Bacteriol.* **174**, 6886–6895.

Nelson, K. and R.K. Selander, 1994 - Intergeneric transfer and recombination of the 6-phosphogluconate dehydrogenase gene (*gnd*) in enteric bacteria. *Proc. Natl. Acad. Sci. USA* **91**, 10227–10231.

Ochman, H. and R.K. Selander, 1984 - Standard reference strains of *E. coli* from natural populations. *J. Bacteriol.* **157**, 690–693.

Postle, K. and R.F. Good, 1983 - DNA sequence of the *Escherichia coli tonB* gene. *Proc. Natl. Acad. Sci. USA* **80**, 5235–5239.

Postle, K. and W.S. Reznikoff, 1978 - *Hind*II and *Hind*III restriction maps of the *attφ80-tonB-trp* region of the *Escherichia coli* genome, and location of the *tonB* gene. *J. Bacteriol.* **136**, 1165–1173.

Reeves, P.R., 1992 - Variation in O-antigens, niche-specific selection and bacterial populations. *FEMS Microbiol. Lett.* **79**, 509–516.

Reeves, P.R., 1993 - Evolution of *Salmonella* O antigen variation by interspecific gene transfer on a large scale. *Trends Genet.* **9**, 17–22.

Rudd, K.E., W. Miller, C. Werner, J. Ostell, C. Tolstoshev and S.G. Satterfield, 1991 - Mapping sequenced *E. coli* genes to a genomic restriction map. *Nucleic Acids Res.* **18**, 313–321.

Rudd, K.E., 1992 - Alignment of *E. coli* DNA sequences to a revised, integrated genomic restriction map. In Miller, J.H., *A Short Course in Bacterial Genetics*, pp. 2.3–2.43. Cold Spring Harbor Laboratory Press, Cold Spring Harbor, NY.

Selander, R.K., D.A. Caugant and T.S. Whittam, 1987 - Genetic structure and variation in natural populations of *Escherichia coli*. In: *Escherichia coli and Salmonella typhimurium Cellular and Molecular Biology*. (Neidhardt, F.C. ed.), pp. 1625–48. American Society for Microbiology, Washington, D. C.

Selander, R.K. and B.R. Levin, 1980 - Genetic diversity and structure in *Escherichia coli* populations. *Science* **210**, 545–547.

Smith, G., 1991, Conjugational recombination in *Escherichia coli*: myths and mechanisms. *Cell* **64**, 19–27.

Smith, J.M., 1995 - Do bacteria have population genetics? In: *Population genetics of bacteria, Symposium 52 of the Society for General Microbiology*, pp. 1–12.

Stevenson, G., B. Neal, D. Liu, M. Hobbs, N.H. Packer, M. Batley, J.W. Redmond, L. Lindquist and P. Reeves, 1994 - Structure of the O antigen of *Escherichia coli* K-12 and the sequence of its *rfb* gene cluster. *J. Bacteriol.* **176**, 4144–4156.

Stewart, G.J., 1989 - The mechanism of natural transformation. In: *Gene Transfer in the Environment*. (Levy, S.B. and Miller, R.V. eds.), pp. 139–64. McGraw-Hill Publishing Co., New York.

Stoltzfus, A.B., 1991 - A survey of natural variation in the *trp-tonB* region of the *E. coli* chromosome. Ph. D. Thesis, The University of Iowa, Iowa City.

Stoltzfus, A., J.F. Leslie and R. Milkman, 1988 - Molecular evolution of the *Escherichia coli* chromosome. I. Analysis of structure and natural variation in a previously in characterized region between *trp* and *tonB*. *Genetics* **120**, 345–358.

Whittam, T.S., 1995 - Genetic population structure and pathogenicity in enteric bacteria. In: *Population genetics of bacteria, Symposium 52 of the Society for General Microbiology*, pp. 217–246.

Wilkins, B.F., 1995 - Gene transfer by bacterial conjugation: diversity of systems and functional specializations. In: *Population genetics of bacteria, Symposium 52 of the Society for General Microbiology*, pp. 51–88.

DNA Sequence Analysis of the Genetic Structure and Evolution of *Salmonella enterica*

Abstract

Comparative sequence analysis indicates that the effective rate of horizontal transfer and recombination in *S. enterica* is low for most housekeeping and invasion (*inv/spa*) genes. Consequently, the species is able to maintain a basically clonal population structure under which lineages are differentially adapted in host-range, disease specificity, and virulence and individual clones may achieve long-term global distribution. But for the hypervariable flagellin *fliC* locus and the *rfb* genes that determine O-antigen structure, genetic exchange among strains is a major source of allelic diversity.

Introduction

The basic goal of bacterial population genetics is to elucidate the factors that determine the genetic structure of natural populations and mediate evolutionary change. In application to pathogenic species, the analysis of genetic variation at the molecular level within and among populations has provided high-resolution methods of strain and species discrimination for clinical and epidemiological microbiology, but the primary contribution of population genetics has been to introduce an essential evolutionary dimension to an understanding of the genetic basis of pathogenesis, host-adaptation, and the origin of new pathogenic forms (Selander and Musser, 1990).

Among the pathogenic bacteria, *Salmonella enterica* is an unusually diverse pathogenic species that presents excellent opportunities for studies of the origin, function, and evolutionary elaboration of both structures and processes. This chapter reviews the recent findings of research on the genetic diversity, population structure, and evolutionary relationships of the salmonellae, with emphasis on information obtained by the comparative nucleotide sequencing of housekeeping, invasion, and flagellin genes.

Subspecific Relationships

For the more than 2,300 serovars of *S. enterica*, seven subspecies are formally recognized on the basis of biochemical variation and genomic DNA hybridiza-

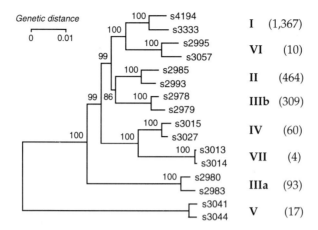

A. Housekeeping Genes 6,294 bp

Genetic distance

I   (1,367)

VI   (10)

II   (464)

IIIb (309)

IV   (60)

VII   (4)

IIIa (93)

V   (17)

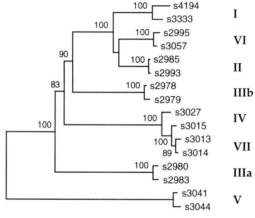

B. Invasion Genes 3,812 bp

I

VI

II

IIIb

IV

VII

IIIa

V

Fig. 1.   A. Neighbor-joining tree for 16 strains of the eight subspecies of *S. enterica*, based on variation in the combined coding sequences of five housekeeping genes, *putP*, *gapA*, *mdh*, *gnd*, and *aceK*. The tree was constructed from a matrix of pairwise genetic distance estimated from the number of substitutions per site (Jukes and Cantor, 1969; Nei and Gojobori, 1986). Subspecies are designated by roman numerals, and the number of serovars assigned to each subspecies (Popoff and Le Minor, 1992) is indicated in parentheses. Bootstrap values based on 1,000 computer-generated trees are indicated at the nodes. B. Neighbor-joining trees for four invasion genes, based on variation in the combined coding sequences. [Adapted from Li *et al.* (1995).]

tion (Le Minor *et al.*, 1986; Popoff and Le Minor, 1992). Additionally, an eighth subspecies (designated as VII) has recently been distinguished for certain strains formerly assigned to subspecies IV (Selander *et al.*, 1991, 1995).

Estimates of the genetic relationships among strains of the eight subspecies, as indexed by variation in the combined nucleotide sequences of five housekeeping genes, proline permease (*putP*) (Nelson and Selander, 1992), glyceraldehyde-3-

DNA sequence analysis of the genetic structure

phosphate dehydrogenase (*gapA*) (Nelson *et al.*, 1991a), malate dehydrogenase (*mdh*) (Boyd *et al.*, 1994), 6-phosphogluconate dehydrogenase (*gnd*) (Nelson and Selander, 1994), and isocitrate dehydrogenase kinase/phosphatase (*aceK*) (K. Nelson, unpublished data) are shown in Fig. 1A. The topology of the tree is consistent with evidence from DNA hybridization and may, therefore, be considered indicative of the actual phylogenetic relationships of the subspecies, notwithstanding the occurrence of a low level of horizontal transfer of gene segments among them (see beyond). That the subspecies I, II, IIIb, and VI - the serovars of which are exclusively or predominantly diphasic in flagellar expression - cluster apart from the monophasic subspecies IIIa, IV, V, and VII suggests the following evolutionary scenario.

Following the divergence of *S. enterica* and *Escherichia coli* from a common ancestor 120–160 million years ago, coincident with the origin of the mammals (Ochman and Wilson, 1987), *E. coli* evolved as a commensal and opportunistic pathogen of mammals and birds. Perhaps 80 million years ago, *E. coli* produced the lineages of the four nominal species of *Shigella* (Tominaga *et al.*, 1994), which, notwithstanding their taxonomic classification, are actually clonal lineages of *E. coli* (Ochman *et al.*, 1983; Karaolis *et al.*, 1994). Meanwhile, the *S. enterica* lineage remained associated with reptiles (which are still the primary hosts of the monophasic subspecies) and evolved as intracellular pathogens through acquisition of the invasion (*inv/spa*) genes and other loci that mediate invasion of host epithelial cells and otherwise distinguish *S. enterica* from *E. coli*. Subsequently, by providing increased ability to circumvent host immune systems, the invention of the mechanism of flagellar antigen phase shifting (diphasic condition) in the *S. enterica* lineage ancestral to subspecies I, II, IIIb, and VI may have been a critical factor permitting an expansion of ecological range to mammals and birds, but as a pathogen rather than a commensal - a niche already long occupied by *E. coli*. Subspecies I became highly specialized for mammals and birds, with some serovars adapting to single host species. Secondarily and inexplicably, given the adaptive advantage that phase shifting would seem to provide, 10% of the serovars of subspecies I and II have reverted to the monophasic condition, usually by loss of expression of phase 2 flagella.

Housekeeping Genes

In the absence of horizontal genetic exchange among strains, bifurcating evolutionary trees based on variation in nucleotide sequences may be interpreted as estimated phylogenies. But even when recombination has occurred and a strict phylogenetic interpretation is, therefore, precluded, tree construction may be a useful method of presenting information on degrees of genetic distance among strains. And discordant features of the topologies of trees for different loci may provide information on the frequency and extent of genetic exchange, which is a major focus of current research in bacterial population genetics because of the important effects of recombination on the genetic structure and mode of evolution of natural populations (Maynard Smith *et al.*, 1993; Whittam, 1995).

Levels of Sequence Diversity

For a sample of 16 strains representing the eight subspecies of *S. enterica*, information on sequence variation in five genes encoding housekeeping proteins are presented in Fig. 2, together with comparable data for four invasion genes. In the figure, d_S is the estimated mean number of synonymous substitutions per synonymous site ($\times 100$) that have occurred between the sequences of pairs of strains, and d_N is the comparable estimate for nonsynonymous (replacement) sites. Among the housekeeping genes, *aceK* is unusually polymorphic with respect to both types of changes.

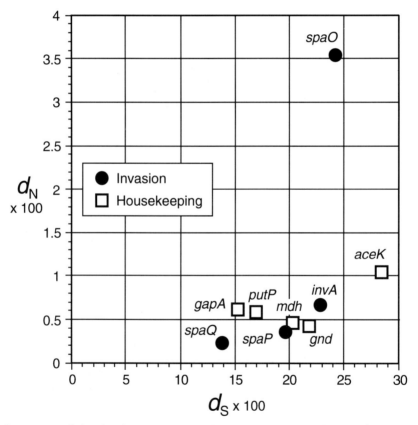

Fig. 2. Sequence variation in nine genes among 16 strains representing all eight subspecies of *S. enterica*. The plotted points indicate mean estimated numbers of substitutions between pairs of strains. See text for definitions of d_S and d_N.

DNA sequence analysis of the genetic structure

Comparisons of individual trees based on the nucleotide sequences of *putP*, *gapA*, *mdh*, and *gnd* (Fig. 3) have revealed several cases in which the order of branching of lineages is discordant. Some of these topological differences are attributable to intragenic recombination events, while others reflect the exchange

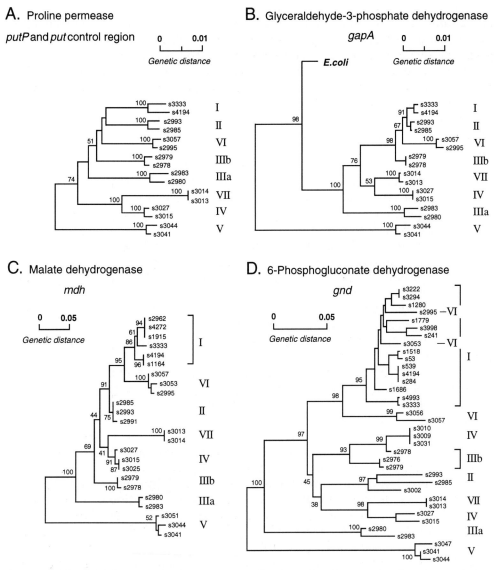

Fig. 3.   Neighbor-joining trees for four genes encoding housekeeping proteins, based on variation at synonymous nucleotide sites. Subspecies are indicated by roman numerals; and bootstrap values based on 1,000 computer-generated trees are indicated at the nodes. [Adapted from Boyd *et al.*, (1994), Nelson *et al.* (1991), and Nelson and Selander (1992, 1994).]

of entire genes (assortative recombination). The DNA segments involved in intragenic recombination, which were identified with the guidance of statistical tests for nonrandom clustering of polymorphic sites (Stephens, 1985; Sawyer, 1989), varied in length from 6 to 1,073 base pairs (bp), but several of them are in the 200–400 bp range.

In the *putP*, *mdh*, and *gnd* trees (Fig. 3A, C, and D), subspecies V clusters with the other seven subspecies; but in the *gapA* tree (Fig. 3B), it forms a branch apart from both the other salmonellae and *E. coli* as a consequence of the presence of a segment of the gene that is almost identical in sequence to that of *Klebsiella pneumoniae* (Nelson and Selander, 1992). Except for this feature, the topologies of the *putP* and *gapA* trees are generally similar, with subspecies I, II, IIIb, and VI in the same relationships. But the positions of the branch leading to IV and VII and that of IIIa are reversed in the two trees. This difference in branching order is attributable to the occurrence of a group of 25 unique polymorphic sites that defines a large segment in the central part of the *putP* sequence in strains of subspecies VII.

The only distinctive feature of the topology of the *mdh* tree (Fig. 3C) is that subspecies I is more similar to VI than to II, whereas I and II cluster together in the trees for *putP* and *gapA*. This difference reflects a recombination event, which was detected by the nonrandom clustering of polymorphic sites in the 5' region of the *mdh* gene.

That segments of substantial length in *putP*, *mdh*, and *gapA* can be clearly identified as recombinant elements in contemporary lineages of *S. enterica* indicates that episodes of intragenic recombination involving these loci are rare. And the simplest explanation for the observation that strains of a given subspecies share the same recombined segments is that these events antedate the time of divergence of the contemporary cell lineages within the subspecies.

Because 6-phosphogluconate dehydrogenase functions in an essential metabolic pathway and the *gnd* locus exhibits a moderate degree of codon bias, the expectation from evolutionary theory is that both nucleotide and amino acid sequences should be relatively conserved. However, in *S. enterica*, the number of allozyme alleles is larger than expected from estimates of total genic diversity (Nelson and Selander, 1994).

For most of 36 strains studied, evolutionary relationships deduced from *gnd* sequences (Fig. 3D) are similar to those indicated by other housekeeping genes. Thus, subspecies V is the most divergent, followed by IIIa. However, assortative recombination has occurred between strains of several subspecies (notably I and VI), and intragenic recombination has also produced positional changes for some strains. For example, the *gnd* sequences indicate a close relationship between the Paratyphi A (s4993) and Typhi (s3333), which is inconsistent with evidence from MLEE (Boyd *et al.*,1993) and the sequences of other genes.

In *E. coli*, recombination at the *gnd* locus—both intragenic and assortative (Bisercic *et al.*, 1991; Dykhuizen and Green, 1991)—has been much more extensive than in *S. enterica* (Nelson and Selander, 1994). Some strains have acquired alleles from species of *Citrobacter and Klebsiella*, and recombination has occurred so frequently that a tree derived from *gnd* sequences bears little resemblance to other gene trees or to a tree based on the results of multilocus enzyme electrophoresis (MLEE) (Selander *et al.*, 1991).

Linkage Interactions between gnd *and rfb*

The most plausible explanation for the unusually high effective rate of recombination in *gnd* is its close linkage to loci that determine the structure of cell-surface macromolecules, including genes of the *rfb* cluster that mediate biosynthesis of the highly antigenic polysaccharide domain (O antigen) of the cell-surface lipopolysaccharide (Bisercic *et al.*, 1991; Dykhuizen and Green, 1991; Nelson and Selander, 1994). Genes of the *rfb* region are believed to be subject to strong frequency dependent selection (Reeves, 1992, 1993); and there is evidence that recombination occurs frequently in the *rfb* region and that some or all of these genes in *S. enterica* and *E. coli* have been recruited from other, distantly related bacteria (Stevenson *et al.*, 1994; Xiang *et al.*, 1993, 1994). The inference is that the frequency of recombination at *gnd* is increased by the action of selection for allelic diversity at neighboring loci, as *gnd* sequences occasionally hitchhike with adaptive recombinants of *rfb* and, perhaps, other genes.

The anomalous position of subspecies IV strains s3010, s3009, and s3031 (Fig. 3D), which are all but identical in *gnd* sequence and also share O antigen 50, may be explained by the transfer of both *gnd* and *rfb* from a strain of IIIb such as s2978, which also expresses O50. And the presence of nearly identical *gnd* and *rfb* sequences in Typhi and Paratyphi A (Nelson and Selander, 1994; Reeves, 1993) clearly indicates co-transfer. For strains of *E. coli*, several examples of the horizontal co-transfer of *rfb* and *gnd* alleles have been identified (Selander *et al.*, 1987; Whittam and Ake, 1993).

Thampapapillai *et al.* (1994) have recently reported the results of an extensive study of sequence diversity in *gnd* among strains of *S. enterica* in which multiple recombination events, some involving co-transfer of parts or all of *gnd* and the *rfb* region, were identified. Several of these events appear to have been mediated by chi-like sequences located near recombination junctions.

Invasion Genes

The invasion of host cells by *S. enterica* is mediated by a large number of genes that map to several chromosomal locations. Homologues of some of these genes occur in *E. coli* (Groisman and Ochman, 1994); but there is a 40-kb segment near 59 min on the *S. enterica* chromosome that is not present in *E. coli* K-12 and contains 15 or more loci, the *inv/spa* genes, whose products are required for the invasion of epithelial cells (Mills *et al.*, 1995). Homologues of these genes, which apparently are involved in the secretion of antigens that promote cell entry, have been identified in a variety of animal and plant pathogens (Galán *et al.*, 1992; Bergman *et al.*, 1994; Eichelberg *et al.*, 1994).

Sequences of four invasion genes—*invA*, *spaO*, *spaP*, *and spaQ*—have recently been obtained for multiple strains of *S. enterica* (Li *et al.*, 1995). Levels of sequence diversity are shown in Fig. 2. The range of variation in d_S and d_N among the invasion genes exceeds that shown by housekeeping genes. The SpaO protein is hypervariable, with 21% of its amino acid positions polymorphic, which is consistent with evidence that it is an exported antigen. However, unlike the flagellin *fliC* gene (see beyond), the *spaO* gene diversity appears to have been generated almost entirely by point mutation, rather than by intragenic recombination. In contrast, the SpaQ protein is unusually well conserved, with only 2.3% of its amino acids polymorphic. Levels of variation in *invA* and *spaP* are relatively normal, although both d_S and d_N are slightly inflated in *invA* by the presence of a recombinant segment, imported from an unidentified source, in the sequences of subspecies IV and VII.

The topology of a tree constructed from the combined sequences of the four *inv/spa* genes (Fig. 1B) is generally similar to the comparable tree for five housekeeping genes (Fig. 1A), with the exception of the position of subspecies II relative to subspecies IIIb and VI and an absence of substantial differentiation between strains of subspecies IV and VII. Because the overall degree of diversification of the invasion genes among the subspecies of *S. enterica* is roughly equivalent to that of the housekeeping genes, the inference is that they were already present in the ancestral form of the species. But the lack of strong differentiation between subspecies IV and VII points to the occurrence of at least one inter-subspecific exchange of part or all of the invasion gene segment. This and other lines of evidence indicates that the chromosome of subspecies VII is a complex mosaic of large segments, some similar in sequence to those of subspecies IV and others highly distinctive in character.

Flagellar Filament Genes

Recombinational Basis of Serovar Diversity

The expression of the same flagellin and/or polysaccharide serotypes by distantly related strains, even those belonging to different subspecies (Table 1), theoretically could reflect the retention of alleles from ancestral populations, convergence in epitope structure, or recombination of horizontally transferred phase 1 flagellin (*fliC*), phase 2 flagellin (*fljB*), or *rfb* genes. On the basis of the discovery, by MLEE analysis, that Enteritidis, Derby, Newport, and some other serovars are polyphyletic assemblages of distantly related strains, horizontal transfer and recombination events involving these genes were postulated to be relatively frequent (Beltran *et al.*, 1988; Selander *et al.*, 1990a, b); and for *fliC*, this hypothesis subsequently was supported by partial sequencing of the gene in strains of Typhimurium (Smith and Selander, 1990) and several other serovars (Smith *et al.*, 1990) and by the discovery of a plasmid-borne *fliC*-like gene (*flpA*) in a triphasic strain of a normally diphasic serovar (Smith and Selander, 1991).

Table 1. Distribution of serovars with phase 1 (*fliC*) serotypes of the g complex among the subspecies of *S. enterica*

Phase 1 serotype[a]	Total no. serovars	No. serovars in indicated subspecies							
		I	II	IIIa	IIIb	IV	V	VI	VII
f, g	14	14							
f, g, m, t	1	1							
f, g, s	4	4							
f, g, t	7	6	1						
g, m	13	13							
g, m, q	1	1							
g, m, [p], s	1	1							
g, m, s	13	12	1						
g, m, s, t	30	2	28						
g, m, t	16	7	9						
g, p	3	3							
g, p, s	1	1							
g, p, u	1	1							
g, q	1	1							
g, s, t	24	20	4						
g, t	27	5	22						
g, z_{51}	35	7		16		10			2
g, z_{62}	5		5						
g, z_{63}	1	1							
m, p, t, [u]	1	1							
m, t	52	23	28						1

[Prepared from data in Popoff and Le Minor (1992).]
[a]Antigenic factors in parentheses are not expressed by all isolates.

As a test of the generality of the horizontal transfer/recombination hypothesis, Li *et al.* (1994) obtained the complete *fliC* sequences of 15 strains of several serovars of subspecies I, II, IV, and VII that express seven combinations of six phase 1 flagellar antigenic factors of the g complex (f, g, m, s, t, and z_{51}). In *S. enterica*, as in other bacteria (Wilson and Beveridge, 1993), the terminal regions of the flagellin molecule (C1 and C2), which are involved in secretion and polymerization, are strongly conserved in both length and amino acid sequence, whereas the central region (V), which is the site of the epitopic variation assayed in serotyping (Joys, 1988; Newton *et al.*, 1991), is hypervariable.

Individual evolutionary trees based on MLEE (indexing the overall genomic relatedness of the strains), the nucleotide sequence of the combined C1 and C2 regions of *fliC*, and the sequence of the V region of the gene are shown in Fig. 4. If the evolution of *fliC* has involved little or no recombination, trees for the V region and the C1 + C2 regions should be topologically concordant. In contrast, horizontal exchange of the V region among strains would be indicated by a clustering of sequences specifying the same flagellin serotype, regardless of the overall genetic relatedness of the strains in which they occur.

Although strains of Enteritidis (En 1) and Othmarschen (Ot 1), which express serotype g,m, are divergent in chromosomal character (Fig. 4A), their *fliC*

A. MLEE (27 loci)

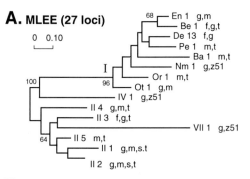

B. *fliC* – Conserved Regions (C1, C2)

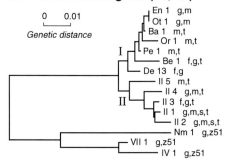

C. *fliC* – Variable Region (V)

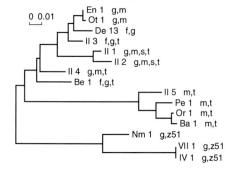

Fig. 4. Evolutionary trees for 15 strains of *S. enterica*. For each strain, the phase 1 flagellin serotype is indicated. A. MLEE tree (based on 27 enzyme loci). Bootstrap values greater than 50% are shown at the nodes. B. Conserved (C1 + C2) regions of the *fliC* gene. Clusters of ETs of sub-species I and II are labeled. Bootstrap values for all nodes are greater than 50%. C. Central variable (V) region of the *fliC* gene. Note that the scale is approximately half that of the conser-ved-sequence tree (B). Subspecies I serovar abbreviations are Ba, Banana; Be, Berta; De, Derby; En, Enteritidis; Nm, Newmexico; Or, Oranienburg; Ot, Othmarschen; and Pe, Pensacola. Roman numerals identify ETs of other subspecies. [Adapted from Li *et al.* (1994).]

DNA sequence analysis of the genetic structure

sequences are nearly identical (Fig. 4B and C). Strains Nm 1, IV 1, and VII 1 (serotype g,z$_{51}$) represent three subspecies, but both their V and C1 + C2 sequences cluster together. ETs Pe 1, Ba 1, Or 1, and II 5 are of serotype m,t. The three subspecies I ETs are not closely allied, and all three are distantly related to II 5. Their C1 + C2 sequences reflect these relationships, but all four ETs form a distinct, tight cluster in the V region tree. This region and part of C2 have been exchanged among the four ETs; and part of this distinctive sequence has also been transferred to ETs Be 1 and II 4.

In sum, the occurrence of each of three flagellin serotypes of the g complex in distantly related strains is clearly attributable to horizontal exchange rather than to convergence in epitope-determining amino acid sequences or retention of ancestral sequences. If antigens of this complex are typical of flagellar antigens in general—and there is no reason to believe they are not—interstrain exchange and recombination is clearly a major evolutionary mechanism generating both allelic variation in *fliC* and serovar diversity in natural populations of the salmonellae.

Evolutionary Loss of Flagella

The serovars Gallinarum and Pullorum, which are invasive pathogens of fowl, are unique among the salmonellae in being obligatorily nonflagellate. MLEE analysis has identified Enteritidis as a close relative, and the sharing of distinctive allozyme alleles at three metabolic enzyme loci and a premature stop codon in the *flgK* gene encoding the first hook-filament junction protein by the ETs of Gallinarum and Pullorum indicates that they are monophyletic and that their most recent common ancestor was nonmotile (Li *et al.*, 1993).

Li *et al.* (1993) found that intact, but silenced, *fliC* genes are present in the nonmotile salmonellae. The genes of strains of some ETs of Gallinarum are identical in sequence to that of Enteritidis, but a nucleotide substitution has created a shared premature stop codon in strains of several ETs. The *fliC* sequences of the Pullorum ETs differ from the standard Enteritidis and Gallinarum sequence in having nonsynonymous substitutions in two or three codons in the V region.

These findings indicate that loss of motility in the avian-adapted salmonellae occurred relatively recently in evolutionary time. Flagella are not expressed *in vivo* by strains of Enteritidis infecting chickens (Chart *et al.*, 1993), and their permanent loss presumably evolved in the Enteritidis-like common ancestor of Gallinarum and Pullorum because motility was for some reason no longer required as the lineage became increasingly restricted in host-range to fowl. Nonsense mutations in *fliC* and *flgK* then began to accumulate when, as a consequence of a mutation in another gene of the flagellar regulon that inhibited flagellar biosynthesis, they were no longer active and subject to purifying selection.

Many isolates of Dublin recovered in recent years from invasive infections in cattle have been nonmotile, although the condition apparently is reversible

(Selander *et al.*, 1992). Like Gallinarum and Pullorum, Dublin is strongly host-adapted and is also a close relative of Enteritidis. It is also of interest that the strongly host-adapted shigellae, as well as most enteroinvasive strains of *E. coli.* are nonmotile, although at least two of the four *Shigella* species carry intact *fliC* genes (Tominaga *et al.*, 1994). Modulation of flagellar biosynthesis may be common strategy of invasive bacterial pathogens, with motility being advantageous under certain environmental conditions (C. Li *et al.*, 1993; Mahenthiralingam *et al.*, 1994) and during colonization but disadvantageous in later stages of infection.

Genetic Structure Of Populations

The Concept of Clonal Structure

For the salmonellae, a basically clonal population structure is evidenced by the presence of strong linkage disequilibrium among alleles at enzyme loci, the association of specific O and H serotypes with only one or a small number of multilocus enzyme genotypes, and the global distribution of certain genotypes (Beltran *et al.*, 1988; Reeves *et al.*, 1989; Maynard Smith *et al.*, 1992; Selander *et al.*, 1990a,b, 1992). *S. enterica* populations are clonal in the sense that the effective (realized) rates of recombination for most chromosomal genes are sufficiently low to permit the mutational diversification of cell lineages in terms of biochemical characteristics and ecological niche relationships, including host distribution, disease specificity, and virulence, and the long-term, if not permanent, maintenance of differentially adapted, widely distributed chromosomal genotypes in populations (Selander *et al.*, 1995). Clonality explains why serotyping is a powerful marker system for recognizing groups of strains with distinct host ranges and pathogenicities, including those of closely related populations such as Dublin and Enteritidis (Selander *et al.*, 1992). At the level of population structure resolved by MLEE, most of the serovars, including most of the common pathogens of humans and domesticated animals, are single ETs or families of closely related ETs; and for many of the medically important serovars, only a single ET is globally predominant at any one time (Table 2).

An evolutionary genetic rational for the prevalence of clonal population structure among pathogenic bacteria has been noted by Falkow (1990). Because pathogenesis is a complex, multifactorial process involving the coordinated action of a large number of virulence-associated loci and genes that permit the pathogen to survive in a variety of habitats, including those that enable it to recognize its hosts and then to avoid, subvert, or nullify their defense systems, there could be little adaptive radiation among pathogenic bacteria if frequent and indiscriminate horizontal genetic transfer and recombination occurred for genes throughout the genome.

DNA sequence analysis of the genetic structure

Table 2. Relative abundance of the commonest ET of *S. enterica* serovars

Serovar	No. of isolates	No. of ETs	Commonest ET	% of isolates of commonest ET
Choleraesuis	85	6	Cs 1	88
Derby[a]				
I	71	2	De 1	93
II	267	3	De 13	61
III	11	1	De 31	100
Dublin	117	3	Du 1	95
Enteritidis	257	14	En 1	93
Gallinarum	56	5	Ga 2	95
Heidelberg	204	8	He	87
Infantis	113	4	In 1	96
Newport[a]				
I	72	7	Np 1	38
II	32	5	Np 11	84
Panama	94	11	Pn 1	77
Paratyphi A	135	6	Pa 1	74
Paratyphi B	123	13	Pb 1	61
Paratyphi C	100	9	Pc 1	60
Pullorum	75	7	Pu 3	51
Typhi	334	7	Tp 1	82
Typhimurium	299	17	Tm 1	83

[Sources of data: Beltran *et al.* (1988), Selander *et al.* (1990a, b, 1992), and Li *et al.* (1993).]
[a]Polyphyletic serovars; see Beltran *et al.* (1988).

Clones of Serovar Typhi

Clonal aspects of the genetic structure of populations of *S. enterica* are well illustrated by the serovar Typhi, which is the agent of human typhoid fever. Both biochemically and genotypically, Typhi is an unusually distinctive and homogenous serovar (Faundez *et al.*, 1990; Franco *et al.*, 1992; Moshitch *et al.*, 1992; Thelfall *et al.*, 1994; Thong *et al.*, 1994). By MLEE analysis, Selander *et al.* (1990b) found that 82% of worldwide isolates were of one genotype (ET 1), with a second clone (ET 2) being represented by 16% of strains, all from western Africa.

Throughout most of the world, Typhi is monomorphic for the d allele at the *fliC* locus encoding the phase 1 flagellin protein. But Indonesian populations are polymorphic for the d allele and a variant j allele (Maher *et al.*, 1986; Franco *et al.*, 1992), which was derived from d by the deletion of a 261-bp segment in the central part of the *fliC* gene (Frankel *et al.*, 1989). Additionally, some Indonesian strains of either phase 1 d or j uniquely express a z_{66} flagellar antigen (Guinée *et al.*, 1981), which presumably is encoded by a phase 2 locus, although they lack the genes that normally mediate phase shifting in *S. enterica* (Moshitch *et al.*, 1992). Inasmuch as the specific deletion that changes d to j may be experimentally produced when Typhi is grown in anti-d serum (Smith *et al.*, 1991), it is likely that it occurs repeatedly in natural populations, where, however, it may normally be disadvantageous because motility is decreased

(Frankel *et al.*, 1989). If so, the problem is to explain why it has managed to reach a frequency as high as 15% in the Indonesian Typhi population (Grossman *et al.*, 1994). An explanation is suggested by the fact that flagellar antigens are the major factors eliciting immune responses after infection with Typhi or vaccine administration (He *et al.*, 1994).

It is probably not coincidental that the frequency of typhoid fever in Indonesia is the highest in the world, with as many as 1,300,000 cases and 20,000 deaths per year (Simanjuntak *et al.*, 1992). Moreover, it is primarily a disease of children, which suggests that the Indonesian population acquires immunity through exposure (Sudarmono and Radji, 1992). Because immunity is serotype-specific, people infected with d allele strains would remain relatively unprotected against infection by strains carrying the j allele, thus accounting for the decrease in the ratio of d/j infections with age (Grossman *et al.*, 1994). Flagellar antigen diversity in Indonesia may well be an example of the maintenance of polymorphism by balancing selection for avoidance of immune responses in the host population.

Inter-locus Variation in Recombination Rate

A generalization emerging from the analysis of gene sequences in populations of *S. enterica* and other bacteria is that the contribution to allelic diversity made by recombination varies markedly among loci encoding proteins of different functional types (Achtman, 1994; Nelson *et al.*, 1991a; Nelson and Selander, 1992; Sibold *et al.*, 1992; Selander *et al.*, 1995; Vásquez *et al.*, 1993), as well as among species and subdivisions of species. As shown in this review, the effective rate of recombination in *S. enterica* is low for genes encoding most metabolic enzymes and other types of housekeeping proteins, as well as for the *inv/spa* virulence genes. In contrast, horizontal transfer and recombination is a major source of allelic diversity for both the highly polymorphic flagellin *fliC* locus and the *rfb* genes that determine O-antigen structure. Entire *fliC* genes and parts or all of the epitope-determining central region have been frequently exchanged within and between subspecies, and many alleles are mosaics of segments derived from several sources. Because flagellin is a highly antigenic and interacts directly with the external environment, recombinant alleles may confer an immediate adaptive advantage to a bacterial cell and, in consequence, be brought to high frequency in local populations by natural selection and then transferred to other lineages. The prevailing view is that the extensive flagellar antigenic polymorphism in *S. enterica* is adaptive in permitting the reinfection of hosts (Brunham *et al.*, 1993); and Reeves (1992) has suggested that genes mediating antigenic variation in flagellin and the cell-surface polysaccharide are subject to niche-specific selection. The observation that sensitivity to flagellotropic bacteriophages may be serotype dependent (Iino, 1977) suggests another possible adaptive basis for flagellin polymorphism; and Skurnik and Toivanen (1994) have proposed that resistance to bacteriophages is also an adaptive basis for O antigen polymorphism.

Table 3. Proteins and polysaccharides for which there is evidence that the encoding or mediating genes are subject to horizontal transfer and intragenic or assortative recombination for which an adaptive basis has been suggested

Protein or structure (gene)	Species	References
Class 1 OMP (*porA*)	*Neisseria meningitidis*	Feavers *et al.* (1992)
Opacity proteins (*opa* family)	*Neisseria meningitidis*	Hobbs *et al.* (1994)
M proteins (*emm* cluster)	*Streptococcus pyogenes*	Harbaugh *et al.* (1993); Whatmore and Kehoe (1994); Bessen and Hollingshead (1994)
Pilin (*pilE* and *pilS*)	*Neisseria gonorrhoeae*	Seifert and So (1988); Seifert *et al.* (1988)
Pili (*pap* and *prs* clusters)	*Escherichia coli*	Plos *et al.* (1989); Arthur *et al.* (1990); Marklund *et al.* (1992)
Capsular polysaccharide (*cap*)	*Haemophilus influenzae*	Kroll and Moxon (1990)
IgA protease (*iga*)	*Neisseria gonorrhoeae* *Neisseria meningitidis* *Haemophilus influenzae*	Halter *et al.* (1989) Lomholt *et al.* (1992); Morelli *et al.* (1994) Poulsen *et al.* (1992)
Penicillin-binding proteins	*Neisseria* spp. *Streptococcus* spp.	Spratt *et al.* (1992); Bowler *et al.* (1994) Dowson *et al.* (1990); Laible *et al.* (1991); Martin *et al.* (1992); Sibold *et al.* (1992)
O antigen (*rfb* cluster)	*Salmonella enterica*	Reeves (1993); Xiang *et al.* (1993, 1994)
Flagellin (*fliC*)	*Salmonella enterica*	Smith *et al.* (1990); Li *et al.* (1994)
R-M enzymes (*hsd*)[a]	*Escherichia coli*	Sharp *et al.* (1992); Murray *et al.* (1993)
Colicin immunity proteins	*Escherichia coli*	Riley (1993)
Pyrogenic exotoxins (*speA*, *speC*)	*Streptococcus pyogenes*	Nelson *et al.* (1991b); Kapur *et al.* (1992); Reda *et al.* (1994)

[Modified from Selander *et al.* (1995).]
[a]R-M, restriction and modification system.

Similar explanations in terms of environmental adaptation apply to a number of genes in other bacteria for which evidence of frequent horizontal transfer and recombination is available (Table 3). Such genes almost without exception encode or mediate the expression of products for which there would seem to be a premium on structural diversity or which confer adaptive traits such as antibiotic resistance (Selander *et al.*, 1995). But for housekeeping or virulence genes that encode polypeptides for which there is no premium on diversity in amino acid sequence per se, it is unlikely that either intragenic or assortative recombination would result in a selective advantage to the recipient cell. And the probable fate of deleterious or selectively neutral recombinants is loss from the population through purifying selection and genetic drift. By comparing the degree of amino acid divergence in 179 homologous proteins in *S. enterica* and *E. coli*, Whittam (1995) has shown that cell-surface proteins, such as flagellins, porins, and pilins, are evolving at nearly three times the rate of cytoplasmic enzymes and proteins that function in transport, DNA replication, and the regulation of transcription, and 10 times faster than ribosomal proteins.

Among the double-stranded DNA bacteriophages of enteric bacteria, recombination, mediated by site-specific invertases, has been a major factor in the evolution of tail-fiber genes, with relatively frequent exchange occurring between otherwise unrelated phage groups (quasispecies) (Sandmeier, 1994). Tail-fiber genes of various phages and certain defective prophages share homologous segments, and individual loci may have a mosaic structure. This locus-specific exchange is adaptive in generating diversity in host-range determinants in the face of strong selective pressure on phages to adapt to mutated host surfaces, which, in turn, are under selective pressure to avoid phage infection. Given the great variation in rate of recombination observed among the genes of *S. enterica* and other bacteria, it would not be surprising to find comparable mechanisms that function to increase the frequency of exchange of certain genes or segments of the chromosome for which selection for diversity is strong.

Acknowledgments

Research leading to this review was supported by Grant AI22144 from the National Institutes of Health.

References

Achtman, M., 1994 - Clonal spread of serogroup A meningococci: a paradigm for the analysis of microevolution in bacteria. *Mol. Microbiol.* **11**, 15–22.

Arthur, M., R.D. Arbeit, C. Kim, P. Beltran, H. Crowe, S. Steinbach, C. Campanelli, R.A. Wilson, R.K. Selander and R. Goldstein, 1990 - Restriction fragment length polymorphisms among uropathogenic *Escherichia coli* isolates: *pap*-related sequences compared with *rrn* operons. *Infect. Immun.* **58**, 471–479.

Beltran, P., J.M. Musser, R. Helmuth, J.J. Farmer III, W.M. Frerichs, I.K. Wachsmuth, K. Ferris, A.C. McWhorter, J.G. Wells, A. Cravioto and R.K. Selander, 1988 - Toward a population genetic analysis of *Salmonella*: genetic diversity and relationships among strains of serotypes *S. choleraesuis, S. derby, S. dublin, S. enteritidis, S. heidelbekrg, S. infantis, S. newport, and S. typhimurium. Proc. Natl. Acad. Sci. USA* **85**, 7753–7757.

Bergman, T., K. Erickson, E. Galyov, C. Persson and H. Wolf-Watz, 1994 - The *lcrB* (*yscN/U*)) gene cluster of *Yersinia pseudotuberculosis* is involved in Yop secretion and shows high homology to the *spa* gene clusters of *Shigella flexneri* and *Salmonella typhimurium. J. Bacteriol.* **176**, 2619–2626.

Bessen, D.E. and S.K. Hollingshead, 1994 - Allelic polymorphism of *emm* loci provides evidence for horizontal gene spread in group A streptococci. *Proc. Natl. Acad. Sci. USA* **91**, 3280–3284.

Bisercic, M., J.Y. Feutrier and P.R. Reeves, 1991 - Nucleotide sequences of the *gnd* genes from nine natural isolates of *Escherichia coli*: evidence of intragenic recombination as a contributing factor in the evolution of the polymorphic *gnd* locus. *J. Bacteriol.* **173**, 3894–3900.

Bowler, L.D., Q.-Y. Zhang, J.-Y. Riou and B.G. Spratt, 1994 - Interspecies recombination between the *penA* genes of *Neisseria meningitidis* and commensal *Neisseria* species during the emergence of penicillin resistance in *N. meningitidis*: natural events and laboratory simulation. *J. Bacteriol.* **176**, 333–337.

Boyd, E.F., K. Nelson, F.-S. Wang, T.S. Whittam and R.K. Selander, 1994 - Molecular genetic basis of allelic polymorphism in malate dehydrogenase (*mdh*) in natural populations of *Escherichia coli* and *Salmonella enterica. Proc. Natl. Acad. Sci. USA* **91**, 1280–1284.

Boyd, E.F., F.-S. Wang, P. Beltran, S.A. Plock, K. Nelson and R.K. Selander, 1993 - *Salmonella* reference collection B (SARB): strains of 37 serovars of subspecies I. *J. Gen. Microbiol.* **139**, 1125–1132.

Brunham, R.C., F.A. Plummer and R.S. Stephens, 1993 - Bacterial antigenic variation, host immune response, and pathogen-host coevolution. *Infect. Immun.* **61**, 2273–2276.

Chart, H., D. Conway and B. Rowe, 1993 - Outer membrane characteristics of *Salmonella enteritidis* phage type-4 growing in chickens. *Epidemiol. Infect.* **111**, 449–454.

Dowson, C.G., A. Hutchison, N. Woodford, A.P. Johnson, R.C. George and B.G. Spratt, 1990 - Penicillin-resistant viridans streptococci have obtained altered penicillin-binding protein genes from penicillin-resistant strains of *Streptococcus pneumoniae. Proc. Natl. Acad. Sci. USA* **87**, 5858–5862.

Dykhuizen, D.E. and L. Green, 1991 - Recombination in *Escherichia coli* and the definition of biological species. *J. Bacteriol.* **173**, 7257–7268.

Eichelberg, K., C.C. Ginocchio and J.E. Galán, 1994 - Molecular and functional characterization of the *Salmonella typhimurium* invasion genes *invB* and *invC*: homology of InvC to the F_0F_1 ATPase family of proteins. *J. Bacteriol.* **176**, 4501–4510.

Falkow, S., 1990 - The 'Zen' of bacterial pathogenicity, p. 3–9. *In* B. H. Iglewski and V.L. Clark (ed.), Molecular basis of bacterial pathogenesis. Academic Press, San Diego.

Faundez, G., L. Aron and F.C. Cabello, 1990 - Chromosomal DNA, iron-transport systems, outer membrane proteins, and enterotoxin (heat labile) production in *Salmonella typhi* strains. *J. Clin. Microbiol.* **28**, 894–897.

Feavers, I.M., A.B. Heath, J.A. Bygraves and M.C.J. Maiden, 1992 - Role of horizontal genetic exchange in the antigenic variation of the class 1 outer membrane protein of *Neisseria meningitidis. Mol. Microbiol.* **6**, 489–495.

Franco, A., C. Gonzalez, O.S. Levine, R. Lagos, R.H. Hall, S.L. Hoffman, M.A. Moechtar, E. Gotuzzo, M.L. Levine, D.M. Hone and J.G. Morris Jr., 1992 - Further consideration of the clonal nature of *Salmonella typhi*: evaluation of molecular and clinical characteristics of strains from Indonesia and Peru. *J. Clin. Microbiol.* **30**, 2187–2190.

Frankel, G., S.M.C. Newton, G.K. Schooknik and B.A.D. Stocker, 1989 - Intragenic recombination in a flagellin gene: characterization of the *H1*:j gene of *Salmonella typhi. EMBO J.* **8**, 3149–3152.

Galán, J.E., C. Ginocchio and P. Costas, 1992 - Molecular and functional characterization of the *Salmonella* invasion gene *invA*: homology of InvA to members of a new protein family. *J. Bacteriol.* **174**, 4338–4349.

Groisman, E.A. and H. Ochman, 1994 - How to become a pathogen. *Trends Microbiol.* **2**, 289–294.

Grossman, D.A., N.D. Witham, D.H. Burr, M. Lesmana, F.A. Rubin, G.K. Schoolnik and J. Parsonnet, 1994 - Flagellar serotypes of *Salmonella typhi* in Indonesia: relationship among mobility, invasiveness, and clinical illness. *J. Infect. Dis.* **171**, 212–216.

Guinée, P.A.M., W.H. Jensen, H.M.E. Maas, L. Le Minor and R. Beaud, 1981 - An unusual H antigen (z_{66}) in strains of *Salmonella typhi. Ann. Microbiol.* (*Inst. Pasteur*) **132A**, 331–334.

Halter, R., J. Pohlner and T.F. Meyer, 1989 - Mosaic-like organization of IgA protease genes in *Neisseria gonorrhoeae* generated by horizontal genetic exchange *in vivo. EMBO J.* **9**, 2737–2744.

Harbaugh, M.P., A. Podbielski, S. Hügl and P.P. Cleary, 1993 - Nucleotide substitutions and small-scale insertion produce size and antigenic variation in group A streptococcal M1 protein. *Mol. Microbiol.* **8**, 981–991.

He, X.-S., M. Rivkina, B.A.D. Stocker and W.S. Robinson, 1994 - Hypervariable region IV of *Salmonella* gene *flic*^d encodes a dominant surface epitope and a stabilizing factor for functional flagella. *J. Bacteriol.* **176**, 2406–2414.

Hobbs, M.M., A. Seiler, M. Achtman and J.G. Cannon, 1994 - Microevolution within a clonal population of pathogenic bacteria - recombination, gene duplication and horizontal genetic exchange in the *opa* gene family of *Neisseria meningitidis. Mol. Microbiol.* **12**, 171–180.

Iino, T., 1977 - Genetics of structure and function of bacterial flagella. *Annu. Rev. Genet.* **11**, 161–182.

Joys, T.M., 1988 - The flagellar filament protein. *Can. J. Microbiol.* **34**, 452–458.

Jukes, T.H. and C.R. Cantor, 1969 - Evolution of protein molecules, p. 21–132. *In* Munro, H.N. (ed.), Mammalian protein metabolism. Academic Press, New York.

Kapur, V., K. Nelson, P.M. Schlievert, R.K. Selander and J.M. Musser, 1992 - Molecular population genetic evidence of horizontal spread of two alleles of the pyrogenic exotoxin C gene (*speC*) among pathogenic clones of *Streptococcus pyogenes*. *Infect. Immun.* **60**, 3513–3517.

Karaolis, D.K.R., R. Lan and P.R. Reeves, 1994 - Sequence variation in *Shigella sonnei*, a pathogenic clone of *Escherichia coli*, over four continents and 41 years. *J. Clin. Microbiol.* **32**, 796–802.

Kroll, J.S. and E.R. Moxon, 1990 - Capsulation in distantly related strains of *Haemophilus influenzae* type b: genetic drift and gene transfer at the capsulation locus. *J. Bacteriol.* **172**, 1374–1379.

Laible, G., B.G. Spratt and R. Hakenbeck, 1991 - Interspecies recombinational events during the evolution of altered PBP 2x genes in penicillin-resistant clinical isolates of *Streptococcus pneumoniae*. *Mol. Microbiol.* **5**, 1993–2002.

Le Minor, L., M.Y. Popoff, B. Laurent and D. Hermant, 1986 - Individualisation d'une septième sous-espèce de *Salmonella*: *S. choleraesuis* subsp. *indica* subsp. *nov. Ann. Inst. Pasteur/Microbiol.* **137B**, 211–217.

Li, C., C.J. Louise, W. Shi and J. Adler, 1993 - Adverse conditions which cause lack of flagella in *Escherichia coli*. *J. Bacteriol.* **175**, 2229–2235.

Li, J., N.H. Smith, K. Nelson, P.B. Crichton, D.C. Old, T.S. Whittam and R.K. Selander, 1993 - Evolutionary origin and radiation of the avian-adapted non-motile salmonellae. *J. Med. Microbiol.* **38**, 129–139.

Li, J., K. Nelson, A.C. McWhorter, T.S. Whittam and R.K. Selander, 1994 - Recombinational basis of serovar diversity in *Salmonella enterica*. *Proc. Natl. Acad. Sci. USA* **91**, 2552–2556.

Li, J., H. Ochman, E.A. Groisman, E.F. Boyd, K. Nelson and R.K. Selander, 1995 - Relationship between evolutionary rate and cellular location among the Inv/Spa invasion proteins of *Salmonella enterica*. *Proc. Natl. Acad. Sci. USA* **92**, 7252–7256.

Lomholt, H., K. Poulsen, D.A. Caugant and M. Kilian, 1992 - Molecular polymorphism and epidemiology of *Neisseria meningitidis* immunoglobulin A1 proteases. *Proc. Natl. Acad. Sci. USA* **89**, 2120–2124.

Mahenthiralingam, E., M.E. Campbell and D.P. Speert, 1994 - Nonmotility and phagocytic resistance of *Pseudomonas aeruginosa* isolates from chronically colonized patients with cystic fibrosis. *Infect. Immun.* **62**, 596–605.

Maher, K.O., J.G. Morris Jr., E. Gotuzzo, C. Ferreccio, L.R. Ward, L. Benavente, R.E. Black, B. Rowe and M.M. Levine, 1986 - Molecular techniques in the study of *Salmonella typhi* in epidemiologic studies in endemic areas: comparison with Vi phage typing. *Am. J. Trop. Med. Hyg.* **35**, 831–835.

Marklund, B.-I., J.M. Tennent, E. Garcia, A. Hamers, M. Båga, F. Lindberg, W. Gaastra and S. Normark, 1992 - Horizontal gene transfer of the *Escherichia coli pap* and *prs* pili operons as a mechanism for the development of tissue-specific adhesive properties. *Mol. Microbiol.* **6**, 2225–2242.

Martin, C., C. Sibold and R. Hakenbeck, 1992 - Relatedness of penicillin-binding protein 1a genes from different clones of penicillin-resistant *Streptococcus pneumoniae* isolated in South Africa and Spain. *EMBO J.* **11**, 3831–3836.

Maynard Smith, J., N.H. Smith, M. O'Rourke and B.G. Spratt, 1993 - How clonal are bacteria? *Proc. Natl. Acad. Sci. USA* **90**, 4384–4388.

Mills, D.M., V. Bajaj and C.A. Lee, 1995 - A 40 kilobase chromosomal fragment encoding *Salmonella typhimurium* invasion genes is absent from the corresponding region of the *Escherichia coli* K-12 chromosome. *Mol. Microbiol.* **15**, 749–759.

Morelli, G., J. del Valle, C.J. Lammel, J. Pohlner, K. Müller, M. Blake, G.F. Brooks, T.F. Meyer, B. Koumaré, N. Brieske and M. Achtman, 1994 - Immunogenicity and evolutionary variability of epitopes within IgA1 protease from serogroup A *Neisseria meningitidis. Mol. Microbiol.* **11**, 175–187.

Moshitch, S., L. Doll, B.-Z. Rubinfeld, B.A.D. Stocker, G.K. Schoolnik, Y. Gafni and G. Frankel, 1992 - Mono- and bi-phasic *Salmonella typhi*: genetic homogeneity and distinguishing characteristics. *Mol. Microbiol.* **6**, 2589–2597.

Murray, N.E., A.S. Daniel, G.M. Cowan and P.M. Sharp, 1993 - Conservation of motifs within the unusually variable polypeptide sequences of type I restriction and modification enzymes. *Mol. Microbiol.* **9**, 133–143.

Nei, M. and T. Gojobori, 1986 - Simple methods for estimating the numbers of synonymous and nonsynonymous nucleotide substitutions. *Mol. Biol. Evol.* **3**, 418–426.

Nelson, K. and R.K. Selander, 1992 - Evolutionary genetics of the proline permease gene (*putP*) and the control region of the proline utilization operon in populations of *Salmonella* and *Escherichia coli. J. Bacteriol.* **174**, 6886–6895.

Nelson, K. and R.K. Selander, 1994 - Intergeneric transfer and recombination of the 6-phosphogluconate dehydrogenase gene (*gnd*) in enteric bacteria. *Proc. Natl. Acad. Sci. USA* **91**, 10227–10231.

Nelson, K., T.S. Whittam and R.K. Selander, 1991a - Nucleotide polymorphism and evolution in the glyceraldehyde-3-phosphate dehydrogenase gene (*gapA*) in natural populations of *Salmonella* and *Escherichia coli. Proc. Natl. Acad. Sci. USA* **88**, 6667–6671.

Nelson, K., P.M. Schlievert, R.K. Selander and J.M. Musser, 1991b - Characterization and clonal distribution of four alleles of the *speA* gene encoding pyrogenic exotoxin A (scarlet fever toxin) in *Streptococcus pyogenes. J. Exp. Med.* **174**, 1271–1274.

Newton, S.M.C., R.D. Wasley, A. Wilson, L.T. Rosenberg, J.F. Miller and B.A.D. Stocker, 1991 - Segment IV of a *Salmonella* flagellin gene specifies flagellar antigen epitopes. *Mol. Microbiol.* **5**, 419–425.

Ochman, H. and A.C. Wilson, 1987 - Evolution in bacteria: evidence for a universal substitution rate in cellular genomes. *J. Mol. Evol.* **26**, 74–86.

Ochman, H., T.S. Whittam, D.A. Caugant and R.K. Selander, 1983 - Enzyme polymorphism and genetic population structure in *Escherichia coli* and *Shigella. J. Gen. Microbiol.* **129**, 2715–2726.

Plos, K., S.I. Hull, R.A. Hull, B.R. Levin, I. Ørskov, F. Ørskov and C. Svandborg-Edén, 1989 - Distribution of the P-associated-pilus (*pap*) region among *Escherichia coli* from natural sources: evidence for horizontal gene transfer. *Infect. Immun.* **57**, 1604–1611.

Popoff, M.Y. and L. Le Minor, 1992 - Antigenic formulas of the *Salmonella* serovars, 6th ed. WHO Collaborating Centre for Reference and Research on *Salmonella*, Institut Pasteur, Paris.

Poulsen, K., J. Reinholdt and M. Kilian, 1992 - A comparative genetic study of serologically distinct *Haemophilus influenzae* type 1 immunoglobulin A1 proteases. *J. Bacteriol.* **174**, 2913–2921.

Reda, K.B.,V. Kapur, J.A. Mollick, J.G. Lamphear, J.M. Musser and R.R. Rich, 1994 - Molecular characterization and phylogenetic distribution of the streptococcal superantigen gene (*ssa*) from *Streptococcus pyogenes*. *Infect. Immun.* **62**, 1867–1874.

Reeves, P.R., 1992 - Variation in O-antigens, niche-specific selection and bacterial populations. *FEMS Microbiol. Lett.* **100**, 509–516.

Reeves, P.R., 1993 - Evolution of *Salmonella* O antigen variation by interspecific gene transfer on a large scale. *Trends Genet.* **9**, 17–22.

Reeves, M.W., G.M. Evins, A.A. Heiba, B.D. Plikaytis and J.J. Farmer III, 1989 - Clonal nature of *Salmonella typhi* and its genetic relatedness to other salmonellae as shown by multilocus enzyme electrophoresis, and proposal of *Salmonella bongori comb. nov. J. Clin. Microbiol.* **27**, 311–320.

Riley, M.A., 1993 - Positive selection for colicin diversity in bacteria. *Mol. Biol. Evol.* **10**, 1048–1059.

Sandmeier, H., 1994 - Acquisition and rearrangement of sequence motifs in the evolution of bacteriophage tail fibers. *Mol. Microbiol.* **12**, 343–350.

Sawyer, S., 1989 - Statistical tests for detecting gene conversion. *Mol. Biol. Evol.* **6**, 526–538.

Seifert, H.S. and M. So, 1988 - Genetic mechanisms of bacterial antigenic variation. *Microbiol. Rev.* **52**, 327–336.

Seifert, H.S., R.S. Ajioka, C. Marchal, P.F. Sparling and M. So, 1988 - DNA transformation leads to pilin antigenic variation in *Neisseria gonorrhoeae*. *Nature* **336**, 392–395.

Selander, R.K. and J.M. Musser, 1990 - Population genetics of bacterial pathogenesis, p. 11–36. *In* B.H. Iglewski and V.L. Clark (ed.), Molecular basis of bacterial pathogenesis. Academic Press, San Diego.

Selander, R.K., D.A. Caugant and T.S. Whittam, 1987 - Genetic structure and variation in natural populations of *Escherichia coli*, p. 1625–1648. *In* F.C. Neidhardt, J.L. Ingraham, K.B. Low, B. Magasanik, M. Schaechter, and H.E. Umbarger (ed.), *Escherichia coli* and *Salmonella typhimurium*: cellular and molecular biology, vol. 2., American Society for Microbiology, Washington, D.C.

Selander, R.K., P. Beltran, N.H. Smith, R.M. Barker, P.B. Crichton, D.C. Old, J.M. Musser and T.S. Whittam, 1990a - Genetic population structure, clonal phylogeny, and pathogenicity of *Salmonella paratyphi* B. *Infect. Immun.* **58**, 1891–1901.

Selander, R.K., P. Beltran, N.H. Smith, R. Helmuth, F.A. Rubin, D.J. Kopecko, K. Ferris, B.D. Tall, A. Cravioto and J.M. Musser, 1990b - Evolutionary genetic relationships of clones of *Salmonella* serovars that cause human typhoid and other enteric fevers. *Infect. Immun.* **58**, 2262–2275.

Selander, R.K., P. Beltran and N.H. Smith, 1991 - Evolutionary genetics of *Salmonella*, p. 25–57. *In* R.K. Selander, A.G. Clark, and T.S. Whittam (ed.), Evolution at the molecular level. Sinauer Associates, Sunderland, Mass.

Selander, R.K., N.H. Smith, J. Li, P. Beltran, K. Ferris, D.J. Kopecko and F.A. Rubin, 1992 - Molecular evolutionary genetics of the cattle-adapted serovar *Salmonella dublin. J. Bacteriol.* **174**, 3587–3592.

Selander, R.K., J. Li, E.F. Boyd, F.-S. Wang and K. Nelson, 1995 - DNA sequence analysis of the genetic structure of populations of *Salmonella enterica* and *Escherichia coli*, p. 1–36. *In* F.G. Priest, A. Ramos-Cormenzana, and R. Tindall (ed.), Bacterial systematics and diversity. Plenum, New York.

Sharp, P.M., J.E. Kelleher, A.S. Daniel, G.M. Cowan and N.E. Murray, 1992 - Roles of selection and recombination in the evolution of type 1 restriction-modification systems in enterobacteria. *Proc. Natl. Acad. Sci. USA* **89**, 9836–9840.

Sibold, C., J. Wang, J. Henrichsen and R. Hakenbeck, 1992 - Genetic relationships of penicillin-susceptible and -resistant *Streptococcus pneumoniae* isolated on different continents. *Infect. Immun.* **60**, 4119–4126.

Simanjuntak, C.H., N.H. Punjabi, F.P. Paleologo, H. Totosudirjo, P. Haryanto, R. Darmowigoto, Soeprawoto [no initials], N.D. Witham, and S.L. Hoffman, 1992 - Vaccine trials for control of typhoid fever in Indonesia, p. 235–241. *In* T. Pang, C.L. Koh, and S.D. Puthucheary (ed.), Typhoid fever. Strategies of the 90's. World Scientific, Singapore.

Skurnik, M. and P. Toivanen, 1994 - *Yersinia enterocolitica* lipopolysaccharide: genetics and virulence. *Trends Microbiol.* **4**, 148–152.

Smith, N.H. and R.K. Selander, 1990 - Sequence invariance of the antigen-coding central region of the phase 1 flagellar filament gene (*fliC*) among strains of *Salmonella typhimurium. J. Bacteriol.* **172**, 603–609.

Smith, N.H. and R.K. Selander, 1991 - Molecular genetic basis for complex flagellar antigen expression in a triphasic serovar of *Salmonella. Proc. Natl. Acad. Sci. USA* **88**, 956–960.

Smith, N.H., P. Beltran and R.K. Selander, 1990 - Recombination of *Salmonella* phase 1 flagellin genes generates new serovars. *J. Bacteriol.* **172**, 2209–2216.

Spratt, B.G., L.D. Bowler, Q.-Y. Zhang, J. Zhou and J. Maynard Smith, 1992 - Role of interspecies transfer of chromosomal genes in the evolution of penicillin resistance in pathogenic and commensal *Neisseria* species. *J. Mol. Evol.* **34**, 115–125.

Stephens, J.C., 1985 - Statistical methods of DNA sequence analysis: detection of intragenic recombination or gene conversion. *Mol. Biol. Evol.* **2**, 539–556.

Stevenson, G., B. Neal, D. Liu, M. Hobbs, N.H. Packer, M. Batley, J.W. Redmond, L. Linquist and P. Reeves, 1994 - Structure of the O antigen of

Escherichia coli K-12 and the sequence of its *rfb* gene cluster. *J. Bacteriol.* **176**, 4144–4156.

Sudarmono, P. and M. Radji, 1992 - Features of typhoid fever in Indonesia, p. 11–16. *In* T. Pang, C.L. Koh, and S.D. Puthucheary (ed.), Typhoid fever. Strategies of the 90's. World Scientific, Singapore.

Thampapapillai, G., R. Lan and P.R. Reeves, 1994 - Molecular evolution in the *gnd* locus of *Salmonella enterica*. *Mol. Biol. Evol.* **11**, 813–828.

Thong, K.L., Y.M. Cheong, S. Puthucheary, C.L. Koh and T. Pang, 1994 - Epidemiologic analysis of sporadic *Salmonella typhi* isolates and those from outbreaks by pulsed-field gel electrophoresis. *J. Clin. Microbiol.* **32**, 1135–1141.

Threlfall, E.J., E. Torre, L.R. Ward, A. Dávalos-Pérez, B. Rowe and I. Gibert, 1994 - Insertion sequence IS*200* fingerprinting of *Salmonella typhi*: an assessment of epidemiological applicability. *Epidemiol. Infect.* **112**, 253–261.

Tominaga, A., M.A.-H. Mahmoud, T. Mukaihara and M. Enomoto, 1994 - Molecular characterization of intact, but cryptic, flagellin genes in the genus *Shigella*. *Mol. Microbiol.* **12**, 277–285.

Vázquez, J.A., L. de la Fuente, S. Berron, M. O'Rourke, N.H. Smith, J. Zhou and B.G. Spratt, 1993 - Ecological separation and genetic isolation of *Neisseria gonorrhoeae* and *Neisseria meningitidis*. *Curr. Biol.* **3**, 567–572.

Whatmore, A.M. and M.A. Kehoe, 1994 - Horizontal gene transfer in the evolution of group A streptococcal *emm*-like genes: gene mosaics and variation in Vir regulons. *Mol. Microbiol.* **11**, 363–374.

Whittam, T.S., 1995 - Genetic population structure and pathogenicity in enteric bacteria, p. 217–245. *In* S. Baumberg, J.P.W. Young, E.M.H. Wellington, and J.R. Saunders (ed.), Population genetics of bacteria. Cambridge University Press, Cambridge.

Whittam, T.S. and S.E. Ake, 1993 - Genetic polymorphisms and recombination in natural populations of *Escherichia coli*, p. 223–245. *In* N. Takahata and A.G. Clark (ed.), Mechanisms of molecular evolution. Sinauer Associates, Sunderland, Massachusetts.

Wilson, D.R. and T.J. Beveridge, 1993 - Bacterial flagellar filaments and their component flagellins. *Can. J. Microbiol.* **39**, 451–472.

Xiang, S.-H., A.M. Haase and P.R. Reeves, 1993 - Variation of the *rfb* gene clusters in *Salmonella enterica*. *J. Bacteriol.* **175**, 4877–4884.

Xiang, S.-H., M. Hobbs and P.R. Reeves, 1994 - Molecular analysis of the *rfb* gene cluster of a group D2 *Salmonella enterica* strain: evidence for its origin from an insertion sequence-mediated recombination event between group E and D1 strains. *J. Bacteriol.* **176**, 4357–4365.

Institute of Molecular Evolutionary Genetics, Pennsylvania State University, University Park, Pennsylvania 16802

Spread of Serogroup A Meningococci: a Paradigm for Bacterial Microevolution

Abstract

Neisseria meningitidis serogroup A bacteria have been subdivided into clonal groupings called subgroups. The global epidemiology of certain subgroups has been investigated and compared with sequence data for variable cell surface or secreted proteins. The results document occasional instances of clonal replacement where recombinant DNA has become established within a bacterial population in a very short period of time.

Bacterial strain collection

A total of about 800 strains of serogroup A *Neisseria meningitidis*, isolated from diverse epidemics since 1915, have been analyzed by multilocus enzyme electrophoresis (MLEE). Initial analyses using 7 cytoplasmic enzymes and 2 outer membrane proteins (OMPs) distinguished 50 electrophoretic types (ETs) differing by at least one allele among 423 isolates from different sources (Olyhoek *et al.*, 1987). Closely related ETs which differed by only 1–2 alleles were grouped into 21 clones belonging to four 'subgroups'. Later work has failed to confirm the existence of the 'clones' (Wang *et al.*, 1992), whereas the subgroup assignments have been supported by various independent analyses. In contrast to this diversity, 75 bacteria isolated from diseased patients and healthy carriers, during (1982–83) and after an epidemic in The Gambia, West Africa, belonged to one single ET within subgroup IV-1 (Crowe *et al.*, 1989). Approximately 70 additional subgroup IV-1 bacteria, isolated between 1963 and 1990 from various countries within the sub-Saharan Sahel region of Africa, allow a comparison of genetic variation within these 3 decades. Over 200 strains of subgroup III serogroup A meningococci, isolated from 2 pandemic waves between 1966 and 1994, have been compared with subgroup IV-1 bacteria for variable cell surface antigens (Achtman *et al.*, 1992). An improved MLEE analysis was performed using 15 cytoplasmic enzymes and 4 OMPs for 290 strains representing the above collection plus an additional 165 strains from additional sources, primarily China (Wang *et al.*, 1992). 84 ETs were recognized which were assigned to the 9 clonal groupings called subgroup I to III, IV-1, IV-1, and V through VIII (Wang *et al.*, 1992).

Epidemiological sources

Subgroup II contains six strains isolated in the 1930's and 1940's in the USA and in the 1960's in Djibouti and may have disappeared. Subgroup IV-2 was isolated from epidemics in World Wars I and II and thereafter from Russia in the 1970 s. Subgroups VII and VIII contain a few bacteria isolated from China between 1956 and 1979 while subgroup VI contains endemic isolates from former East Germany, Scandinavian countries and Russia. The limited numbers of bacteria available from these subgroups suggests that, with time, additional subgroups may be identified when endemic isolates from a greater variety of countries are tested. In contrast, the epidemiology of the other subgroups described below is well defined and numerous isolates are available.

Subgroup I: The following is a reinterpretation of the data presented by Olyhoek *et al.* (1987) forced by the recognition that the subgroup is the basic unit of epidemic spread in serogroup A organisms (Wang *et al.*, 1992). The oldest subgroup I strain available was isolated in the UK in 1941. In the early 1960's, subgroup I bacteria were isolated from an epidemic in Niger and from endemic disease in Algeria, Chad and among US army personnel stationed in West Germany. In 1967, epidemic disease caused by subgroup I flared in North Africa and the Mediterranean and spread by 1968–1972 throughout West Africa. In the early 1970's, subgroup I caused outbreaks among native Americans in Canada followed by outbreaks among 'Skid Road' inhabitants in the Pacific Northwest of the United States (Counts *et al.*, 1984; Olyhoek *et al.*, 1987). Epidemics in Nigeria and Rwanda in the late 1970's were caused by subgroup I (Olyhoek *et al.*, 1987) as was an outbreak among Maoris and Pacific Islanders in New Zealand in 1985 (Schwartz *et al.*, 1989) and an outbreak among aboriginals in central Australia in the late 1980's (Patel *et al.*, 1993) (D. A. Caugant, pers. comm.). During the 1970's, subgroup I meningococci were isolated globally from endemic disease (Olyhoek *et al.*, 1987).

Subgroup IV-1: Subgroup IV-1 is associated with different epidemiological patterns than subgroups I or III. Almost all endemic isolates from West Africa since the early 1960's belong to subgroup IV-1 (Olyhoek *et al.*, 1987) despite two waves of epidemic disease caused by subgroup I in the 1960's and 1970's. In addition, some isolates from an epidemic in Niger in the early 1960's and all isolates from epidemics in West Africa in the early 1980's belonged to subgroup IV-1 (Olyhoek *et al.*, 1987). All subgroup IV-1 bacteria have been isolated in West Africa (Olyhoek *et al.*, 1987; Wang *et al.*, 1992), except for 4 strains isolated in India (Bjorvatn *et al.*, 1992).

Subgroup V: Similar to subgroup IV-1, subgroup V bacteria have only been isolated in China, where they caused epidemic disease in the 1970's and were occasionally isolated in the 1980's (Wang *et al.*, 1992). The epidemiology of these two subgroups shows that even epidemic bacteria are not necessarily able to spread extensively between continents, for unknown reasons.

Subgroup III: Subgroup III bacteria were first isolated from China during a huge epidemic in the mid-1960's and spread to cause epidemics in Moscow

(1969), an outbreak in Norway (1969), and epidemics in Finland and Brazil (mid-1970's) (Achtman *et al.*, 1992; Wang *et al.*, 1992). These bacteria were also responsible for most of the endemic meningococcal disease in Sweden during the 1970's and beginning of the 1980's, but they did not cause any epidemics or outbreaks there (Salih *et al.*, 1990). During the 1970's, subgroup III disappeared from China, to be replaced by subgroup V, but they reappeared in China (and in Nepal) in the early 1980's. Thereafter in 1987, they caused an epidemic in Mecca, Saudi Arabia during the annual Haj pilgrimage (Moore *et al.*, 1988, 1989). Healthy pilgrims carried these bacteria back to their countries of origin, including the USA, UK and France but subgroup III disappeared from most countries within a few years. In contrast, epidemics caused by subgroup III did break out in eastern Africa in 1988 and have continued to affect one African country after another since then (Achtman, 1995a).

The mechanisms responsible for epidemic disease are unknown but several theories based on coinfection with viruses or other bacteria (summarized in (Achtman, 1995a, 1995b; Cartwright, 1995) have been proposed. The results presented above show that it will be difficult to apply population genetic models based on steady state competition to epidemic bacteria.

Genetic variation

The serogroup A subgroups consists of related ETs which differ by a few alleles in MLEE. Such variation is often assumed to reflect evolutionary changes during clonal descent of bacteria derived from a common ancestor. However, the work needed to identify electrophoretic variation is sufficiently laborious that only limited numbers of strains can be investigated. We have used an alternative, less labor-intensive, approach to screen for variation, namely analysis of cell-surface antigens detected by reactivity with monoclonal antibodies (MAbs). Numerous bacteria have been screened for epitopes within pilin, the PorA and PorB porins (also called Class 1 and 3 proteins, respectively), Opa and Opc proteins (collectively called Class 5 proteins), and IgA1 protease (IgA1P). Variation was then analyzed by DNA sequencing, some of which has not yet been published. The results reveal that genetic variation differs with the antigen and with the subgroup and indicate that epidemic spread results in loss of antigenic variation and reduction of clonal diversity. The results with PorA (Wang *et al.*, 1992; Suker *et al.*, 1994) are reviewed in M. Maiden's chapter elsewhere in this volume.

Opc protein

A formerly undescribed Class 5 outer membrane protein, formerly called 5C but now called Opc, was expressed by some of the subgroup IV-1 meningococci from The Gambia (Crowe *et al.*, 1989). The purified Opc protein consists of a trimer or tetramer of 28 KDal subunits (Achtman *et al.*, 1988). The *opc* gene is expressed after cloning in *Escherichia coli* and the recombinant Opc protein is localized on the cell surface (Olyhoek *et al.*, 1991). Expression of Opc enables meningococci to adhere to and invade endothelial or epithelial cells (Virji *et al.*, 1992, 1993). Binding to the apical surface of endothelial cells is dependent on serum factors, such as vitronectin, which bind through their RGD sequences to eukaryotic β-integrins (Virji *et al.*, 1994). The Opc protein is expressed at varying levels by different colonies of the same strain, varying from non-detectable to being one of the major outer membrane proteins. When a single colony is spread on a plate to single colonies, several will differ from the majority phenotype in regard to Opc expression and variation is correlated with changes in the length of a poly-cytidine stretch within the Opc promoter (Sarkari *et al.*, 1994). Poly-C stretches of 12–13 nucleotides are correlated with very efficient transcription and protein expression, stretches of 11 or 14 with intermediate expression and either shorter or longer poly-C stretches with lack of expression.

Meningococcal DNA was subjected to hybridization with the cloned *opc* gene: all serogroup A meningococci gave a positive signal as did many serogroup B, C, 29E, Y and W strains. However, some serogroup B and C bacteria, in particular all ET-37 complex strains, did not give a signal and lack an *opc* gene (Sarkari *et al.*, 1994). PCR products from 110 meningococci containing an *opc* gene have been tested for restriction site polymorphism within the 819 bp region encoding *opc* and the 293 bp region upstream of the coding region. Variant RFLP patterns were identified and sequenced as were representatives of each of the serogroup A subgroups (Seiler, A., *et al.*, man. in prep.) The results show about 1% sequence variation within the coding region, including non-synonymous changes, and 4% within the upstream non-coding region. (None of these sequence polymorphisms affect the site recognized by monoclonal antibody B306 and it is anticipated that this antibody will recognize all Opc protein variants in meningococci.) Some strains contain a 250 bp insert at a particular nucleotide within the upstream region, and that insert is itself subject to about 10% sequence variation. Although at first glance, these results resemble those expected of evolutionary variation by slow accumulation of mutations, much of the sequence polymorphism occurs in mosaic blocks with different combinations of the same nucleotides and it seems as if the rearrangement of these sequence variants reflects recombinational exchange. The insertion is also present or absent in otherwise identical alleles indicating that it too is subject to recombinational exchange.

Among serogroup A meningococci, the same allele of *opc* was found in all subgroups except subgroup IV-2, where it differed by 1 nucleotide. No sequence differences were found within the 293 bp upstream region, except for a 1 nucleotide difference in subgroups V and VII, which were identical, and another single nucleotide difference in subgroup IV-2. These results are compatible with the notion that all serogroup A meningococci are descended from one common ancestor, which contained a primordial *opc* allele, and that only limited evolution has occurred or been maintained since then. Interestingly, one subgroup IV-2 variant, isolated in Britain in 1942, has been identified in which the whole

1.1 Kb region has been replaced by a different allele containing numerous nucleotide exchanges as well as the 250 bp insert in the upstream region. Because this *opc* allele was only found once while other subgroup IV-2 bacteria isolated both considerably earlier and later followed the pattern described above, this variant seems not to have spread extensively.

The Opc protein is immunogenic in humans (Rosenqvist *et al.*, 1993) and bactericidal antibodies were stimulated after immunization with an outer membrane vesicle vaccine. It might have been expected that an immunogenic protein would be under selection pressure and more sequence variation should have been observed. Two possible explanations are i) that the *opc* gene has only recently been introduced into meningococci and has not yet had time to evolve and ii) that variable expression of Opc prevents bactericidal antibodies from being effective because only few of the infecting bacteria express sufficient Opc for the antibodies to be effective.

Opa proteins

opa genes consist of conserved sequences surrounding two highly variable regions, called HV1 and HV2, which are exposed on the cell surface. Whereas 11 or 12 *opa* genes are present on the chromosome of *N. gonorrhoeae*, meningococci only contain 3 or 4 (Aho *et al.*, 1991; Hobbs *et al.*, 1994). Serogroup A meningococci from The Gambia contained 3 *opa* genes, called *opaA*, *opaB* and *opaD* (Hobbs *et al.*, 1994), in addition to *opc. opaA* and *opaB* have an identical HV1 region while *opaB* and *opaD* have an identical HV2 region. In addition, a 9 bp repeat is duplicated in tandem within *opaB*. Individual Opa proteins were screened by SDS PAGE for size differences and by reactivity with MAbs recognizing specific HV regions. Within The Gambia, almost all Opa proteins were indistinguishable from OpaA, OpaB or OpaD but an exceptional protein was found (5e) which migrated differently (Achtman *et al.*, 1991). This *opa* gene consisted of a variant *opaB* in which the tandem 9 bp duplication had been resolved, with the corresponding loss of 3 amino acids (Hobbs *et al.*, 1994). Sequencing of other variant strains revealed 1 strain in which *opaB* had translocated to the locus of *opaA*, replacing it and yielding a chromosome with *opaD* plus 2 copies of *opaB*. In still another strain, DNA had been imported from an unknown source, leading to an altered *opaD* locus containing novel HV1 and HV2 regions. The novel HV1 region had then translocated to replace that of *opaB*. Unpublished results (Cannon, J.C., pers. comm.) confirm that most other serogroup A meningococci isolated from The Gambia possessed indistinguishable *opa* genes from those present in the reference strain.

The Opa proteins expressed by subgroup IV-1 bacteria differed with the country of origin (Achtman, 1994). One strain isolated in Ghana in 1970 possessed an indistinguishable *opaA* gene but possessed an *opaF* allele at the *opaD* locus and an *opaG* allele at the *opaB* locus. *opaF* differs from *opaD* in the HV2 region, which is almost identical to that of an *opa* gene in *N. gonorrhoeae* strain MS-11. *opaG* differs from *opaB* in the HV1 region, which is almost identical to that of an *opa* gene in serogroup C meningococci of the ET-37 complex (Hobbs *et al.*, 1994).

More recent analyses (Malorny, B. *et al.*, man. in prep.) have concentrated on *opa* genes from subgroup III and other subgroup IV-1 strains from different countries. Subgroup III serogroup A meningococci isolated prior to the Mecca epidemic of 1987 variably expressed Opa proteins formerly called 5a, 5f and/or 5h while those isolated during or after that epidemic expressed 5a, 5f and/or 5i (Achtman *et al.*, 1992). Proteins indistinguishable from 5f and 5h were also expressed by some subgroup IV-1 strains isolated in the 1960's (Achtman *et al.*, 1988). The sequences of these *opa* genes, *opaF* and *opaH*, have now been determined. *opaF* is indistinguishable to that described above while *opaH* is a novel, formerly undescribed gene. Subgroup III meningococci contain 4 *opa* alleles (plus *opc*) and the sequences of the *opa* genes from the bacteria isolated prior to Mecca correspond to *opaA*, *opaF*, *opaH* plus a new gene, *opaJ*. The former 3 sequences are identical to those in subgroup IV-1 bacteria from the 1960's, indicating that such sequences can be inherited over very long periods of time, and that subgroup III and IV-1 are descended from a common ancestor. The *opa* genes have also been sequenced from one subgroup III strain isolated after the Mecca epidemic. *opaA* and *opaJ* are unchanged. *opaF* differs by 1 nucleotide and *opaH* has been replaced by a novel gene, *opaI*. The mechanisms leading to nucleotide exchange are unclear but the genetic replacement can only have happened by import of foreign DNA in the mid-1980's. OpaH (5h) was never expressed by any subgroup III meningococci isolated in Africa after 1988 and it is amazing that such a genetic recombination event can have been fixed within this short period of time.

IgA1 Protease

IgA1 protease is a highly immunogenic (Brooks *et al.*, 1992) protein secreted by all meningococci and gonococci. Within serogroup A meningococci, MAbs to 3 variable epitopes distinguished 6 antigenic variants, which were uniform within individual subgroups, except subgroup III (Morelli *et al.*, 1994). Subgroup III bacteria isolated prior to the Mecca epidemic expressed one serological variant of IgA1P while bacteria isolated later expressed a different variant. During the few months after the Mecca outbreak, 4 strains were isolated which still expressed the ancestral serological variant. Two of these four strains also expressed OpaH while the two others expressed neither OpaH nor OpaI and have not yet been tested by DNA techniques.

The 3 Kb segment of the *iga* gene encoding the mature IgA1 protease has been sequenced from 4 meningococci (Morelli *et al.*, man. in prep.) and shows minor sequence variation throughout the gene. The *iga* sequences from meningococci isolated prior to Mecca and post Mecca differ in two regions by numerous nucleotides, indicating that at least one and possibly two recombinational events have occurred. T-track comparisons of numerous *iga* genes from post-Mecca subgroup III meningococci showed no differences: all contained the recombinant sequence (Morelli *et al.*, man. in prep.). However, diversity was found within 6 strains isolated in China in 1966. 2 of the sequences contain a T at a position where the other 6 and subsequent isolates possessed a C. Thus, at least two sequential events of clonal replacement have occurred in these bacteria, with bacteria isolated after 1966 all possessing the C nucleotide and bacteria isolated post-Mecca containing the recombinant sequence.

Clonal expansion and replacement

The most surprising aspect of the work described above is the speed with which serogroup A populations can be replaced by variants which differ in one or more alleles. These results contrast with the relative uniformity of these bacteria within any one epidemic or most epidemic waves. Several examples have also been described where sequences have been uniform since the evolution of the individual subgroups. Yet, over just a few years, other genes can be totally replaced leading to a uniform recombinant population.

The phenomenon of epidemic spread has been reviewed elsewhere (Achtman, 1994, 1995b) and the differences to periodic selection emphasized. Although the role of selection in clonal replacement remains uncertain, I believe that spread of only few bacteria from country to country coupled with a high rate of recombination during epidemics is at least as likely to explain clonal replacement as are selection pressures (Achtman, 1994, 1995b).

The analysis of genetic phenomena in meningococci complements analyses of bacterial populations that do not spread rapidly and that do not seem to possess efficient methods of genetic exchange. Our data with meningococci illustrate several of the phenomena predicted by population biologists (see chapters by Milkman and Selander in this volume) and show that these occur continuously within relatively short periods of time, decades rather than millennia. Correlation with the epidemiology of infectious disease may allow a better understanding of microevolution in bacteria and meningococci may well be a paradigm for studying such phenomena.

References

Achtman, M., M. Neibert, B.A. Crowe, W. Strittmatter, B. Kusecek, E. Weyse, M.J. Walsh, B. Slawig, G. Morelli, A. Moll and M. Blake, 1988 - Purification and characterization of eight class 5 outer membrane protein variants from a clone of *Neisseria meningitidis* serogroup A. *J. Exp. Med.* **168**, 507–525.

Achtman, M., R.A. Wall, M. Bopp, B. Kusecek, G. Morelli, E. Saken and M. Hassan-King, 1991 - Variation in Class 5 protein expression by serogroup A meningococci during a meningitis epidemic. *J. Infect. Dis.* **164**, 375–382.

Achtman, M., B. Kusecek, G. Morelli, K. Eickmann, J. Wang, B. Crowe, R.A. Wall, M. Hassan-King, P.S. Moore and W. Zollinger, 1992 - A comparison of the variable antigens expressed by clone IV-1 and subgroup III of *Neisseria meningitidis* serogroup A. *J. Infect. Dis.* **165**, 53–68.

Achtman, M., 1994 - Clonal spread of serogroup A meningococci. A paradigm for the analysis of microevolution in bacteria. *Mol. Microbiol.* **11**, 15–22.

Achtman, M., 1995a - Global epidemiology of meningococcal disease. 159–175.

Achtman, M., 1995b - Epidemic spread and antigenic variability of *Neisseria meningitidis*. *Trends Microbiol.* **3**, 186–192.

Aho, E.L., J.A. Dempsey, M.M. Hobbs, D.G Klapper and J.G. Cannon, 1991 - Characterization of the *opa* (class 5) gene family of *Neisseria meningitidis*. *Mol. Microbiol.* **5**, 1429–1437.

Bjorvatn, B., M. Hassan-King, B. Greenwood, R.T. Haimanot, D. Fekade and G. Sperber, 1992 - DNA fingerprinting in the epidemiology of African serogroup A *Neisseria meningitidis*. *Scand. J. Infect. Dis.* **24**, 323–332.

Brooks, G.F., C.J. Lammel, M.S. Blake, B. Kusecek and M. Achtman, 1992 - Antibodies against IgA1 protease are stimulated both by clinical disease and by asymptomatic carriage of serogroup A *Neisseria meningitidis*. *J. Infect. Dis.* **166**, 1316–1321.

Cartwright, K., 1995 - Meningococcal carriage and disease. In: Meningococcal Disease, K. Cartwright (Ed.), *John Wiley & Sons*, Chichester, pp. 115–146.

Counts, G.W., D.F. Gregory, J.G. Spearman, A.L. Barrett, G.A. Filice, K.K. Holmes and J.M. Griffiss, 1984 - Group A meningococcal disease in the U. S. Pacific Northwest: Epidemiology, clinical features, and effect of a vaccine control program. *Rev. Infect. Dis.* **6**, 640–648.

Crowe, B.A., R.A. Wall, B. Kusecek, B. Neumann, T. Olyhoek, H. Abdillahi, M. Hassan-King, B.M. Greenwood, J.T. Poolman and M. Achtman, 1989 - Clonal and variable properties of *Neisseria meningitidis* isolated from cases and carriers during and after an epidemic in the Gambia, West Africa. *J. Infect. Dis.* **159**, 686–700.

Hobbs, M.M., A. Seiler, M. Achtman and J.G. Cannon, 1994 - Microevolution within a clonal population of pathogenic bacteria: recombination, gene duplication and horizontal genetic exchange in the *opa* gene family of *Neisseria meningitidis*. *Mol. Microbiol.* **12**, 171–180.

Moore, P.S., L.H. Harrison, E.E. Telzak, G.W. Ajello and C.V. Broome, 1988 - Group A meningococcal carriage in travelers returning from Saudi Arabia. *JAMA*, **260**, 2686–2689.

Moore, P.S., M.W., Reeves, B. Schwartz, B.G. Gellin and C.V. Broome, 1989 - Intercontinental spread of an epidemic group A *Neisseria meningitidis* strain. *Lancet*, **ii**, 260–263.

Morelli, G., J. del Valle, C.J. Lammel, J. Pohlner, K. Müller, M. Blake, G.F. Brooks, T.F. Meyer, B. Koumaré, N. Brieske and M. Achtman, 1994 - Immunogenicity and evolutionary variability of epitopes within IgA1 protease from serogroup A *Neisseria meningitidis*. *Mol. Microbiol.* **11**, 175–187.

Olyhoek, A.J.M., J. Sarkari, M. Bopp, G. Morelli and M. Achtman, 1991 - Cloning and expression in *Escherichia coli* of *opc*, the gene for an unusual class 5 outer membrane protein from *Neisseria meningitidis. Microb. Pathog.* **11**, 249–257.

Olyhoek, T., B.A. Crowe and M. Achtman, 1987 - Clonal population structure of *Neisseria meningitidis* serogroup A isolated from epidemics and pandemics between 1915 and 1983. *Rev. Infect. Dis.* **9**, 665–692.

Patel, M.S., A. Merianos, J.N. Hanna, K. Vartto, P. Tait, F. Morey and S. Jayathissa, 1993 - Epidemic meningococcal meningitis in central Australia, 1987-1991. *Med. J. Aust.* **158**, 336–340.

Rosenqvist, E., E.A. Høiby, E. Wedege, B. Kusecek and M. Achtman, 1993 - The 5C protein of *Neisseria meningitidis* is highly immunogenic in humans and induces bactericidal antibodies. *J. Infect. Dis.* **167**, 1065–1073.

Salih, M.A.M., D. Danielsson, A. Bäckman, D.A. Caugant, M. Achtman and P. Olcén, 1990 - Characterization of epidemic and non-epidemic *Neisseria meningitidis* serogroup A strains from Sudan and Sweden. *J. Clin. Microbiol.* **28**, 1711–1719.

Sarkari, J., N. Pandit, E.R. Moxon and M. Achtman, 1994 - Variable expression of the Opc outer membrane protein in *Neisseria meningitidis* is caused by size variation of a promoter containing poly-cytidine. *Mol. Microbiol.* **13**, 207–217.

Schwartz, B., P.S. Moore and C.V. Broome, 1989 - Global epidemiology of meningococcal disease. *Clin. Microbiol. Rev.* **2 Suppl.** S118–S124.

Suker, J., I.M. Feavers, M. Achtman, G. Morelli, J. Wang and M.C.J. Maiden, 1994 - The *porA* gene in serogroup A meningococci: evolutionary stability and mechanism of genetic variation. *Mol. Microbiol.* **12**, 253–265.

Virji, M., K. Makepeace, D.J.P. Ferguson, M. Achtman, J. Sarkari and E.R. Moxon, 1992 - Expression of the Opc protein correlates with invasion of epithelial and endothelial cells by *Neisseria meningitidis. Mol. Microbiol.* **6**, 2785–2795.

Virji, M., K. Makepeace, D.J.P. Ferguson, M. Achtman and E.R. Moxon, 1993 - Meningococcal Opa and Opc proteins: their role in colonization and invasion of human epithelial and endothelial cells. *Mol. Microbiol.* **10**, 499–510.

Virji, M., K. Makepeace and E.R. Moxon, 1994 - Distinct mechanisms of interactions of Opc-expressing meningococci at apical and basolateral surfaces of human endothelial cells; The role of integrins in apical interactions. *Mol. Microbiol.* **14**, 173–184.

Wang, J., D.A. Caugant, X. Li, X. Hu, J.T. Poolman, B.A. Crowe and M. Achtman, 1992 - Clonal and antigenic analysis of serogroup A Neisseria meningitidis with particular reference to epidemiological features of epidemic meningitis in China. *Infect. Immun.* **60**, 5267–5282.

R. Hakenbeck

Evolution of Penicillin-Binding Protein Genes of Sensitive Streptococci into Resistance Determinants of *Streptococcus pneumoniae*

Abstract

Different clones of penicillin-resistant strains can be recognized which have spread, within a country, across borders and even intercontinentally. The genes encoding penicillin-binding proteins, the primary targets for β-lactam antibiotics, have mosaic structure in all resistant isolates examined, and encode PBP variants with low affinity to β-lactams. Commensal, sensitive streptococcal species have been identified as origin of the mosaic blocks, and there is evidence that these genes have been changed via point mutations into resistance determinants. The mosaic PBP genes can be identical in different clones, related in related clones, or highly variable within a clone, demonstrating a different history of gene transfer.

Introduction

Several parameters have to be studied in order to understand evolution and spread of penicillin-resistant *Streptococcus pneumoniae*, a problem of growing concern worldwide (Schutze *et al.*, 1994). This paper summarizes data on clonal distribution of resistant *S. pneumoniae*, and discusses sequence analysis of genes involved in resistance development in this and other related streptococcal species.

Determination of the clonal structure is one of the prerequisites for understanding the dynamics of occurrence and spread of such strains. Although several reports have been published since the problem of antibiotic resistant pneumococci has been recognized, the results are often biased by a selective collection of a few strains, obtained from a few hospitals and only over a short period of time. Nevertheless, the predominance of a few clones associated with various serotypes in some countries became obvious, such as serotype 6A in South Africa, serotype 19A in Hungary, and serotype 9V, 6B and 23F in Spain (Muñóz *et al.*, 1992; Sibold *et al.*, 1992). In addition, single isolates which are genetically unrelated are frequently encountered in every sample analyzed, already demonstrating that resistance in the pneumococcus has emerged on multiple occsaions. A rapid way for identifying clones in a large number of strains is based on the characterization of PBP properties by using antibodies that distinguish between epitope variants of PBP1a and 2b of resistant isolates in combination of PBP profiles revealed after labeling with radioactive β-lactam followed by SDS-polyacrylamide gel electrophoresis and fluorography (Hakenbeck *et al.*, 1991a; Hakenbeck *et al.*, 1991b). Such clones were confirmed on the basis of multilocus enzyme electrophoresis (MLEE) (Sibold *et al.*, 1992), pulsed-field gel electrophoresis of chromosomal DNA (Lefevre *et al.*, 1993), and fingerprinting of PBP genes (Coffey *et al.*, 1991).

No data on clonal structure are available from strains collected before the 1980es, and it is assumed on the mere basis of quantity, i.e. a high percentage of resistant strains in a geographic area, that resistant strains emerged e.g. in the countries mentioned above and have spread from there into other countries with lower numbers of resistant isolates. Already a classical example of such a development is the sudden occurrence of serotype 6B isolates in Iceland in the late 80s followed by a dramatic increase of such strains that represent the same clone which is predominant in Spain only within a few years (Soares *et al.*, 1993). There is, however, no proof for such assumptions, and it cannot be excluded that the same clone exists in many different locations over a long period of time, and that for unknown reasons proliferation is favoured at certain times in certain areas.

Penicillin-resistance in clinical isolates of streptococci is mediated by alterations in penicillin-binding proteins (PBPs), the target enzymes for β-lactam action (Hakenbeck, 1995). PBPs are inhibited by β-lactam antibiotics upon forming a covalent penicilloyl-complex via a serine residue in their active center. PBP-variants in resistant strains have a reduced penicillin affinity, and consequently a much higher concentration is required for inhibiting their enzymatic functions, and the biological activity of the drug is also reduced. Four of the six pneumococcal PBPs have been shown to be phenotypically altered in resistant isolates (Laible *et al.*, 1991). The three penicillin-binding proteins PBP2x, 2b and 1a, have been characterized as mosaic genes in all resistant isolates examined so far, where divergent blocks of approximately 20% divergence have replaced homologous sequences of the sensitive strain (Laible *et al.*, 1991; Martin *et al.*, 1992; Dowson *et al.*, 1989). This strongly suggests that gene transfer events are required for evolution of these genes into resistance determinants, a concept that has emerged through early analysis of non-β-lactamase producing penicillin resistant *Neisseria* sp. where similar mechanisms are operating (Spratt *et al.*, 1991).

The degree of divergence may be controlled by two factors: i- the recombination is markedly reduced if DNA of more than 20% divergence is used in transformation experiments (Humbert *et al.*, 1995); ii- the changes in the amino acid sequence of the PBP need to be tolerable for the cell, since their important biosynthetic functions have to be maintained. Nevertheless, resistant isolates contain chemically altered peptidoglycan and this property is transferred together with penicillin resistance into sensitive recipient strains, indicating that changes in penicillin affinity also affect substrate specificity of at least one of the PBPs (Garcia-Bustos and Tomasz, 1990; Garcia-Bustos *et al.*, 1995).

Comparison of a wide variety of genes from different resistant *S. pneumoniae* isolates indicates that more than five different species contribute to the gene pool from which pneumococci can recruit homologous sequences. In penicillin resistant *Neisseria gonorrhoeae* and *N. meningitis*, such sequences apparently originate from commensal species that are naturally higher penicillin resistant (Spratt *et al.*, 1991). However, no such naturally resistant commensal streptococci exist that could account for MIC levels that exceed 1 μg/ml easily in resistant isolates. On the other hand, commensals with very high levels of penicillin resistance are reported with increasing frequency (Guiot *et al.*, 1994). We hope that with more available sequence information of a wide variety of species and strains, the evolutionary history can be further clarified.

Clones of resistant *S. pneumoniae* in Europe

We have analyzed resistant clinical isolates in several countries in Europe (Reichmann *et al.*, 1995): Spain and Hungary, which were the first European countries reporting on high rates of penicillin and multiple resistant isolates (Fenoll *et al.*, 1991; Marton, 1992), France where an increase of resistant strains is observed since the late 80s (Geslin *et al.*, 1992), and Germany and Finland where resistance is below 10% (Reinert *et al.*, 1994; Schutze *et al.*, 1994). Fig. 1 shows different patterns seen for different clonal groups as determined by multi-locus enzyme electrophoresis. Circles represent clones found in the various countries, small circles indicate that only one member of such isolate was detected. The same pattern (black, white or dark grey) is used for identical clones connected by lines, dotted lines between different clones indicate a close genetic relationship.

Members of a serotype 9V clone have been isolated in Spain since 1987, and the frequency of serotype 9V resistant isolates in France increased from 1988 where the first such isolate was recorded to 15% in 1993 (Geslin *et al.*, 1993). Type 9V strains from both countries are one clone, and a member of this clone has also been isolated in Germany, curiously from a Spanish child (Gasc *et al.*, 1995; Hakenbeck *et al.*, 1994) (Fig. 1, top).

The penicillin and multiresistant serotype 23F clone, which has been identified in the US (Muñóz *et al.*, 1992) and South Africa (Sibold *et al.*, 1992), was found in every country, even in Hungary, the only example we have seen so far where members of the same clone appeared in a West and an East European country (Fig. 1, middle) (Reichmann *et al.*, 1995). The 23F isolate from Hungary has been isolated in the early 90s, and could have been imported via facilitated and increased travel activities between West and East European countries. However, as stated above, we have no means to come to a final conlusion on this subject. A closely related 23F clone, that differed only by one allele and had slightly different MICs for penicillin, was observed in Germany, members of which were

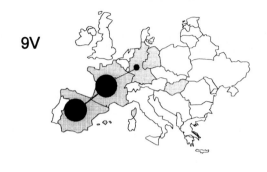

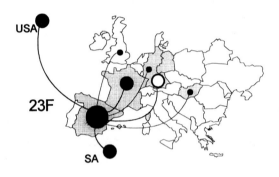

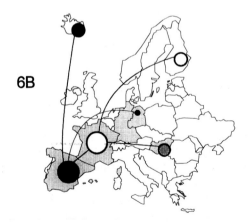

Fig. 1. Relationship between penicillin-resistant *S. pneumoniae* strains. See text for explanation.

Evolution of penicillin-binding protein genes

isolated in various West German cities. Again we do not know whether this clone has evolved only recently. In this context it is remarkable that all resistant isolates from West Germany examined were either single isolates or related to clones from Western European countries, whereas resistant strains obtained from Jena that were isolated before 1989 were either single or related to a clone in Hungary, strongly suggesting that this picture is a result of restricted travel activities before 1989. Another three genetically distinct serotype 23F clones were recognized in this study, consisting of isolates from Finland, Hungary and former East Germany, and France and West Germany.

The pattern of serotype 6B isolates is still different (Fig. 1, bottom). A group of closely related serotype 6B clones was identified, with each clone being found in one country only. These were a type 6B clone from Finland described before (Hakenbeck *et al.*, 1991a), a 6B clone in France which was identical in its MLEE profile but distinct in PBP properties compared to the Finish isolates, a group of 6B isolates from Hungary, and the multiresistant Spanish 6B clone, one member of which was isolated in West Berlin. It will be interesting to follow the dynamics of these clones in the future.

Mosaic PBP genes in Spanish clones

Penicillin-resistant isolates of the three serotypes 9V, 6B and 23F, belong to three distinct clones which cluster at different position in the dendogram shown in Fig. 2, a compilation of a recent survey of resistant *S. pneumoniae* in Europe (Reichmann *et al.*, 1995). Isolates, respectively clones are indicated by number of the electrophoretic type (ET), serotype, and origin (Sp, Spain; F, France; Fi, Finland, G, Germany, Cz, Czech Republic, Hu, Hungary). Nevertheless, fingerprinting analysis of the *pbp1a, 2x* and *2b* genes strongly suggested that the 9V isolates contain identical PBP genes compared to the 23F clone (Coffey *et al.*, 1991). Indeed, the *pbp2x* genes are 100% identical not only within the mosaic block but also in the 'sensitive' region which is expected if chromosomal DNA fragments are exchanged as indicated in Fig. 2. DNA sequences of *pbp2x* genes (Sibold *et al.*, 1994) and also of *pbp1a* genes (Martin *et al.*, 1992) of members of the 6B and 23F clone revealed that long segments of the mosaic blocks in both genes are identical to those in the corresponding genes of the 23F clone, and identity meant almost 100% identity indeed. However, different borders of the mosaic blocks and short divergent regions indicated that the mosaic genes must have been introduced into these two clones independent from each other, and the 'sensitive' sequence parts differed also. Thus, resistance development in Spain involves one main genetic source, and incluced interspecies gene transfer in respect to the type 23F and 9V clone, and intraspecies gene transfer in respect to those two and the 6B clone.

The class of mosaic gene that occurs in the major Spanish clones is also found in a wide variety of resistant *S. pneumoniae* as well as other streptococci isolated in different countries and continents (Reichmann, König and Hakenbeck,

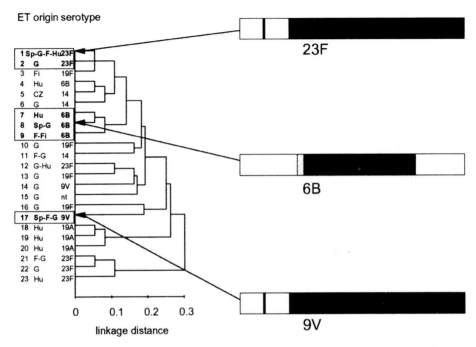

Fig. 2. Cluster analysis, based on multilocus enzyme electrophoresis, of European penicillin-resistant *S. pneumoniae* strains. Composition of mosaic structure of 3 *pbp2x* genes present in Spanish strains.

unpublished results). Thus, this gene is widely distributed and enough time has elapsed to allow for divergence ranging from a few nucleotides up to a few percent. Still another feature was detected in Hungarian 19A isolates, the only case so far where a high degree of variation in mosaic structure of PBP genes was seen within a clone (Reichmann and Hakenbeck, unpublished results).

Origin of divergent sequences in pneumococcal PBP genes

As mentioned above, no naturally resistant commensal streptococcal species exists to our knowledge that could account for PBPs as resistance determinants for the highly penicillin resistant pneumcoocci. It was nevertheless surprising to find *pbp2x* genes from perfectly penicillin sensitive *S. oralis* and *S. mitis* that were less than 4% divergent from mosaic blocks in homologous genes of resistant *S. pneumoniae* (Sibold *et al.*, 1994) (König and Hakenbeck, unpublished results), i.e. they differed by only a few amino acids. Similarly, the mosaic block of *pbp2b* genes in several resistant *S. pneumoniae* also consisted of *S. mitis* DNA (Dowson *et al.*, 1993). Fig. 3 documents the relationship between an *S. oralis*

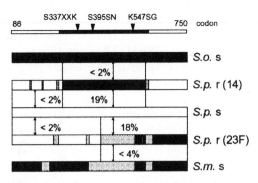

Fig. 3. Schematic representation of the mosaic structure of *pbpx* genes from penicillin-sensitive streptococci and penicillin-resistant *S. pneumoniae* strains. The shading indicates related sequences. s, sequence of genes from sensitive or resistant (r) strains. Light grey, unrelated sequences of unknown origin. Abbreviations *S. mitis* (*S.m.*), *S. oralis* (*S.o.*), *S. pneumoniae* (*S.p.*) serotype 14 and 23 F. See text for further explanation.

pbp2x gene to a resistant *S. pneumoniae* type 14 strain isolated in the Czech Republic in 1987 (Laible *et al.*, 1991). In this figure, very similar sequences are shown by identical pattern (black, white, or shaded). The general design of the PBP2x is shown on top, with the central penicillin-binding domain drawn in black. The three homology boxes that are common to all PBPs are also indicated; the SXXK sequence contains the active site serine and is in the sensitive streptococci STMK and in most resistant *S. pneumoniae* isolates SATK. The % divergence in nucleotide sequence is also shown. One should point out that the *S. oralis* sequence is that from a South African isolate, and that this class of mosaic genes is the one which is widely distributred and found in the three Spanish clones as described above. *S. mitis* related *pbp2x* genes were found in a French isolate of serotype 23F, member of a clone of intermediate penicillin resistance that can be frequently be isolated in France meanwhile (Fig. 3) (Reichmann *et al.*, 1995), and is often found in mosaic genes of Hungarian 19A isolates (Reichmann, König and Hakenbeck, unpublished results). It is curious that both, the Hungarian 19A clone and the French 23F clone, also share other properties (Reichmann *et al.*, 1995): they cluster distinct from the Spanish clones (see Fig. 2), and both contain a PBP3 with unusual higher electrophoretic mobility suggesting a common ancestor.

Only the gene of the resistant pneumococci transferred readily cefotaxime resistance into sensitive strains, *S. pneumoniae* as well as *S. mitis*, demonstrating that a few amino acids account for the phenotypic difference, and that the gene functions as a resistance determinant in different species. The amino acid changes that distinguish the sensitive from the resistant gene were generally not necessarily shared by mosaic *pbp2x* genes of other resistant pneumococcal clones, confirming the flexibility of resistance development documented in *pbp2x* of laboratory mutants (Laible and Hakenbeck, 1991) and also documenting a distinct evolutionary history within this class of mosaic genes. Most remarkably, however, was the fact that even the *pbp2x* gene of the sensitive *S. mitis* and *S. oralis* could be transformed into sensitive *S. pneumoniae* recipients, and that such transformants were slightly less susceptible to β-lactams than any one of the parental strains (Sibold *et al.*, 1994). These results in addition to sequence data obtained with *pbp2x* genes of various transformants point out several issues important if one attempts to deduce the evolutionary history of a mosaic gene retrospectively.

i- mosaic genes exist in sensitive streptococci. This is true for the *S. mitis pbp2x* gene compared to the *S. oralis* gene, and was also seen in *S. pneumoniae* transformants obtained with *pbp2x* of the sensitive *S. mitis* in the laboratory (Fig. 3). Thus, alterations contributing to the evolution of a PBP gene into a resistance determinant could in principle occur before or after transfer into another species resulted in a mosaic structure.

ii- the history of a mosaic gene can only be deduced if both, donor and recipient, are known. This sounds trivial and in fact is, but it is nevertheless important to realize that the donor DNA does not necessarily constitute the central mosaic block of a mosaic gene resulting from transformation experiments, but that also the reverse situation can occur where donor sequences represent 3' and 5' flanking regions of a central sequence block of the recipient gene (Fig. 4A).

iii- the *S. pneumoniae* transformants obtained with the *pbp2x* gene of the sensitive *S. oralis* or *S. mitis* were slightly higher resistant than each of the parental strains, but no mutation could be detected in their (mosaic) *pbp2x* genes. Thus it appears that the mosaic structure per se can contribute to changes in penicillin susceptibility. It also shows that a homologous PBP gene apparently functions perfectly well in a different species, at least under laboratory conditions, without further modification.

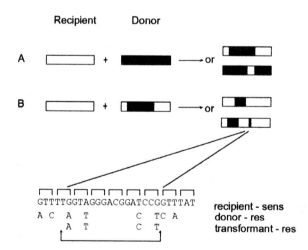

Fig. 4. Examples of the formation of mosaic BPB genes. B. shows a mosaic constructed in the laboratory containing multiple recombinationable events. See text for further explanation.

iv- the apparent recombination sites in mosaic *pbp2x* genes constructed in the laboratory were identical to those found in *pbp2x* of (unrelated) resistant clinical isolates containing even different divergent sequences. This shows that apparent identical borders in different mosaic genes are not necessarily an indication of evolutionary relatedness.

v- one curiosity was noted that could explain the higher degree of divergence between sensitive sequences of different mosaic genes (around 4%), compared to sequences of genes from unrelated sensitive isolates (less than 1%). As shown in Fig. 4B, the transfer event where the *pbp2x* gene from a resistant type 6B pneumococcus was introduced into a sensitive strains involved more than one apparent recombination event, resulting in a very short region of divergence in addition to a longer mosaic block (Sibold *et al.*, 1994). The short block does not result in an amino acid change at this site, excluding the possibility that selection plays a role. It also shows that recombination does not necessarily occur in regions of high homology; instead, apparent recombination sites do occur between two altered nucleotides. Since the enzymes responsible for recombination are not known yet, the molecular mechanism responsible for such structures is also not known.

We believe that *β*-lactam resistant commensal streptococci represent a potent reservoir for resistance determinants—altered PBP genes—readily available to the pneumococcus. In order to understand molecular epidemiology of PBP genes, such strains which are often not recognized since they usually do not cause disease should be included in future studies.

References

Coffey, T.J., C.G. Dowson, M. Daniels, J. Zhou, C. Martin, B.G. Spratt and J.M. Musser, 1991 - Horizontal transfer of multiple penicillin-binding protein genes, and capsular biosynthetic genes, in natural populations of *Streptococcus pneumoniae*, *Mol. Microbiol.* **5**, 2255–2260.

Dowson, C.G., T.J. Coffey, C. Kell and R.A. Whiley, 1993 - Evolution of penicillin resistance in *Streptococcus pneumoniae*; the role of *Streptococcus mitis* in the formation of a low affinity PBP2B in *S. pneumoniae*, *Mol. Microbiol.* **9**, 635–643.

Dowson, C.G., A. Hutchison and B.G. Spratt, 1989 - Extensive re-modelling of the transpeptidase domain of penicillin-binding protein 2B of a penicillin-resistant South African isolate of *Streptococcus pneumoniae*, *Mol. Microbiol.* **3**, 95–102.

Fenoll, A., C.M. Bourgon, R. Muñóz, D. Vicioso and J. Casal, 1991 - Serotype distribution and antimicrobial resistance of *Streptococcus pneumoniae* isolates causing systemic infections in Spain, 1979-1989 - *Rev. Infect. Dis.* **13**, 56–60.

Garcia-Bustos, J.F., B. Chait and A. Tomasz, 1995 - Altered peptidoglycan structure in a pneumococcal transformant resistant to penicillin, *J. Bacteriol.* **170**, 2143–2147.

Garcia-Bustos, J. and A. Tomasz, 1990 - A biological price of antibiotic resistance: major changes in the peptidoglycan structure of penicillin-resistant pneumococci, *Proc. Nat. Acad. Sci. U.S.A.* **87**, 5415–5419.

Gasc, A.M., P. Geslin and A.M. Sicard, 1995 - Relatedness of penicillin-resistant *Streptococcus pneumoniae* serogroup 9 strains from France and Spain, *Microbiology* **141**, 623–627.

Geslin, P., A. Buu-Hoi, A. Fremaux and J.F. Acar, 1992 - Antimicrobial resistance in *Streptococcus pneumoniae*: an epidemiological survey in France, 1970–1990 - *Clin. Infect. Dis.* **15**, 95–98.

Geslin, P., A. Frémaux and G. Sissia, 1993 - Epidemiologie de la résistance de *Streptococcus pneumoniae* aux bêta-lactamines en France et dans le monde, in, Carbon, C., Chastang, C., and Decazes, J.M. (eds.), *Infection à pneumocoqes de sensibilité diminueé aux bêta-lactamines*. Springer Verlag: Paris, p. 55–71.

Guiot, H.F.L., L.J.A. Corel and J.M.J.J. Vossen, 1994 - Prevalence of penicillin-resistant viridans streptococci in healthy children and in patients with malignant haematological disorders, *Eur. J. Clin. Microbiol. Infect. Dis.* **13**, 645–650.

Hakenbeck, R., 1995 - Target mediated resistance to β-lactam antibiotics: *Biochem. Pharmacol.* **50**, 1121–1127.

Hakenbeck, R., T. Briese, L. Chalkley, H. Ellerbrok, R. Kalliokoski, C. Latorre, M. Leinonen and C. Martin, 1991a - Antigenic variation of penicillin-binding proteins from penicillin resistant clinical strains of *Streptococcus pneumoniae*, *J. Infect. Dis.* **164**, 313–319.

Hakenbeck, R., G. Laible, T. Briese, C. Martin, L. Chalkley, C. Latorre, R. Kalliokoski and M. Leinonen, 1991b - Highly variable penicillin-binding proteins in penicillin-resistant strains of *Streptococcus pneumoniae*, in, Dunny, G.M., Cleary, P.P., and McKay, L.L. (eds.), *Genetics and Molecular Biology of Streptococci, Lactococci, and Enterococci*. American Society for Microbiology: Washington, DC 20005, p. 92–95.

Hakenbeck, R., P. Reichmann and C. Sibold, 1994 - Evolution and spread of β-lactam resistant *Streptococcus pneumoniae*, *Klin. Labor.* **40**, 230–235.

Humbert, O., M. Prudhomme, R. Hakenbeck, C.G. Dowson and J.-P. Claverys, 1995 - Homeologous recombination and mismatch repair during transformation in *Streptococcus pneumoniae*: saturation of the Hex mismatch repair system, *Proc. Nat. Acad. Sci. U.S.A.* **92**, 9052–9056.

Laible, G. and R. Hakenbeck, 1991 - Five independent combinations of mutations can result in low-affinity penicillin-binding protein 2x of *Streptococcus pneumoniae*, *J. Bacteriol.* **173**, 6986 6990.

Laible, G., B.G. Spratt and R. Hakenbeck, 1991 - Inter-species recombinational events during the evolution of altered PBP 2x genes in penicillin-resistant clinical isolates of *Streptococus pneumoniae*, *Mol. Microbiol.* **5**, 1993–2002.

Lefevre, J.C., G. Faucon, A.M. Sicard and A.M. Gasc, 1993 - DNA fingerprinting of *Streptococcus pneumoniae* strains by pulsed-field gel electrophoresis, *J. Clin. Microbiol.* **31**, 2724–2728.

Martin, C., C. Sibold and R. Hakenbeck, 1992 - Relatedness of penicillin-binding protein 1a genes from different clones of penicillin-resistant *Streptococcus pneumoniae* isolated in South Africa and Spain, *EMBO J.* **11**, 3831–3836.

Marton, A., 1992 - Pneumococcal antimicrobial resistance: the problem in Hungary, *Clin. Infect. Dis.* **15**, 106–111.

Muñóz, R., J.M. Musser, M. Crain, D.E. Briles, A. Marton, A.J. Parkinson, U. Sorensen and A. Tomasz, 1992 - Geographic distribution of penicillin-resistant clones of *Streptococcus pneumoniae*: characterization by penicillin-binding protein profile, surface protein A typing, and multilocus enzyme analysis, *Clin. Infect. Dis.* **15**, 112–118.

Reichmann, P., E. Varon, E. Günther, R.R. Reinert, R. Lütticken, A. Marton, P. Geslin, J. Wagner and R. Hakenbeck, 1995 - Penicillin-resistant *Streptococcus pneumoniae* in Germany: genetic relationship to clones from other European countries, *J. Med. Microbiol.* **43**, 377–385.

Reinert, R.R., A. Queck, A. Kaufhold, M. Kresken and R. Lütticken, 1994 - Antibiotic sensitivity of *Streptococcus pneumoniae* isolated from normally sterile body sites: first results of a multicenter study in Germany, *Infection* **22**, 113–114.

Schutze, G.E., S.L. Kaplan and R.F. Jacobs, 1994 - Resistant pneumococcus: a worldwide problem, *Infection* **22**, 233–237.

Sibold, C., J. Henrichsen, A. König, C. Martin, L. Chalkley and R. Hakenbeck, 1994 - Mosaic *pbpX* genes of major clones of penicillin-resistant *Streptococcus pneumoniae* have evolved from *pbpX* genes of a penicillin-sensitive *Streptococcus oralis*, *Mol. Microbiol.* **12**, 1013–1023.

Sibold, C., J. Wang, J. Henrichsen and R. Hakenbeck, 1992 - Genetic relationship of penicillin-susceptible and -resistant *Streptococcus pneumoniae* strains isolated on different continents, *Infect. Immun.* **60**, 4119–4126.

Soares, S., K.G. Kristinsson, J.M. Musser and A. Tomasz, 1993 - Evidence for the introduction of a multiresistant clone of serotype 6B *Streptococcus pneumoniae* from Spain to Iceland in the late 1980s - *J. Infect. Dis.* **168**, 158–163.

Spratt, B.G., C.G. Dowson, Q.-Z. Zhang, L.D. Bowler, J.A. Brannigan and A. Hutchison, 1991 - Mosaic genes, hybrid penicillin-binding proteins, and the origins of penicillin-resistance in *Neisseria meningitidis* and *Streptococcus pneumoniae*, in, *Perspectives on Cellular Regulation: From Bacteria to Cancer*. Wiley-Liss, Inc. p. 73–83.

Max-Planck Institut für molekulare Genetik, Ihnestr. 73, D-14195 Berlin
Tel.: +49-30-8413 1340
Fax: +49-30-8413 1385
E-mail: hakenbeck@mpimg-berlin-dahlem.mpg.de

Peter Reeves

Specialised Clones and Lateral Transfer in Pathogens

Bacterial populations are clonal and we have heard from others something of the population structure. I will concentrate on the adaptive nature of clones. This is largely overlooked in many studies which treat the population as undifferentiated in this sense; but we should remember that widespread interest in bacterial clones began with the observation by the Ørskovs that pathogenic *Escherichia coli* had the characteristics of clones, with isolates over a long period of time and from a wide area having an identical set of characters including mode of pathogenicity, host range and O-antigen specificity (Ørskov and Ørskov, 1976; Ørskov and Ørskov, 1977). They also noted that only some O-antigens were commonly found in such pathogenic clones. The clones the Ørskovs studied are a good example of niche adapted clones. However the clonal nature of bacterial populations and their adaptive nature was appreciated in a practical sense before that, as the science of epidemiology is predicated both on the clonal nature of bacterial populations and the fact that clones differ in pathogenesis. In my lab we are interested in clones and their relationships and suggest that for many species at least clones are adapted to specific niches within the broad niche of the species (Reeves, 1992).

The two concepts of clonal structures can be seen by reference to Fig. 1. The classical model which was discussed earlier by Roger Milkman (Milkman, 1996) is illustrated in the lower diagram. Each enclosed area represents a clone, which starts from a single organism after mutation to give a a widely favorable motivating allele which initiates a round of periodic selection and displacement of other clones (Milkman and Bridges, 1990). Clones eventually decrease in size as there is a succession of clones. Clones 1 to 3, still extant at the top of the time frame shown, derive from a single parent clone, as do clones 4 to 6. All six clones have a common ancestor one further generation back and all clones shown have common ancestor yet one more generation back. In general the parent clone is not indicated precisely, but clones extant at time 6 are lightly shaded and their parent clones (now level 2 clones) have darker shading, and so on for the next two levels. As seen at time 6: clones 1 through 13 are all level 1 clones, clones 1 through 3 comprise a level 2 clone, clones 1 through 6 another level 3 clone, and all 13 clones comprise a level 4 clone which originated at time 2. The clone shown in black with its progeny clones represents the level 4 clone through time. The diagram is clearly an oversimplification as for example it does

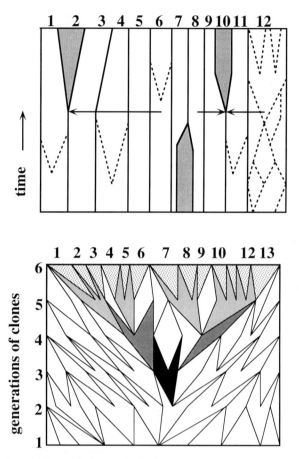

Fig. 1. Models for bacterial populations. Vertical axes represent time and horizontal axes bacterial numbers. Enclosed spaces represent clones. Top: Niche-adapted clone model. Bottom: Clonal frame model. For details see text. After Reeves (1992).

not show development of variation within a clone and clones are shown as starting synchronously across the space illustrated.

In the top diagram of Fig. 1 is a alternative view of clones. Clones, considered now to be adaptive, have a long life because periodic selection in one clone is not likely to displace other clones. A clone will survive until its niche disappears or it is displaced by a clone better adapted to that niche. One clone is shown as being lost; and two clones arise in the diagram, clone 2 by transfer of an adaptive allele from a cell of clone 6 to a cell of clone 1, and clone 10 by recombination between organisms of clones 8 and 12 in which both contribute substantially. Only transfer related to birth of clones is shown. Dotted lines indicate rounds of periodic selection confined to single clones, which retain relatively constant populations in comparison to the predictions of the clonal frame model. I have discussed elsewhere the way in which natural selection will act in a population of this sort (Reeves, 1992). In presenting an alternative model I am not arguing that my preferred model is totally correct and the other totally wrong, but suspect that aspects of both will survive when we better understand bacterial populations. However I want to focus on adaptive clones and the model in the top panel is appropriate for that.

There can be little doubt of the existence of clones adapted to specific niches. *E. coli* and *S. enterica* are well characterised species each with clones adapted to specific niches. Consider the range of pathogenic modes and the host specificity of many clones of *E. coli*, or compare the Typhi and Typhimurium clones of *S. enterica* (Note that Selander *et al.* (1990) recognised one clone of serovar Typhimurium but two closely related clones of serovar Typhi).

Maynard Smith (1993) has analysed multi-locus enzyme electophoresis data of several bacterial species to determine the degree of clonality, finding them to range from clonal at all levels (individual isolates, electrophoretic types (ETs) or major genetic divisions) to panmictic at all levels. *Neisseria mengitidis* for example was found to be panmictic when clusters of ETs are considered but clonal when individual isolates are considered. It is said to have an epidemic population structure, which is essentially panmictic but marked by short lived epidemic clones of which one, ET5, comprised 156 of the 688 isolates. It was suggested that this particular association of electromorphs will reduce in frequency (due to recombination) and eventually fail to mark the epidemic. It is most important from our point of view to consider the time frame for such changes. ET5 has been in existence now for 20 years, which is a substantial number of bacterial generations. Even in so called panmictic species one may have to go back decades or more to eliminate ancestors which contribute more than say 20% of their genome. In contrast in outbreeding eucaryotic species the contribution of individual ancestors is halved for each generation one goes back.

Recombination in bacteria generally involves transfer of a small segment of DNA and in a clonal population can be likened to lateral transfer of genes between species. We are interested in the extent to which niche adaptation can maintain species diversity in the face of recombination and it is possible that even in 'panmictic' bacteria recombination rates per generation may still be too low relative to selection levels to prevent clonal adaptation (see Reeves (1992) for discussion).

The O-antigen

We have undertaken several studies which impinge on clonal adaptation and I will present some of that work. Let us start with the O-antigen, a surface polysaccharide which, like many bacterial polysaccharides is made of repeats of an oligosaccharide unit, in this case called the O-unit. This O-unit usually varies even within a species in the sugars present and in the linkages between them. We have worked mostly with *S. enterica* which has approximately 50 O-unit forms, of which some are shown in Fig. 2. By way of background I should point out that *S. enterica* is strongly clonal.

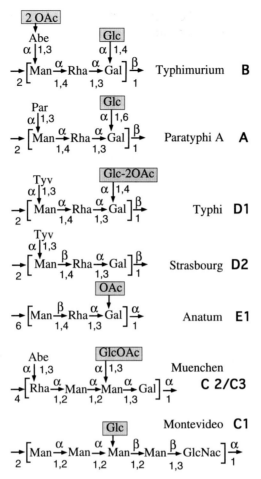

Fig. 2. Structures of the repeat units of six *S. enterica* O antigens. Each defines a group (A, B etc.) and one serovar of each group is named. Gal, galactose; Man, mannose; Rha, rhamnose; Abe, abequose; Par, paratose; Tyv, tyvelose; GlcNac, N-acetyl glucosamine. Shading indicates residues not always present and determined by genes outside of *rfb*. These residues are thought to be added after completion of the main O unit.

Seven subspecies have been recognised by biotyping and recent work from Selander's lab in particular has shown that in general all strains of a given subspecies group together in studies on sequence variation in house-keeping genes (Boyd *et al.*, 1994; Selander, 1996). This tells us that whole gene transfer is very infrequent over the time-frame of subspeciation. However a look at the distribution of O-antigen types shows that they do not fit this pattern at all as most are present in several subspecies (Table 1). There must have been extensive transfer of O-antigen genes between subspecies.

We know that of the approximately 50 O-antigens in *S. enterica* and 170 reported in *E. coli* only 3 are common to both species. We suggest that since

Table 1. Distribution of O-antigen types over a number of *S. enterica* subspecies. Taken from Thampapillai (1994).

Serovar	Subspecies	O Antigen
Typhimurium LT2	I	B
Paratyphi B	I	B
Choleraesuis	I	C1
Tennessee	I	C1
Glostrup	I	C2
Muenchen	I	C2
Typhi	I	D1
Strasbourg	I	D2
Canoga	I	E3
Senftenberg	I	E4
Berkeley	I	43
Dahlem	I	48
Sofia	II	B
9,12: mt: e,n,x	II	D1
Lindrick	II	D1
1,9,12: mst: 5z42	II	D1
Haarlem	II	D2
Westpark	II	E1
Springs	II	40
Freemantle	II	42
Phoenix	II	47
Ar 10a10b: 17,20	IIIa	40
Ar 1,3:1,3,11	IIIa	44
Ar 38: 1,v: z53,z54	IIIb	38
Ar 26:27-21	IIIb	47
Ar 5,29: 33-31	IIIb	48
38: z4,z23	IV	38
Houten	IV	43
43: z4 : z23	IV	43
Brookfield	V	66
Balboa	V	48
Marseille	VI	F
41 : b:1,7	VI	41
Vrindaban	VI	45

divergence of these two species there has been an almost complete turnover. As discussed below we believe that new forms are obtained from other species and presumably old forms are lost. We suggest that each clone is adapted to a specific niche, essentially a host or group of hosts and perhaps a specific mode of interaction with the host. As circumstances change a given surface structure may become non-ideal, generating selection pressure for substitution of the O-antigen which will occur by either by recombination within the species or by capture from outside. We should however remember that the time frame is very long with *E. coli* and *S. enterica* thought to have diverged about 140m years ago (Ochman and Wilson, 1987) and the subspecies may go back a significant fraction of that 140m years. The distribution of O-antigens among subspecies is then due to the same forces that lead to capture of new forms from other species.

The genes for O-antigen synthesis are grouped together in the *rfb* gene cluster. Functions common to other pathways are often encoded elsewhere but with few exceptions all those specific to O-unit synthesis are in the *rfb* cluster, which maps at the same place in both *E. coli* and *S. enterica*. We have undertaken an extensive study of the genetic basis of this variation, mostly in *S. enterica* but also in *E. coli* and *Yersinia pestis* (see Reeves (1993) for review). Building on the work of Nikaido (Nikaido *et al.*, 1967) who had localised many of the *rfb* genes of laboratory strain LT2, we cloned and sequenced the whole LT2 *rfb* cluster and over time identified all the genes. We repeated this for several other O-antigen forms of *S. enterica*. The *rfb* region of LT2 is shown in Fig. 3 together with its G + C content. It can be seen that the G + C content varies but none of the *rfb* DNA has 51% G + C typical of *S. enterica*, although the cluster is flanked by such DNA. We believe that the deviation of G + C content from 51% indicates that the DNA originated in species other than *S. enterica*, or for much

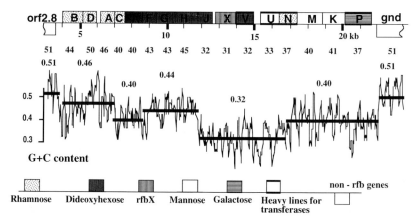

Fig. 3. The *rfb* gene cluster of *S. enterica* group B strain LT2. The *rfb* genes genes are indicated by letters and flanking genes by orf number or gene symbol. The four transferase genes are indicated by heavy lines and the relevant sugar for both nucleotide sugar pathway and sugar transferase genes is indicated by shading as shown in the key below. The graph gives the G + C content of 100 bp spans, and the G + C content of individual *rfb* genes is shown above the graph.

of it outside the Enterobacteriaceae. The variation in G + C content within the *rfb* cluster suggests that the cluster was assembled from several sources and only later transferred to, or as I prefer to think of it, was captured by, *S. enterica*.

Fig. 4 shows the genetic organisation of several *rfb* clusters. Although it is not shown they also have atypical and varying G + C contents. Groups A, B, C2/C3, D1, D2 and E1 are related both chemically and genetically. The level of the shading for each gene indicates the level of amino acid identity of the encoded protein. The genes found are essentially those expected. There are genes for the pathways and transferases which are needed for synthesis and only in group E1 is one gene not accounted for. In groups A, B and D1 the *rfc* gene for polymerisation maps elsewhere but this is now seen as atypical and for the others it maps within the cluster. Each cluster has a gene for a protein with about 12 predicted transmembrane segments. We have named them *rfbX* and as the sequence varies greatly suggest that *rfbX* encodes a protein for the predicted flipping of the O-unit on its undecaprenol carrier, from cytoplasmic face where it is synthesised to periplasmic face of the cytoplasmic membrane where polymerisation occurs. This step should be present in all cases but be specific to the O-unit.

Two things stand out in the comparison of the clusters. The genes of each cluster are in the same order: rhamnose pathway genes, abequose pathway genes (if present), *rfbX*, a group of transferase genes, mannose pathway genes and the galactose transferase gene common to all as all start synthesis by transfer of

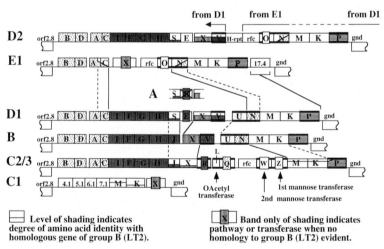

Fig. 4.   *Rfb* region from 7 groups of *S. enterica*: Genes for different functions are indicated by using shading as in Fig. 3. The level of shading indicates amino acid identity to the homologous gene of Group B. Most *rfb* genes are identified and the letters given but some of group C1 have orf numbers. The transferases indicated (Liu *et al.*, 1993, 1995) are those which transfer sugar to oligosaccharide from nucleotide sugar. Lines between groups connect breaks in homology. Group A has the Group D1 *rfb* cluster with the *rfbE* gene non functional. The postulated origin of the GroupD *rfb* cluster by recombination between group D1 and group E1 *rfb* clusters is shown (Xiang *et al.*, 1994). See Reeves (1993) for other references.

galactosyl phosphate to undecaprenol phosphate. The other striking thing is that some genes, such as *rfbB* have essentially the same sequence in all of these related groups, whereas other genes such as *rfbD*, also in the rhamnose pathway, can be either similar or very different while yet others such as the transferases with different specificity have very little similarity between forms. We suggest that the common order indicates that the clusters are homologous and derive from a single ancestral cluster. The sequence difference between *rfbM* and *rfbK* of groups B and C2 is about 28% at amino acid level and that between *rfbJ* of the two groups is 36%. This suggests divergence of the *rfbK* and *rfbM* genes long before *E. coli* and *S. enterica* diverged an estimated 140mY, with the *rfbJ* divergence being even more ancient (Brown *et al.*, 1992).

How do we account for these observations?

Some of the differences relate to functional differences between groups, in this case presence or absence of abequose and different transferases. We know little of the origins of this variation but note that the genes involved are always grouped in the centre of the *rfb* cluster. These genes, which determine the polymorphism, are those on which natural selection acts to maintain the diversity and while each is selected for in at least one of the niches occupied, will not be lost by random genetic drift. We propose that during the whole of the period of divergence (only part of which was in *S. enterica*) there was genetic exchange involving the other genes and that the sequences underwent random genetic drift in concert, in a manner analogous to concerted evolution of genes present in multiple copies within a species. Indeed this will also apply to genes generally present in the species if the population model shown in the top section of Fig. 1 with long lived clones is valid (Reeves, 1992) and the ability to exchange small segments of DNA has been proposed as a definition of a species in procaryotes (DuBose *et al.*, 1988).

To return to *rfbM*, *rfbK*, *rfbD* and *rfbJ*, each of these genes, which have undergone major sequence divergence without as far as we are aware any functional divergence, is adjacent to the central group of genes which determine the functional differences between clusters (treating *rfbN* and *rfbK* together). We suggest that in each case divergence by chance proceeded to a level where the recombination needed for them to drift in concert became unlikely and that they continued to drift. This can only happen to DNA adjacent to the genes with functional differences as otherwise recombination in the DNA flanking the segment which had started to diverge would allow random genetic drift to occur in concert. We conclude then that the divergence observed for *rfbJ* puts a minimum period for divergence of the group B and group C2/C3 *rfb* clusters (Brown *et al.*, 1992).

Before leaving this discussion of O-antigen variation in *S. enterica* I must emphasise that those we have discussed form a related family. While the other groups studied by ourselves and others all appear to have undergone lateral transfer, their origins do not seem to be closely associated with those of the family of O-antigens discussed today. Group C1 is shown in Fig. 4 as an example of the many forms which are not in this family.

Is there any evidence to support the claim that O-antigen variation confers adaptation to specific niches? It has to be said that there is not as much as we would like. The O-antigen is known to be essential for pathogenicity in most gram negative pathogens, but there have been few studies on the role of O-antigen specificity, one of the more comprehensive being by the groups of Loreta Leive and Helena Makela which does indicate an adaptive role for O-antigen specificity (Jimenez-Lucho *et al.*, 1990).

We do have one case where we can perhaps speculate in more detail on inter-species gene capture of O-antigen genes. *E. coli* Sonnei (more usually referred to as *Shigella sonnei*, but clearly a member of the species *E. coli*) has the characteristics of a clone and recent work of ours has confirmed that (Karaolis *et al.*, 1994b). It has an O-antigen which is not found otherwise in *E. coli*, but is identical to that of serotype 17 of *Plesiomonas shigelloides*. The *rfb* genes of Sonnei are unusual in being on a plasmid and it has recently been shown that they will probe the *rfb* genes of *P. shigelloides*. serotype O17 (Viret *et al.*, 1993). Houng *et al.*, (1996) showed that for at least a few hundred base pairs the sequences are identical. Now S. sonnei and indeed all the Shigellae and many other human pathogenic clones of *E. coli* are thought to have relatively recently adapted to the diarrhoea mode of pathogenesis in humans (Fenner, 1970; McKeown, 1988). This is because the nature of the infection and transmission makes them unlikely to be successful in a hunter gatherer society. We have then a clone of *E. coli* which has occupies a newly available niche, and has on a plasmid *rfb* genes which may well be essentially identical to those of a form found in a rather distantly related species. It is perhaps reasonable to deduce that in the new niche the O-antigens already available in *E. coli* were less suitable than some present in other species, and that when by chance the *rfb* region of *P. shigelloides* serotype O17 entered *E. coli* on a plasmid it was retained, perhaps with modification of regulatory or other aspects. One would anticipate that if we came back in perhaps 10,000 years time the gene capture

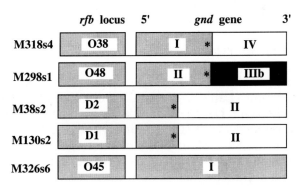

Fig. 5. Representation of postulated recombination events involving both the *rfb* gene cluster and *gnd* gene. Shaded regions represent sequences thought to have been derived by transfer from another subspecies with the subspecies of origin indicated. Where two donors are implicated two levels of shading are used. The subspecies of each strain is appended to its name. Taken from Thampapillai (1994).

```
         1222333444556666666667 77777777 7778888888888999999000000011111111112222333
         9459029468230122455670 44444455 6671478888992368891556783455558991467012
         2657340153240817804095 45678901 2819941258177391707038436825892475502280

S41s1    ......................  CCTGGTGG ...GTTCGA.TAAACTGC.TCTGGCACTCTGTGACAAA..
M46s1    ......................  CCTGGTGG ...GTTCGA.TAAACTGCATCTGGCACTCT.TGACAAA..
M318s4   CATTTATTCTCTTCCCGATCCT  CCTGGTGG TACTCCTTGTCCGGTCATGGGCACTGTCTCACACTCGGTA
M319s4   TCCCCGCGTCTGCATTAGCTTC  CCTGGTaG GGT......C........A...........G......CG
M320s4   TCCCCGCGTCTGCATTAGCTTC  CCTGGTaG GGT......C..CCC...A..................CG
```

Fig. 6.   Recombination in the *gnd* gene of *S. enterica* M318. The M318 *gnd* sequence is shown in bold together with those of the two most closely related subspecies I and subspecies IV strains, named as in Fig 4. Only those bases which differ in these strains are shown and the deduced recombination event is evident. The chi like sequence postulated to have been involved in recombination is also shown (bases 744 to 751). Taken from Thampapillai (1994).

may have been completed with these *rfb* genes integrated into the chromosome in the typical *E. coli* position next to *gnd* (see Fig. 2).

There is also support for intraspecies transfer of the *rfb* locus in the sequence of the *gnd* gene (Fig. 2). In a recent study (Thampapillai *et al.*, 1994) we observed that for several *S. enterica* strains the *gnd* gene did not group with that of other strains of the same subspecies. This is of course quite atypical for *S. enterica*. In Fig. 5 we see five cases where the *gnd* sequence does not fit that expected for the subspecies. In four cases the *gnd* gene appears to be chimeric, with the 5′ end atypical for the subspecies but in three of the four cases the 3′ end typical for the subspecies. In each of the four recombinant genes just upstream of the junction there is a one base variant of the 8 base chi site, the recognition sequence for RecBCD recombination. In all five cases it is reasonable to conclude that there has been a recombination event in which all or part of the *rfb* cluster was transferred together with all or part of the adjacent *gnd* gene. The sequence is shown for M318 in Fig. 6 and one can clearly see the junction, in this case between subspecies I and subspecies IV derived DNA. The selective pressure was presumably provided by the *rfb* cluster, with the *gnd* gene providing the evidence.

The overall level of lateral gene transfer

We have also looked at the overall extent of gene transfer in *S. enterica* using subtractive hybridisation (Lan and Reeves, 1996). We mixed DNA from two strains, one (the subtracter DNA) labelled with biotin and, after denaturation and hybridisation, removed with streptavidin DNA of the subtractor strain, together with any of the Sau3A cut DNA of the target strain which had hybridised to it. The subtraction was repeated three times with fresh subtracter DNA and the residual DNA, which is now essentially target strain DNA not present in the subtractor strain, was amplified by PCR. We used *S. enterica* LT2 for target DNA (a derivative without the pSLT plasmid) and four other strains of the same species for subtracter DNA. The four preparations of LT2 DNA amplified after subtraction were found as expected to hybridise to target DNA but not to respective subtracter DNA in Southern blots. The proportion of the chromosome involved was estimated by doing Southern blots against a large number of cosmids of LT2 DNA. We found that approximately 20% of the DNA present in a subspecies V strain is absent in LT2, with lesser amounts for the other more closely related strains. We undertook various tests to show that this residual DNA had not simply diverged in sequence but was not present in the subtractor strain. We conclude that 20% of DNA has undergone lateral transfer. This will include intraspecies transfer as for the *rfb* cluster discussed above but is still a much higher level of lateral transfer than we had expected.

Remember that house-keeping genes have general congruent trees and appear not to undergo lateral transfer. How do we explain the discrepancy? We cloned and sequenced 39 of the Sau3A fragments and found that only 6 were identifiable by searching against the databases. These included one potential phage derived gene, a restriction modification gene and four metabolic pathway or uptake genes. We suggest that much of the DNA variation between clones is in their metabolic pathway genes. Perhaps the outcome should not have surprised us. Farmer *et al.* (1985) have listed 47 biochemical reactions of 84 Enterobacteriaceae, including subspecies of *S. enterica*. There is a wide variation in metabolic properties of species, which is even wider as in general the reactions recorded are those which are both easily detected and useful for taxonomic distinctions. It is clear that many properties are present or absent in a given species while others are present in some strains. This type of pattern is well documented and is used extensively in bacterial classification. Some properties such as utilisation (uptake) of citrate are present in *S. enterica* and absent in *E. coli*. Utilisation of lactose shows in general the reverse pattern but is present in some subspecies of *S. enterica*, while dulcitol shows yet another distribution. Where it has been studied, presence or absence of function generally correlates with presence or absence of the genes. The pattern indicates extensive lateral transfer of these periferal components of metabolism, while the central housekeeping pathways are, as observed above, generally not subject to such transfer. Only myo-inositol utilisation shows the pattern expected for the 20% of DNA found in our subspecies I target but not in our subspecies V subtractor strain, but this reflects both the limited selection in the table and limited knowledge. The intention is to point to the substantial intra- and inter-specific variation in metabolic pathways which is probably part of the adaptation of clones to specific niches.

Vibrio cholerae

We have also looked at specific clones in an attempt to observe the dynamics of clonal evolution. I have already referred to *E. coli* Sonnei, but would like to concentrate now on *V. cholerae*. It is an interesting organism for such a study. There have been seven recorded pandemics in which cholera has erupted over many countries (see Barua (1992) for review), although Blake (1994) suggests that it may be reasonable to consider the first six as a single continuing pandemic as the divisions between them are indistinct, and explosive expansions of the seventh pandemic could have been considered separate pandemics according to the methods used previously. The seventh started in 1961 and is still with us. The sixth ended in 1923, leaving nearly 40 years in which cholera, although still causing outbreaks, was not at pandemic levels. The seventh pandemic originated in Indonesia and in a few years spread widely in Asia. These are the hallmarks of a new clone, and this is supported by the work of several groups which has shown that there is very little variation in seventh pandemic isolates (see Wachsmuth *et al.* (1994) for review). The seventh pandemic was easily distinguished from isolates from the sixth pandemic which still persisted, as it was of the El Tor biotype (see below). *V. cholerae* also occurs in natural environments such as muds and waters, mostly marine or brackish, and also in association with crustacea or molluscs. It is interesting that these isolates show considerable variation, with for example 140 O-antigen forms, only one of which has been found until recently in pathogenic isolates.

We undertook to study evolution within the seventh pandemic clone and its relationship to other clones. We expected relatively little variation within the clone so needed a method likely to be effective in such circumstances and chose ribotyping. Ribotyping is a form of restriction fragment length polymorphism analysis in which ribosomal RNA or DNA is used for Southern blotting. There are 7 copies of the rRNA genes in *E. coli* and probably the same number in *V. cholerae*. The enzymes used cut within the *rrn* loci and one observes 14 bands although some are not always easily seen. The variation is thought to be mostly in the restriction sites in the flanking DNA as the *rrn* loci are rather strongly conserved. The method is used mostly to 'fingerprint' clones and had been used before with *V. cholerae* (Koblavi *et al.*, 1990). We extended the number of enzymes used and found sufficient variation in 45 seventh pandemic isolates from 1961 to 1993 to study development of the clone.

We used the data to identify restriction sites which were present or absent in any strain. Unfortunately we don't know anything else about these sites and specifically do not know in which genes they are located. We were however able to draw trees using the 1961 isolate to root the tree as it must be close the original form. As can be seen from Fig. 7 the original form was the only one isolated for the first few years and it is still present. We then have 21 African and Asian isolates of a significantly different form first seen in a 1966 isolate and surviving to the present, also giving rise to a group of related ribotypes found only in Africa from 1971. This parallels what is known of the history of the pandemic. After starting in 1961 in Indonesia, the seventh pandemic spread through much of southern and south-eastern Asia, followed by a lull from 1966 and an upsurge in 1970-1971 (Barua, 1992) which spread to Africa. Our data suggest that the development of the form which gave rise to the upsurge was accompanied by changes in ribotype. This may not be due simply to accumulation of random neutral changes as the original forms are still isolated after more

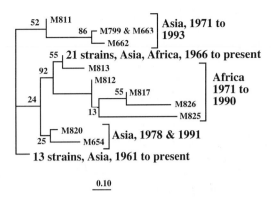

than 30 years, but due to recombination. We also looked at the ribotypes of strains from the sixth pandemic, some strains which caused small outbreaks between the pandemics and the so-called US gulf strains. Ribotyping enabled us to observe differences but the differences are too great for us to relate band changes to sites or to draw convincing trees.

We therefore turned to DNA sequence. Remarkably, although the genetics of *V. cholerae* was studied quite extensively and of course there has been a remarkable amount of work on the molecular biology of pathogenesis, only one housekeeping gene, *asd*, has been sequenced. We sequenced this gene from three sixth pandemic and 13 seventh pandemic strains and from a set of environmental strains of different O-antigen groups and countries of origin. We also sequenced it from a *Vibrio mimicus* strain for use as outgroup and were able to derive a tree from the data (Fig. 8). There is no variation within either sixth or seventh pandemic clones but the clones differ at 1.62% of bases. This is greater than the average pairwise variation of 1.41% (if three *V. cholerae* strains with all or part *V. mimicus* like sequence are omitted). The sixth and seventh pandemic clones are seen to group with different environmental strains, suggesting that they arose independently from unrelated environmental strains. As might be expected (Mooi, 1996) the *asd* sequence of O139 strains is identical to that of the seventh pandemic strains. The picture we see for *V. cholerae* is of an environmental species with considerable neutral sequence variation which on at least two occasions has developed the capacity to become pathogenic for humans . However these conclusions should be treated as tentative as they are as yet based on the *asd* gene only.

It is interesting to look at some aspects of the biology of *V. cholerae* and cholera, the disease it causes. The disease is found naturally only in humans and is thought to have only arisen when villages and water supplies were established (Fenner, 1970; McKeown, 1988). In effect it is only when our species systemati-

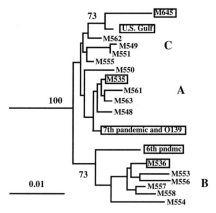

Fig. 8. Relationships of *V. cholerae* strains as indicated by sequence of bases 1 to 931 of the *asd* gene. *V. mimicus* was used as outgroup Strains with V. mimicus like sequence omitted and names of O1 strains enclosed in boxes. Bootstrap values as for Fig 6. Taken from Karaolis (1995).

cally contaminated drinking water with sewage that the niche was created for *V. cholerae* to become the pathogen for which the species is named. Clearly the environmental strains occupy the original and still predominant niche for *V. cholerae*. What is that niche? *V. cholerae* in the environment is often thought of a free living organism which gets concentrated by filter feeders such as molluscs. However all strains have a haemolysin and chitinase which suggests that they normally associate with marine invertebrates, perhaps using these proteins to undertake limited invasion as it is not generally a pathogen for these hosts. The two pandemic clones both have the major *ctx* toxin genes in the cassette described earlier by Mekalanos (1995) and also have the toxin coregulated pilus. The toxin genes are very similar in sequence in the two pandemic clones (Olsvik *et al.*, 1993) and as the *asd* sequences suggest that the clones are not closely related we conclude that the seventh pandemic strain obtained its *ctx* cassette from the sixth pandemic strain. However the *tcp* genes are very different in sequence (Rhine and Taylor, 1994) and were presumably independently derived. It is also possible that the seventh pandemic clone obtained its *rfb* (O-antigen) genes from the sixth pandemic strains as they are extremely similar in sequence (Rhine and Taylor, 1994).

There are some other aspects which deserve comment. *V. cholerae* is often divided first into classical and El Tor biotypes and separately into O1 and non-O1 strains. These distinctions can now be seen to be of not much further use. Some of the properties which define the El Tor form are found in most clones. It was the early focus on sixth pandemic isolates, which are rather atypical, which made the distinction useful. We can now see that the classical biotype (fifth and sixth pandemic strains) has in effect lost the haemolysin and acetoin formation (Voges Proskauer test) properties present in most *V. cholerae*. Thus, the 'classical' biotype is atypical, not the El Tor. Many seventh pandemic isolates now have some classical biotype properties, most isolates since 1966 for example being non-haemolytic (Barrett and Blake, 1981): we can conclude that the properties being lost are those that are not needed in the new human pathogen niche. It so happened that the first *V. cholerae* isolates studied were from the sixth pandemic long after it had become pathogenic. It was only later that normal *V. cholerae* were isolated from the environment and the biotype distinction served to differentiate environmental from pandemic isolates. It was understandable in retrospect that the seventh pandemic, arising as it has from an environmental source, should be of the El Tor biotype and of course equally understandable that this came as a surprise at the time.

The O1/non-O1 distinction is also not particularly useful. The O1 O-antigen of both pandemic strains is also found in environmental strains but is not characteristic of a group of related clones with pathogenic potential but rather spread among a range of different clones in a manner reminiscent of the distribution of O-antigens in *S. enterica* as discussed above (Table 1). The distinctions can be especially confusing when for example comparison of groups of sixth and seventh pandemic strains is taken to represent a comparison of El Tor and classical biotypes. But once again I stress that these conclusions are at present based largely on variation in the *asd* gene.

General conclusions

We have looked at studies of O-antigen polymorphism, the extent of lateral transfer in *S. enterica* and of clonal structures in *V. cholerae*. Each gives a different perspective on clonal adaptation. The extensive knowledge of virulence factors present in particular clones of many species and the data on O-antigen distribution strongly support the concept of niche adaptive clones, and the specific clones we have looked at appear to be niche adapted. This implies a limited level of recombination and limited scope for species wide periodic selection, both of which would dilute clonal specialisation. However recombination was seen to be important in generating that adaptation in the case studies of *S. enterica* and *V. cholerae*. The critical factor will be the frequency of recombination. The subtractive DNA study suggested that the amount of DNA involved in lateral transfer may be as much as 20% even within a species, and in this context it should be noted that subspecies V is at the borderline of species status as some consider it to be a separate species. The *V. cholerae* study allowed us to speculate on the dynamics of the evolution of specific clones.

We still have long way to go in understanding bacterial populations but an indication of how far we have come already can be seen by looking at a quotation from that great geneticist Theodosius Dobzhansky

'The subdivision of the mass of clones into species *Escherichia coli*, *Salmonella typhosa*, and *S. enteritidis* is purely a matter of taste; one might just as well regard all of them as a single species' (Dobzhansky, 1951).

This was written just before discovery of the structure of DNA (Watson and Crick, 1953), and serves to highlight the contribution of molecular genetic analysis.

References

Barrett, T.J. and P.A. Blake, 1981 - Epidemiological usefulness of changes in hemolytic activities of *Vibrio cholerae* biotype El Tor during the seventh pandemic. *J. Clin. Microbiol.* **13**, 126–129.

Barua, D., 1992 - History of Cholera. In *Cholera*. Barua, D. and Greenough III, W.B. (eds.), New York:Plenum, Ch. 1, pp. 1–36.

Blake, P.A., 1994 - Historical perspectives on pandemic cholera. In *Vibrio cholerae and cholera, molecular to global perspectives*. Wachsmuth, I.K., Blake, P.A. and Olsvik, Ø. (eds.), Washington:ASM Press, pp. 357–370.

Boyd, E.F., K. Nelson, F.-S. Wang, T.S. Whittam and R.K. Selander, 1994 - Molecular genetic basis of allelic polymorphism in malate dehydrogenase (*mdh*) in natural populations of *Escherichia coli* and *Salmonella enterica*. *Proc. Natl. Acad. Sci. USA* **91**, 1280–1284.

Brown, P.K., L.K. Romana and P.R. Reeves, 1992 - Molecular analysis of the *rfb* gene cluster of *Salmonella* serovar Muenchen (strain M67): genetic basis of the polymorphism between groups C2 and B. *Mol. Microbiol.* **6**, 1385–1394.

Dobzhansky, T., 1951 - *Genetics and the origin of species*. New York: Columbia.

DuBose, R.F., D.E. Dykhuizen and D.L. Hartle, 1988 - Genetic exchange among natural isolates of bacteria: recombination within the *phoA* gene of *E. coli*. *Proc. Natl. Acad. Sci. USA* **85**, 7036–7040.

Farmer, J.J., Betty R. Davis, F.W. Hickman-Brenner, ALMA McWhorter, G.P. Huntley-Carter, M.A. Asbury, Conradine Riddle, H.G. Wathen-Grady, C. Elias, G.R. Fanning, A.G. Steigerwalt, Caroline M. O Hara, G.K. Morris, P.B. Smith and Don J. Brenner, 1985 - Biochemical Identification of New Species and Biogroups of Enterobacteriaceae Isolated from Clinical Specimens. *J. Clin. Microbiol.* **21**, 46–76.

Fenner, F., 1970 - The effects of changing social organisation on the infectious diseases of man. In *The impact of civilization on the biology of man*. Boyden, S.W. (eds.), Toronto:University of Toronto Press, pp. 48–68.

Houng, 1996 - The roles of IS630 sequence in the expression of the formI antigen of *Shigella sonnei*: molecular and evolutionary aspects. In *Ecology of pathogenic bacteria*. Van der Zeijst, B.A.M., W.P.M. Hoekstra, J.D.A. van Embden and A.J.W. van Alphen (eds.), North-Holland, Amsterdam/Oxford/New York/Tokyo.

Jimenez-Lucho, V., L.L. Leive and K.A. Joiner, 1990 - Role of O-antigen of lipopolysaccharide in *Salmonella* in protection against complement action. In *The Bacteria*. Iglewski, B.H. and Clark, V.L. (eds.), Vol. 11. Academic Press, pp. 339–354.

Karaolis, D.K.R., R. Lan and P.R. Reeves, 1994a - Molecular evolution of the 7th pandemic clone of *Vibrio cholerae* and its relationship to other pandemic and epidemic *V. cholerae* isolates. *J. Bacteriol.* **176**, 6199–6206.

Karaolis, D.K.R., R. Lan and P.R. Reeves, 1994b - Sequence variation in *Shigella sonnei* (Sonnei), a pathogenic clone of *Escherichia coli*, over four continents and 41 years. *J. Clin. Microbiol.* **32**, 796–802.

Specialised clones and lateral transfer in pathogens

Karaolis, D.K.R., R. Lan and P.R. Reeves, 1995 - The sixth and seventh cholera pandemics are due to independent clones separately derived from environmental, nontoxigenic, non-O1 *V. cholerae. J. Bacteriol.* **177**, 3197–3198.

Koblavi, S., F. Grimont and P.A.D. Grimont, 1990 - Clonal diversity of *Vibrio cholerae* 01 evidenced by rRNA gene restriction patterns. *Res. Microbiol.* **141**, 645–657.

Lan, R. and P.R. Reeves, 1996 - Gene transfer is a major factor in bacterial evolution. *Mol. Biol. Evol.* **13**, 47–55.

Liu, D., A.M. Haase, L. Lindqvist, A.A. Lindberg and P.R. Reeves, 1993 - Glycosyl transferases of O-antigen biosynthesis in *S. enterica*: identification and characterization of transferase genes of groups B, C2 and E1. *J. Bacteriol.* **175**, 3408–3413.

Liu, D., L. Lindquist and P.R. Reeves, 1995 - Transferases of O-antigen biosynthesis in Salmonella enterica: dideoxhexosyl transferases of groups B and C2 and acetyltransferase of group C2. *J. Bacteriol.* **177**, 4084–4088.

Maynard Smith, J., N.H. Smith, M. O'Rourke and B.G. Spratt, 1993 - How clonal are bacteria? *Proc. Natl. Acad. Sci. USA* **90**, 4384–4388.

McKeown, T., 1988 - *The origins of human disease.* Oxford: Basil Blackwell.

Mekalanos, J.J., 1996 - Molecular cross talk between bacteria and their hosts. In *Ecology of pathogenic bacteria.* Van der Zeijst, B.A.M., W.P.M. Hoekstra, J.D.A. van Embden and A.J.W. van Alphen (eds.), North-Holland, Amsterdam/Oxford/New York/Tokyo.

Milkman, R., 1996 - Recombination and DNA sequence variation in *E. coli.* In *Ecology of pathogenic bacteria.* Van der Zeijst, B.A.M., W.P.M. Hoekstra, J.D.A. van Embden and A.J.W. van Alphen (eds.), North-Holland, Amsterdam/Oxford/New York/Tokyo.

Milkman, R. and M.M. Bridges, 1990 - Molecular evolution of the *Escherichia coli* chromosome. III: Clonal Frames. *Genetics* **126**, 505–517.

Mooi, F.R., 1996 - Genetics of the novel epidemic V. cholerae strain O139; evidence for horizontal transfer. In *Ecology of pathogenic bacteria.* Van der Zeijst, B.A.M., W.P.M. Hoekstra, J.D.A. van Embden and A.J.W. van Alphen (eds.), North-Holland, Amsterdam/Oxford/New York/Tokyo.

Nikaido, H., M. Levinthal, K. Nikaido and K. Nakane, 1967 - Extended deletions in the histidine-rough-B region of the *Salmonella* chromosome. *Proc. Natl. Acad. Sci. USA* **57**, 1825–1832.

Ochman, H. and A.C. Wilson, 1987 - Evolution in bacteria: evidence for a universal substitution rate in cellular genomes. *J. Mol. Evol.* **26**, 74–86.

Olsvik, Ø., J. Wahlberg, B. Petterson, M. Uhlen, T. Popovic, I.K. Wachsmuth and P.I. Fields, 1993 - Use of automated sequencing of polymerase chain reaction-generated amplicons to identify three types of cholera toxin subunit B in *Vibrio cholerae* O1 strains. *J. Clin. Microbiol.* **31**, 22–25.

Ørskov, F. and I. Ørskov, 1976 - Special *Escherichia coli* serotypes among enterotoxigenic strains from diarrhoea in adults and children. *Med. Microbiol. Immunol.* **162**, 73–80.

Ørskov, I. and F. Ørskov, 1977 - Special O:K:H serotypes among enterotoxigenic *Escherichia coli* strains from diarrhoea in adults and children. *Med. Microbiol. Immunol.* **103**, 99–110.

Popoff, M.Y. and L. Le Minor, 1992 - *Antigenic formulas of the Salmonella serovars, 6th revision*. Paris, France: WHO Collaborating Centre for Reference and Research on *Salmonella*. Institut Pasteur, Paris.

Reeves, P.R., 1992 - Variation in O antigens, niche specific selection and bacterial populations. *FEMS Microbiol. Lett.* **100**, 509–516.

Reeves, P.R., 1993 - Evolution of *Salmonella* O antigen variation by interspecific gene transfer on a large scale. *Trends Genet.* **9**, 17–22.

Rhine, J.A. and R.K. Taylor, 1994 - TcpA pilin sequences and colonization requirements for O1 and O139 *Vibrio cholerae. Mol. Microbiol.* **13**, 1013–1020.

Selander, R.K., 1996 - DNA sequence analysis of the genetic structure of *Salmonella enterica* and *Escherichia coli*. In *Ecology of pathogenic bacteria*. Van der Zeijst, B.A.M., W.P.M. Hoekstra, J.D.A. van Embden and A.J.W. van Alphen (eds.), North-Holland, Amsterdam/Oxford/New York/Tokyo.

Selander, R.K., P. Beltran, N.H. Smith, H. Reiner, F.A. Rubin, D.J. Kopecko, K. Ferris, B.T. Tall, A. Cravioto and J.M. Musser, 1990 - Evolutionary genetic relationships of clones of *Salmonella* serovars that cause human typhoid and other enteric fevers. *Infect. Immun.* **58**, 2262–2275.

Thampapillai, G., R. Lan and P.R. Reeves, 1994 - Molecular variation at the *gnd* locus of 34 natural isolates of *Salmonella enterica*: DNA sequence: evidence for probable chi-dependent interallelic recombination. *Mol. Biol. Evol.* **11**, 813–828.

Viret, J.-F., S.J. Cryz Jr., A.B. Lang and D. Favre, 1993 - Molecular cloning and characterisation of the genetic determinants that express the complete *Shigella* serotype D (*Shigella sonnei*) lipopolysaccharide in heterologous live attenuated vaccine strains. *Mol. Microbiol.* **7**, 239–252.

Wachsmuth, I.K., Ø. Olsvik, G.M. Evins and T. Popovic, 1994 - Molecular epidemiology of cholera. In *Vibrio cholerae and cholera, molecular to global perspectives*. Wachsmuth, I.K., Blake, P.A. and Olsvik, O. (eds.), Washington:ASM Press, pp. 357–370.

Watson, J.D. and F.H.C. Crick, 1953 - Genetic implications of the structure of DNA. *Nature* **171**, 964–967.

Xiang, S.H., M. Hobbs and P.R. Reeves, 1994 - Molecular analysis of the *rfb* gene cluster of a group D2 *salmonella enterica* strain: evidence for its origin from an insertion sequence-mediated recombination event between group E and D1 strains. *J. Bacteriol.* **176**, 4357–4365.

E.R. Moxon and P.B. Rainey

Pathogenic Bacteria; the Wisdom of their Genes

Abstract

To counteract the extensive repertoire of polymorphisms and immune mechanisms of their hosts, pathogenic bacteria have evolved several mechanisms for generating phenotypic diversity. In addition to classical gene regulation (phenotypic acclimation), population diversity is achieved through intragenomic mechanisms which alter the sequence or conformation of DNA. These include homopolymeric tracts and short repeats which affect the activity (transcription or translation) of genes, especially those which direct the interactions of the bacterium with the host environment. These hypermutable loci generate phenotypic diversity which is random in time but programmed with respect to location in the genome, thereby maximising polymorphisms within a clonal bacterial population while minimising the deleterious effects of increased genetic load.

So entrenched in contemporary society is the idea that microbes cause specific diseases, we are liable to forget that, barely a hundred years ago, the concept was novel and controversial. Germ theory and the ensuing golden era of microbiology remain one of the milestones in the history of medicine. A century later, microbial disease has undergone a revolution galvanised by the application of the new genetics. Molecular and cell biology are transforming our ideas on epidemiology, pathogenesis, diagnosis, treatment and prevention of microbial diseases.

The impact of molecular genetics and cell biology can be well illustrated with respect to three bacterial genera *Haemophilus influenza*, *Neisseria meningitidis* and *Streptococcus pneumoniae* which together account for most cases of pyogenic meningitis. Acute bacterial meningitis is a global problem of some magnitude. Most cases occur in young children at a time when their central nervous system is undergoing its critical period of development. Thus, in addition to mortality, there is considerable morbidity occurring in those children who contract meningitis but who, through the use of antibiotics and sometimes intensive care, are able to survive. Although this may be the majority in the Western world, death is the rule rather than the exception elsewhere, for example tropical Africa where there are regular epidemics of meningococcal meningitis.

Bacteria causing meningitis: their candidacy for a 'Nobel Prize for Microbes'

Incidently, and as an historical footnote, the bacteria responsible for meningitis have played a not inconsiderable part in shaping the molecular era. It was in the Ministry of Health in London that the pathologist, Fred Griffith, carried out his experiments with pneumococci in which he showed that avirulent, capsule deficient organisms could be transformed to virulence by exposure to killed, encapsulated virulent pneumococci. After a hiatus of some twenty years, the transforming principle was recognised as nucleic acid by Avery and his colleagues at the Rockefeller (Avery *et al.*, 1994). In 1953, the structure of DNA was solved and, in the late 60s, a crucial step was the isolation of restriction enzymes from *Haemophilus influenzae*; their exploitation to construct a physical map of the SV40 virus ushered in the era of recombinant DNA. So, to stretch a point, the organisms responsible for meningitis have been of major significance in the history of molecular biology and in the technology of the new genetics.

Bacterial meningitis: a paradigm for the study of pathogenesis

Based on clinical observations and experimental studies, there is now a reasonable picture of the pathogenesis of *H. influenzae* meningitis. *H. influenzae* colonizes the respiratory tract efficiently, and most commensal strains of *H. influenzae* lack capsule, findings consistent with studies showing that this surface polysaccharide does not enhance, in fact decreases, the efficiency with which *H. influenzae* associates with epithelial cells or mucus. In experiments using human organ cultures, the propensity of *H. influenzae* to associate with mucus is very striking and suggests there are mechanisms which effect specific binding to receptors within mucus. *H. influenzae* elaborates cell wall components, such as lipopolysaccharide, and a low-molecular-weight factor, possibly a glycopeptide, that impair and ultimately disrupt ciliary function and cause damage to the respiratory epithelium (Wilson and Moxon, 1988). These events apparently predispose *H. influenzae* to associate with and damage the respiratory mucosa, mechanisms that could facilitate both localized and systemic disease.

There is evidence that adherence to and internalization by epithelial cells is enhanced by both fimbrial and nonfimbrial determinants, but their role in invasion and the occurrence of bacteraemia is uncertain. Studies of human organ cultures indicate that *H. influenzae* penetrates regions of damage where the integrity of the respiratory epithelial barrier has been breached. Subsequently, the bacteria appear to reach the blood by entering directly into endothelial cells rather than by the lymphatic route; *H. influenzae* is endocytosed by and translocates across human endothelial cells (Moxon, 1992a; Virji *et al.*, 1991).

It is useful to distinguish the separate events involved in invasiveness since different virulence determinants are implicated. Whereas the evidence that capsule enhances survival of *H. influenzae* in blood is unequivocal, capsule apparently does not facilitate translocation across cellular barriers. *In vitro*, both endothelial and epithelial cells internalize encapsulated strains less efficiently than they do capsule-deficient variants, although translocation of both occurs. However, capsule could enhance transmission from one host to another and could also facilitate survival within cells. There are major deficits in our understanding of the mechanisms by which *H. influenzae* enters the blood and, in particular, why encapsulated type b strains cause clinically significant episodes of bacteraemia so much more often than do other strains.

The most compelling explanation for the virtual monopoly of type b strains in causing meningitis is that these strains resist the intravascular clearance mechanisms more efficiently than do strains of the other serotypes or those lacking capsule. Both clinical and experimental data indicate that the duration and magnitude of bacteraemia are critical to the occurrence of meningitis. In rats and primates, there is a strong correlation between the number of bacteria in the blood and the probability of meningitis (Moxon, 1992a).

In the pathogenesis of meningitis in the rat model, a further characteristic of bacteraemia must be accommodated in any comprehensive description of the mechanisms leading to CNS invasion. After intranasal inoculation, the population of organisms in the blood is derived from a very small number of progenitor organisms, often a single bacterium. Thus, *in vivo* replication of *H. influenzae* must be highly efficient if the ~18 generations required to reach concentrations of $\geqslant 10^5$/ml of blood are to occur within several hours. Indeed, calculation of the effective mean generation time (replication minus clearance) necessary to achieve these numbers indicates that doubling of organisms must occur about every 50 min. This is in agreement with serial measurements of the magnitude of bacteraemia. The balance of evidence favours the blood (or perhaps vascular endothelium) as the most likely site. Consistent with this, after an intravenous injection of small numbers of type b organisms (<10), serial blood cultures showed immediate exponential bacterial growth until concentrations of 10^5–10^7 bacteria/ml were reached. These data suggest that there must be efficient, intravascular proliferation of type b organisms (Moxon, 1992a).

The fact that the pathogenesis of bacteraemia involves the survival and proliferation of a single organism argues that there is a 'bottleneck' followed by clonal expansion and that the overwhelming majority of organisms are ultimately denied representation in the population of bacteria that infect the blood and the meninges. At what stage does this bottleneck occur? After intranasal inoculation of rats with about equal numbers of isogenic variants (distinguished by susceptibility or resistance to streptomycin), early blood cultures (>6 h after inoculation) showed that both variants were present. However, blood cultures obtained later (>12 h after challenge) yielded predominantly one or the other variant but not both. Thus, the bottleneck apparently occurs after translocation of bacteria from the nasopharynx to the blood (Moxon and Murphy, 1978).

The sequence of events, therefore, appears to be an early bacteraemia occurring within minutes to an hour after intranasal challenge, a latent period in which bacteraemia is undetectable (or nearly so) and proliferation of organisms resulting in high level bacteraemia. This three-stage profile of the pathogenesis of experimental bacteraemia conforms to a general pattern observed by several investigators. Apparently, in experimental *H. influenzae* infection, the third stage involves the emergence of a rare bacterial clone that eludes the host's clearance mechanism and sets up high-level bacteraemia - an event compatible with the occasional type b organism persisting in and escaping from some intracellular site of sequestration. Such a bacterium, it might reasonably be supposed, has been subjected to strong selective effects and may also have undergone phenotypic shifts favourable to survival.

The third stage of bacteraemia generates the necessary (but not sufficient) conditions for CNS invasion. The balance of evidence supports the choroid plexus as the site of bacterial entry, although a critical product of the number of bacteria and the duration of bacteraemia is required to facilitate bacterial entry into the CNS. Finally, there is the triggering of the host response through the interaction of biologically active mediators, such as lipopolysaccharide and cell wall glycopeptides, to produce inflammation and cellular damage.

The pathogenic personality and the molecular basis of virulence

Upon this platform of observations on the pathogenesis, the tools of molecular and cell biology have been applied to extricate the molecular details of the host-microbial interactions. Stanley Falkow, one of the pioneers of the application of molecular genetics to bacterial pathogens, has captured the essence of the molecular revolution in microbial disease through his revised version of Koch's postulates (Falkow, 1988). The modern goal is to identify the genes (or groups of genes) responsible for virulence, isolate these genes through recombinant DNA technology and amplify them *in vitro* through cloning or the use of polymerase chain reaction and prove their essential role by using genetically defined strains. For example by inserting either the wild-type or mutated genes into the microbe in question and assaying for virulence. From investigations that were limited to studies on virulence phenotype, the molecular version of Koch's postulates has now opened the door to the study of virulence genotype and, as a result, an opportunity to understand the fundamentals of the pathogenic personality. What, in molecular terms is virulence? In the context of meningitis and, indeed, the pathogenesis of most microbial diseases, the molecular analysis of microbial host interactions can be conveniently broken down into a triad of factors which together make up the complex entity referred to as virulence: 1) genes which determine tropism for the host and for a particular niche; 2) genes which are permissive for the microbe to survive clearance and replicate in the host; 3) genes which determine tissue damage (cytotoxicity) (Table 1).

Let us, very briefly, exemplify these three attributes of the pathogenic personality using examples from the bacteria causing meningitis. Most bacteria possess adhesins which facilitate interactions with a particular host and, within that host, particular tissues. Our example here is the pilus or fimbria which acts as a biological grappling hook; specific domains on the subunit polypeptide engage

Table 1.

Molecular Basis of Virulence	
Tropism	host and tissue specificity
Multiplication	mean generation time: factors include scavenging for nutrients, evading host clearance
Cytotoxicity	damage to host tissues

with specific receptors, in the case of the *H. influenzae* fimbria, lactosyl ceramide, found on human epithelial cells (Van Alphen *et al.*, 1991).

As an example of a determinant which facilitates survival and replication within the host, we have the capsular polysaccharides which protect microbes against bacterial lysis and opsonophagocytosis, activities mainly carried out by complement, antibodies and cells of the monocyte/macrophage family. Efficient clearance requires serum antibody to the capsule. In the absence of specific antibodies, *H. influenzae* multiply voraciously in the intravascular compartment and disseminate to sites such as the CNS to cause meningitis. Induction of serum antibodies through immunisation has resulted in the virtual elimination of disease from several countries in Europe and from North America (Shapiro, 1993; Booy *et al.*, 1994).

Elaboration of microbial toxins results in tissue injury either directly, as in the case of true toxins, or through the triggering of inflammation, as in the case of endotoxins. To quote Lewis Thomas (Thomas, 1974): 'It is the information carried by bacteria that we cannot abide. For example, they display lipopolysaccharide endotoxin in their walls, and these macromolecules are read by our tissues as the very worst of bad news. When we sense lipopolysaccharide, we are likely to turn on every defence at our disposal; we will bomb, defoliate, blockade, seal off, and destroy all the tissues in the area. Leucocytes become more actively phagocytic, release lysosomal enzymes, turn sticky, and aggregate together in dense masses, occluding capillaries and shutting off the blood supply. Complement is switched on at the right point in its sequence to release chemotactic signals, calling in leucocytes from everywhere. Vessels become hyper-reactive to epinephrine so that physiological concentrations suddenly possess necrotising properties. Pyrogen is released from leucocytes, adding fever to haemorrhage, necrosis and shock.'

Genetics can pinpoint the molecular basis of tropism, multiplication in the host and cytoxicity, the key components of virulence. The molecular analysis of virulence has also uncovered subtleties in the workings of those genes which are essential to a deeper understanding of the interactions and the co-evolution of hosts and microbes.

Evolutionary biology of virulence

Any student of infectious diseases faces the challenge of understanding the virulence of microbes and its implications for their evolution and that of their hosts. It is worth emphasising not just the molecular basis of virulence—the triad of tropism, multiplication within host tissues, and cytotoxicity—but also that mutuality is of the essence. When we say that a microbe is virulent, we must necessarily ask 'for which host' and conversely, if a host is susceptible, 'to what microbe?' There is currently a strong motivation to seek answers to these questions which inform us at the molecular level.

On the one hand, one can construct plausible rationales for the role of many virulence factors, especially toxins; for example, the toxins of cholera and pertussis bacteria may facilitate their transmission. But the biological advantage of many virulence factors, including the polysaccharide capsules and invasins of the bacteria causing meningitis, is not so obvious. After all, strains of *H. influenzae*, which lack the genetic basis for expression of capsule, are enormously successful commensals. Indeed, there seems little intuitive wisdom in causing meningitis, which merely kills the host and is, literally, a 'dead-end' for the bacterium. Perhaps then the molecular analysis of pathogenic bacteria can give us insight into what Stephen Wills has engagingly called 'the wisdom of the gene' (Wills, 1989). We will attempt this by examining some ideas on the evolution of virulence behaviour which emphasise the role of phenotypic variation, adaptive behaviour and hypermutation of pathogenic bacteria.

A challenge for infecting bacteria; life without sex

Evolutionary biologists have for some time taken a keen interest in the interactions of microbe and host and the ensuing conflicts which determine their co-evolutionary trajectory. This mutuality has attracted such colourful metaphors as gene for gene arms races (Dawkins and Krebs, 1979) or the Red Queen hypothesis (Van Valen, 1973). Populations of a particular species of bacteria, or other microparasites such as viruses, can outnumber those of their host because of their relatively rapid generation time but, since they divide by binary fission, give rise to a clonal population. Intuitively, there would seem to be a need for a clonal population to have mechanisms for generating phenotypic diversity as a strategy for surviving the gauntlet of varying microenvironments, the repertoire of polymorphisms and the eclectic immune clearance mechanisms which are characteristic of hosts. This is particularly relevant to certain acute infections in which the inoculum transmitted from one host to another is subjected to a bottleneck and where it has been shown that the entire population of infecting bacteria is derived from a single organism, or a very small number (Moxon, 1978).

Mechanisms for generating phenotypic diversity

During the course of an infectious episode with a particular species of bacteria, classical point mutations (transitions or transversions) occur relatively infrequently. Also, the contribution of horizontal transfer of genes (sex) would be so rare as to be negligible despite the latter's crucial evolutionary importance in the long term. Nonetheless, intraclonal polymorphisms within bacterial populations are extensive. Over the past decade, there has been an explosion of knowledge detailing the rich panoply of molecular mechanisms through which pathogenic microbes generate phenotypic diversity (Figure 1). Some of these are examples of phenotypic acclimation (classical gene regulation). This is well exemplified by catabolite repression and two component signalling mechanisms, histidine protein kinases; environmental signals, such as those experienced when a bacteria translocates from an extracellular to an intracellular environment, effect changes in phenotype. In contrast to these programmed or discriminate mechanisms, there are the many examples of genetically determined antigenic variation which result from mutational events. Many of these would seem to provide the opportunistic strategies through which clonal populations can furnish the diversity upon which selection can act. By opportunistic, we are emphasising the requirement for bacteria to evolve mechanisms with which to cope with sudden and unpredictable environmental fluxes, situations which in an evolutionary sense are novel or have not been previously experienced. This has been referred to by Gunsalus as the 'biology of anticipation' (Ornston *et al.*, 1990). Pathogenic bacteria face the same challenges as do the genomes of all biological systems; how to attain the optimal constraints on genetic change while maintaining the potential for rapid diversification. An example of this strategy, which can be considered as a biological paradigm of how organisms cope with the unpredictable, is exemplified by the evolution of hypermutable loci. Because the probability of these mutations is stochastic with respect to time but not location, these loci generate phenotypic diversity at high frequency while minimising the deleterious effects of increased genetic load. We have referred to these hypermutable sequences as *contingency loci* to emphasise their role in facilitating the

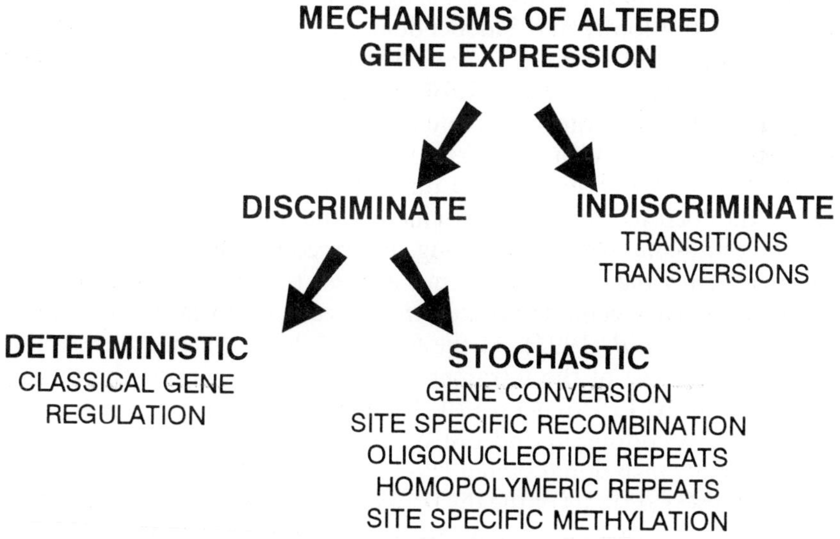

Fig. 1. Mechanisms of altered gene expression (Rainey, 1993).

adaptive behaviour of bacteria when confronted with sudden and unpredictable challenges to their survival (Moxon *et al.*, 1994).

Many hypermutable contingency loci consist of short repeats or homopolymeric tracts positioned either within genes or in important adjacent regions which are involved in transcription, e.g. promoters. These sequences influence the activity of these genes because the repeats are subject to polymerase slippage so that the number of copies of the repeated nucleotides increase or decrease (Moxon and Maskell, 1992b). This introduces frame shifts altering translation or the efficiency with which target sites bind transcriptional factors. In most of the examples which have been described to date in pathogenic bacteria, the altered activity of genes subject to slipped strand mispairing occurs in one out of every 100–1000 bacteria per generation when the rates are studied *in vitro*.

Antigenic variation of core lipopolysaccharides of Haemophilus influenzae

LPS is a macromolecule that is unique to Gram-negative bacteria, and it is the major component of the outer leaflet of the cell envelope. LPS consists of lipid A, which is anchored in the cell envelope, and core saccharide, which extends out from the cell surface. LPS is known to be a major virulence determinant of *H. influenzae*. Phenotypic variation in *H. influenzae* cell-surface LPS provides a further example of random variation generated by high frequency mutations. In this case, however, the variation is not due to a transcriptional mechanism like that responsible for fimbriae phase variation. Rather, the phenotypic expression of several LPS core saccharide structures can be reversibly lost or gained despite continuous synthesis of mRNAs for the enzymes of LPS biosynthesis. The switch is instead effected at the level of translation of these mRNAs, which is turned on and off by frame-shift mutations (Weiser *et al.*, 1989). As the different core saccharide structures switch randomly and independently of each other, a population of *H. influenzae* founded by a single clone and residing within a single host can generate an extensive repertoire of variant LPS epitope.

The molecular basis of the variable expression of one of these saccharide structures, galα(1-4)galβ (Virji *et al.*, 1990) has been studied in some detail. When colonies of *H. influenzae* were blotted on to nitrocellulose filters and allowed to react with a monoclonal antibody specific for the structure galα(1-4)galβ, individual colonies showed either strong, intermediate, or undetectable binding. Mutants have been isolated which do not express the digalactoside structure and one of these maps to a gene designated *lic2*, a gene essential for synthesis of the digalactoside (High *et al.*, 1993). At the 5′ end of the *lic2* gene, there are multiple tandem repeats (ca. 16) of the tetramer 5′-CAAT-3′. However, the number of CAAT repeats varies; loss or gain of CAAT, usually a single repeat, moves upstream initiation codons in and out of frame with the remainder of the gene, thereby creating a translational switch (Weiser *et al.*, 1989; Weiser *et al.*, 1990) and resulting in variable synthesis of the digalactoside. Similar to the phase variation of fimbriae, the presumed mechanism for the frame shift is slipped-strand mispairing (Levinson and Gutman, 1987), a *recA*-independent mechanism capable of mediating high-frequency random changes in nucleotide sequence. It should also be noted that the resulting mutation and its potential for fortuitously adaptive changes in phenotype can occur either during the replication process or through mismatch repair; the latter mechanism is potentially important with respect to the behaviour of bacteria under stress and perhaps in a non-replicating state (stationary phase). It may be significant that the region immediately up-stream of *lic2* is especially rich in AT nucleotides (High *et al.*, 1993). This would tend to facilitate strand separation and increase the likelihood of slipped-strand mis-pairing; such a region would be prone to the effects of altered supercoiling, since changes in superhelicity are known to affect transcriptional efficiency. There is accumulating evidence in support of a role for global regulation of gene expression through changes in supercoiling (Higgins and Dorman, 1990).

A typical characteristic of contingency loci is that they affect the activity of genes responsible for the expression of surface molecules which are important in the interactions of the bacterium with its host. Through a few such key genes, whose activities are subject to these mutational hot spots, this high frequency phenotypic variation influences such characteristics as antigenicity, motility, chemotaxis, attachment to host-cells, acquisition of nutrients, and sensitivity to antibiotics while concurrently minimising the deleterious effect that high mutation rates would impose on house-keeping functions of the genome (Figure 2). But propitiously, homopolymeric tracts or short nucleotide repeats could also provide a mechanism which lends itself to some degree of environmental responsiveness. For example, changes in supercoiling would be particularly likely to influence regions of DNA such as short tandem repeats which undergo strand separation, exposure of single stranded DNA, changes in orientation of sequence and alternative DNA structures. It is well established that changes in the environment can affect the topology of DNA and changes in super-coiling can affect the activity of genes.

Contingency loci

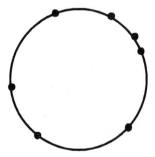

Fig. 2. A bacterial genome, double stranded circular DNA, is depicted with several hypermutable loci [●] which result in altered activity of genes. These contingency loci result in changes in phenotype which occur at high frequency [about 1:100–1000 bacteria per generation] and typically affect the activity of genes which interact with environment. These mutational events are random in time and therefore generate heterogeneity within a clonal population of replicating bacteria. They are non-random in location and therefore maximise intraclonal polymorphisms while minimising deleterious effects on the genome as a whole.

The concept that cells should be at their most mutable when conditions are unfavourable to an organism is appealing. Indeed, stress-induced mutagenesis is not a new concept. McClintock captured the idea quite beautifully: 'These ...... responses, now known to occur in many organisms, are significant for appreciating how a genome may reorganise itself when faced with a difficulty for which it is unprepared.' (McClintock, 1993)

The conventional view is that the environment selects among pre-existing variants; mutations arise without regard for their utility. But, intuitively, it is evident that it could be advantageous for organisms to evolve mechanisms through which the environment could influence the genetic mechanisms which generate phenotypic variation and upon which selection acts. Have mechanisms evolved which result in mutations which arise when, and even because, they are advantageous?

In a letter to Nature in 1988, Cairns, Overbaugh and Miller pointed out that the classical Luria-Delbruck experiments were not designed nor were they able to detect mutants that arose during or following the imposition of lethal selection (Cairns et al., 1988). Two types of data were presented which, they suggested, provided some evidence to suggest that 'cells may have mechanisms for choosing which mutations will occur.' First, fluctuation tests in which *Escherichia coli* organisms deficient in lactose gave distributions of lac + mutants which suggested that they arose only in response to selection. Second, plate tests in which lac + organisms accumulated over time when lac − cells were incubated in the presence of added lactose, but failed to do so when lactose was not present. This class of mutations has been given various names, including directed, adaptive, non-random and selection induced (Foster, 1993). Can we countenance ideas 'suggesting that cells may have mechanisms for choosing which mutations will occur' (Cairns et al., 1988)? In the ensuing years, these and some later data have been the subject of spirited, at times heated, controversy involving evolutionary biologists and bacterial geneticists who have debated whether or not the occurrence of 'directed mutations' was real and if so, the molecular mechanisms giving rise to them (Lenski and Mittler, 1993). There is now convincing evidence that some mutations do occur in non-replicating bacterial populations after the imposition of changes to their external environment, such as the provision of a novel nutrient. Further and importantly, these mutations appear to be different from mutants which are present in the population prior to the addition of a selective agent (Rosenberg et al., 1994; Foster and Trimarchi, 1994). No entirely satisfactory model which would explain directed mutations has yet been advanced. But does the behaviour of 'stationary phase' bacteria plated on to simple laboratory media have relevance to the biology of infectious disease and the evolution of commensal and virulence behaviour? The link between directed mutations in *E. coli* on the one hand and hypermutation in contingency loci of pathogenic microbes on the other stems from observations that the mechanism involved in both instances involves frame shifts in small nucleotide repeats or homopolymeric tracts presumptively through polymerase slippage.

It has been a central tenet of molecular biology that there is independence of genetic information from events occurring outside or even inside the cell. Indeed, it has been argued that 'the very nature and structure of the genetic code and the way it is transcribed implies that no information from outside can ever penetrate the inheritable genetic message' (Judson, 1979). Thus, it has been argued that specific mutations do not occur at higher rates when they are beneficial than when they are neutral or disadvantageous. So, with respect to the proposition that organisms can selectively enhance mutations in specific genes in response to signals from the environment, would not such a mechanism challenge the fundamental tenets of Darwinian theory that mutations are random with respect to their selective utility?

In an insightful essay, Keller argues that the meaning of randomness in mutations provides the key to this escape (Keller, 1992). To quote B.D. Davis on randomness: 'Used to mean an undirected process, occurring by chance in any gene, this term has become firmly embedded in classical genetics. But equally clearly, randomness in the strict mathematical sense, as equal probability, does not apply to the genome at the level of nucleotides or of short sequences surrounding a site of mutation. The notion of biased randomness is thus not a radical one; it has been with us since the discovery of fine structure genetics, with its recognition of mutational hot spots.' (Davis, 1989)

It does not seem unreasonable to extend the notion to DNA sequences subject to influence by the environment. There is no evidence that external signals can instruct bacterial cells to make specific mutations - the most unorthodox of the proposed mechanisms to explain directed mutations and the one which made the issue rather controversial (Cairns *et al.*, 1988). Rather, it would seem that variants generated by specialised, hypermutable sequences (contingency loci) are programmed (directed) in that they have evolved so as to alter the activity of a few, strategically important genes. Indeed, that directed mutations might appear to result from environmental instruction is testimony to the power of an event (mutation) which is stochastic in time and in the direction of the phenotypic switch, but programmed (evolved) in its assignment to specific chromosomal locations. Thus, the concept of hypermutable 'contingency loci' offers a neo-Darwinian explanation for adaptive mutations in which there is no requirement for any novel molecular mechanisms or a 'reverse flow of information' (Cairns *et al.*, 1988). The trial and error model proposed by Hall can be adapted so that the hypermutable state is localised to particular regions of the genomes of each bacterium (Hall, 1990). The slow repair and error prone tendency of the stressed bacterium mean that errors occur at particularly high rates (MacPhee, 1993). If the cell achieves success, it exits and resumes growth. This seems to be particularly apposite to pathogenic bacteria in which hypermutation through repetitive DNA, in principle environmentally responsive, offers the advantage of the biology of anticipation at a minimal cost to the fitness provided by the evolution of biological memory (housekeeping genes). It also suggests a good explanation for the bottleneck which occurs in the pathogenesis of menigitis (Moxon and Murphy, 1978); indeed, it would appear that in many infections, there is a stage when the progression of infection depends upon clonal expansion of a few microbes, even a single founder organism.

Perspective

Despite our preoccupation with disease, business as usual for pathogenic microbes is the commensal state, an opportunity for residence, multiplication and transmission. In this paper, we have examined the molecular basis of some of the phenotypic variation occurring in certain pathogenic bacteria. We have suggested that pathogenic bacteria have mechanisms that promote extensive phenotypic variation while maintaining their genomes more or less intact and that these contingency strategies are a component of the evolution of the pathogenic personality. For some host-adapted bacterial pathogens responsible for invasive infections, virulence reflects the evolution of a repertoire of mechanisms which maximise their success to colonise the mucosal surfaces, such as the respiratory tract, and to promote opportunities for transmission to another human host. For example, invasion of host epithelial cells may enhance successful residence in the host and allow sequestration of bacteria from host clearance mechanisms which act in the extracellular environment. Although this attribute also facilitates systemic invasion and the potential for killing its host, this occurrence is a relatively rare event and so the host-microbial strategy approximates closely to that of balanced parasitism. Disease is an incidental and accidental consequence of the relentless drive of microbes to perpetuate their selfish genes. Pathogenicity is the flip side of a coin which constitutes the currency of survival.

References

Avery, O.T., C.M. McCleod and M. McCarty, 1944 - Studies on the chemical nature of the substance inducing transformation of pneumococcal types. Induction of transformation by a desoxyribonucleic acid fraction isolated from pneumococcus type III. *J. Exp. Med.* **79**, 137–158.

Booy, R., S. Hodgson, L. Carpenter, R.T. Mayon-White, M.P.E. Slack, J.A. Macfarlane, E.A. Haworth, M. Kiddle, S. Shribman, J. St. Clair Roberts and E.R. Moxon, 1994 - Efficacy of the *Haemophilus influenzae* type b conjugate vaccine PRP-T. *Lancet* **344**, 364–366.

Cairns, J., J. Overbaugh and S. Miller, 1988 - The origin of mutants. *Nature* **335**, 142–145.

Davis, B.D., 1989 - Transcriptional bias: A non-Lamarckian mechanism for substrate-induced mutations. *Proc. Natl. Acad. Sci. USA* **86**, 5005–5009.

Dawkins, R. and J.R. Krebs, 1979 - Arms races within and between species. *Proc. R. Soc. Lond. B* **205**, 489–511.

Falkow, S., 1988 - Molecular Koch's postulates applied to microbial pathogenicity. *Rev. Infect. Dis.* **10** (suppl), 274–276.

Foster, P.L. and J.M. Trimarchi, 1994 - Adaptive reversion of a frameshift mutation in Escherichia coli by simple base deletions in homopolymeric runs. *Science* **265**, 407–409.

Foster, P.L., 1993 - Adaptive mutation: the uses of adversity. *Ann. Rev. Microbiol.* **47**, 467–504.

Hall, B.G., 1990 - Spontaneous point mutations that occur more often when advantageous than when neutral. *Genetics* **126**, 5–16.

Higgins, C.F. and C.J. Dorman, 1990 - DNA supercoiling: a role in the regulation of gene expression and bacterial virulence. In *Bacterial Proteins Toxins.* Edited by Rappuoli R. *et al.* New York, Gustav Fischer, 293–301.

High, N.J., M.E. Deadman and E.R. Moxon, 1993 - The role of a repetitive DNA motif ('5-CAAT-3') in the variable expression of the *Haemophilus influenzae* lipopolysaccharide epitope Galα(1-4)β Gal. *Mol. Microbiol.* **9**, 1275–1282.

Judson, H., 1979 - The eighth day of creation: the makers of the revolution in biology. Simon and Schuster, New York.

Keller, E.F., 1992 - Question of directive mutation. Perspectives in Biology and Medicine **35**, 292–306.

Lenski, R.E. and J.E. Mittler, 1993 - The directed mutation controversy and neo-Darwinism. *Science* **259**, 188–194.

Levinson, G. and G.A. Gutman, 1987 - Slipped-strand mispairing: a major mechanism for DNA sequence evolution. *Mol. Biol. Evol.* **4**, 203–221.

MacPhee, D.G., 1993 - The directed mutation affair. Today's Life Science, 10–14.

McClintock, B., 1993 - The significance of responses of the genome to challenge. Nobel Lecture, 8th December 1993.

Moxon, E.R., 1992a - Molecular basis of invasive *Haemophilus influenzae* type b disease. *J. Infect. Dis.* **165**, S77–S81.

Moxon, E.R., P.B. Rainey, M.A. Nowak and R.E. Lenski, 1994 - Adaptive evolution of highly mutable loci in pathogenic bacteria. *Curr. Biol.* **4**, 24–33.

Moxon, E.R. and P.A. Murphy, 1978 - Haemophilus influenzae bacteremia and meningitis resulting from survival of a single organism. *Proc. Natl. Acad. Sci. USA* **75**, 1534–1536.

Moxon, E.R. and D. Maskell, 1992b - *Haemophilus influenzae* lipopolysaccharide: the biochemistry and biology of a virulence factor. In: C. Hormaeche, C.W. Penn and C.J. Smyth (eds). Molecular biology of bacterial infection: current status and future perspectives. *SGM Symposium* **49**, 75–96.

Ornston, L.N., E.L. Neidle and J.E. Houghton, 1990 - Gene rearrangements, a force for evolutionary change; DNA sequence arrangements, a source of genetic constancy. In The Bacterial Chromosome. Eds. K. Drlica and M. Riley. American Society for Microbiology, Washington DC, 325.

Rainey, P.B., E.R. Moxon and I.P. Thompson, 1993 - Intraclonal polymorphism in bacteria. In Advances in Microbial Ecology (Vol. 13). Ed. J.G. Jones. Plenum Press, New York, 267.

Rosenberg, S.M., S. Longerich, P. Gee and S.H. Reuben, 1994 - Adaptive mutation by deletions in small mononucloetide repeats. *Science* **265**, 405–407.

Shapiro, E.P., 1993 - Infections caused by *Haemophilus influenzae* type b. The beginning of the end? (editorial comment) *JAMA* **269**(2), 227–231.

Thomas, L., 1974 - Lives of a Cell. Notes of a Biology Watcher. New York: Viking Press, 78–79.

Van Alphen, L., L. Geelen van den Broek, L. Blaas, M. van Ham and J. Dankert, 1991 – Blocking of fimbria-mediated adherence of Haemophi lusin-fluenzae by sialyl gangliosides. *Infect. Immun.* **59**, 4473–4477.

Van Valen, L., 1973 - A new evolutionary law. *Evol. Theory* **1**, 1–30.

Virji, M., H. Kayhty, D.J.P. Ferguson, C. Alexandrescu and E.R. Moxon, 1991 – Interactions of *Haemophilus influenzae* with cultured human endothelial cells. *Microbial. Pathog.* **10**, 231–245.

Virji, M., J.N. Weiser, A.A. Lindberg and E.R. Moxon, 1990 - Antigenic similarities in lipopolysaccharides of *Haemophilus* and *Neisseria* and expression of digalactoside structure also present on human cells. *Microb. Pathog.* **9**, 441–450.

Weiser, J.N., D.J. Maskell, P.D. Butler, A.A. Lindberg and E.R. Moxon, 1990 - Characterisation of repetitive sequences controlling phase-variation of *Haemophilus influenzae* lipopolysaccharide. *J. Bacteriol.* **172**, 3304–3309.

Weiser, J.N., J.M. Love and E.R. Moxon, 1989 - The molecular mechanism of phase variation of *H. influenzae* lipopolysaccharide. *Cell* **59**, 657–665.

Wills, C., 1989 - The Wisdom of the genes. New Pathways in Evolution. Oxford University Press.

Wilson, R. and E.R. Moxon, 1988 - Molecular mechanisms of *Haemophilus influenzae* pathogenicity in the respiratory tract. In: Donachie W., Griffiths E., Stephen J., eds. Bacterial Infections of Respiratory and Gastrointestinal Mucosae. Washington DC: IRL Press. 1988; **24**, 29–38.

Posters

Of Leptospiral Lps and Heat Shock Proteins: where does *Leptospira* fit in?

Ben Adler, Susan Ballard, Solly Faine, Marina Harper and Tu Vinh

The genes encoding the rhamnose biosynthesis locus involved in LPS biosynthesis in *Leptospira interrogans* serovar *copenhageni* were cloned and sequenced. Analysis revealed a gene order of *rfbDCBA*, with the translated protein sequences showing up to 57% identity with the homologous proteins in *Salmonella* and *Shigella*. The cloned locus could restore normal LPS phenotype to an *rfbB*::Tn*5* mutant of *S. flexneri*.

The *dnaK* and *groE* operons of serovar *copenhageni* were cloned and sequenced. Both revealed the presencve of a CIRCE type repetitive upstream element which appeared to control the regulation of the operons at transcriptional level. There was no evidence for a sigma-32 based regulatory sustem. The *dnaK* operon had an organisation similar to that of *Bacillus subtilis*, with a gene order of *orf1*, *grpE*, *dnaK* and *dnaJ*.

Phylogenetic analysis of the sequences indicated an early evolutionary divergence of *Leptospira* and resembled the taxonomic position determined by 16S rRNA sequences.

Department of Microbiology, Monash University, Clayton 3168, Melbourne, Australia.

In Search of the Holy Grail: The Quest for Universal Lipid A Binding and Neutralizing Ligands for Treatment of Severe Gram-negative Infections

B.J. Appelmelk, A. Y. Qing, E.J. Helmershorst, J.J. Maaskant, P.R. Abraham, L.G. Thijs and D.M. MacLaren

Introduction

Adehesion of microorganisms, including Gram-negative bacteria, to host epithelial cells may be followed by penetration through the epithelial lining, invasion into the bloodstream and finally, dissemination to lungs, liver, brain tissue and other organs. This process may have severe consequences for the host, since bacterial lipopolysaccharide (LPS, endotoxin) is a very potent inducer of cytokines like tumour necrosis factor (TNF) and interleukins (IL-1, -6, -8). The overinduction of these cytokines causes the clinical symptoms of sepsis and septic shock and leads to inadequate tissue perfusion, multiple organ failure, and ultimately, death. Mortality due to Gram-negative sepsis and shock remains high despite the availability of potent antibiotics: the bacteria may be killed by antibiotics but the endotoxin remains active! Hence, the novel strategies to lower mortality of Gram-negative infections have focused on ways of inactivating endotoxin. As lipid A (LA) is the toxic part of LPS these attempts have focused on preparing LA-binding ligands. LA is structurally the most conserved part of LPS and thus an additional advantage of the anti-LA approach is that potentially, a single ligand (monoclonal antibody or peptide) may be prepared active against all or the majority of strains belonging to the species most often involved in Gram-negative sepsis and shock, i.e. *Escherichia coli*, *Pseudomonas aeruginosa*, *Klebsiella pneumoniae*.

Subject

The immunochemical properties of four currently known groups of LA ligands will be described, i.e., three groups of LA binding monoclonal antibodies (Mabs), and a non-antibody LA ligand: recombinant/bactericidal permeability increasing protein (rBPI$_{23}$).

Results

The **first** group of anti-LA Mabs recognizes the hydrophilic part of LA. Binding requires a non-substituted C'60H in LA and affinity for Re- and other R-and S- LPS was very low. These Mabs (IgG and IgM) do not display hydrophobic interactions and do not bind to non-lipid A antigens, i.e. they are monoreactive.

The **second** group of Mabs (IgM) displays hydrophobic properties, binds also to single-stranded (ss) DNA, phospholipids and proteins, i.e. Mabs are polyreactive. Binding of these Mabs to bacteria involved interaction with outer membrane proteins; affinity for LPS was very low. The **third** group of LA Mabs (IgM) are anti-Kdo Mabs in disguise. They bind to LA, Kdo, ssDNA and phospholipids, i.e., they are also polyspecific. Due to their Kdo (a common epitope) specificity, these Mabs bind with high affinities to some but not all LPS of *E. coli*, *Klebsiella* and *Psuedomonas*. They are functionally active in passive hemolysis.

The **fourth** group comprises antibacterial peptides like $rBPI_{23}$, which binds well to all lipid As ($n = 8$) and all Re-, R- and S- LPS tested ($n = 200$). Thus, unique for BPI is its ability to bind to lipid A even when the C'60H group is substituted with Kdo. Other peptides have been reported in the literature that have binding- and neutralizing properties similar to $rBPI_{23}$, for example polymyxin B and derivatives thereof and a LA-binding polypeptide present in amoebocytes of the horseshoe crab *Limulus polyphemus* and oligopeptide derivatives thereof.

Summary

LA Mabs are a heterogenous group of antibodies. Immunochemically speaking, none of the various LA Mabs looks promising as an immunotherapeutic agent. In contrast, $rBPI_{23}$ is a universal LA/LPS ligand.

Future

For the future is will be crucial to understand on a molecular scale, i.e. three-dimensionally, the manner in which LPS-neutralizing peptides interact with LA and to define what structural element(s) in a peptide are crucial for neutralization. To this end we have synthesized a variety of small (less than 30 amino acids) LA-binding peptides. These novel peptides, that bind to and neutralize LA, are currently under investigation in a variety of *in vitro* and *in vivo* assay systems.

Department of Medical Microbiology and Medical Intensive care Unit, Vrije Universiteit, Amsterdam, the Netherlands

The Pathogenicity of *Taylorella equigenitalis*

N.M.C. Bleumink-Pluym, D.J. Houwers and B.A.M. van der Zeijst

Taylorella equigenitalis is the causative agent of contagious equine metritis (CEM), a sexually transmitted disease of horses.

Comparison of 16S ribosomal gene sequences showed that *Bordetella bronchiseptica, Alcaligenes xylosoxidans* and *Alcaligenes faecalis* are its closest relatives, which is surprising in view of the differences in the G + C contents of the genomes.

In 32 *T. equigenitalis* strains studied, the capacity to invade and replicate intracellularly varied considerably, indicating that strains differ in their virulences.

The N-terminal amino acid sequences of the immunodominant 39kDa outer membrane protein was determined. Homologies were found with porins of *Bordetella pertussis* (89%), *Neisseria gonorrhoeae* (75% with P1A) and *Neisseria meningitidis* (75% with class 3).

Universiteit Utrecht, Utrecht, the Netherlands.

Actinobacillus pleuropneumoniae in Swine: Pathogenesis, Antigens and Vaccination

Han van den Bosch

Porcine pleuropneumoniae is an important disease in fattening pigs, caused by *A. pleuropneumoniae* (App). At present 13 different serotypes have been described, based on differences in CPS and LPS.

The 23 different App serotypes express one or two of three different RTX toxins, designated ApxI, ApxII and ApxIII (1). Within each serotype a remakably consistent Apx toxin profile was found in field isolates from all over the world, both with regard to genotype and phenotype (2). Four different toxin profiles could be distinguished: 1) ApxI and ApxII in serotypes 1, 5a, 5b, 9 and 11; 2) ApxII and ApxIII in serotypes 2, 3, 4, 6 and 8; 3) ApxII in serotypes 7 and 12; 4) ApxI in serotype 10.

Besides an OMP-A homologous outer membrane protein (OMP), all App serotypes and 99% of field isolates express a common 42kDa-OMP. By sequence comparisons this 42kDA-OMP appeared to be homologous to the P2-OMP of *H. influenzae* type b (3).

A vaccine (Actinoporc^{TM}) was composed by including purified ApxI, ApxII and ApxIII toxoids and purified 42kDa-OMP in an aqueous adjuvant formulation (Diluvac^{TM} Forte). The vaccine appeared to induce almost complete protection in pigs with regard to morbidity, mortality and development of typical lung lesions, against aerosol challenge with several App serotypes. Since the vaccine was shown to induce protection against challenge with at least one representative of all 4 toxin profiles, it was concluded as very likely that the vaccine will protect against all App serotypes.

References

1. Frey, J. et al. 1993 - *Actinobacillus pleuropneumoniae* RTX-toxins: uniform designation of haemolysins, cytolysins, pleurotoxin and their genes. J. Gen. Microbiol. **139**, 1723–1728.
2. Beck, M., J. F. van den Bosch, I.M.C.A. Jongenelen, P.L.W. Loeffen, R. Nielsen, J. Nicolet and J. Frey, 1994 - RTX toxin genotypes and phenotypes in *Actinobacillus pleuropneumoniae* field strains. *J. Clin. Microbiol.* **32**, 2749–2754.

3. van den Bosch, J.F., A.N.B. Pubben, F.G.A. van Vugt and R.P.A.M. Segers, 1994. Synergistic effect of a P2-homologous outer membrane protein and ApxI toxin in protection against *Actinobacillus pleuropneumoniae*. In: H.A.P. '94, Edinburgh, p. 36.

Intervet International BV, P.O. Box 31, 5830 AA Boxmeer, the Netherlands

Swedish β-lactam Resistant *Enterococcus faecium* mostly belong to a Cluster of Closely Related Strains

Sara Hæggman and Lars G. Burman

Introduction

Enterococci highly resistant to crucial agents such as aminoglycosides, β-lactams and vancomycin represent an emerging worldwide threat. Whereas ampicillin resistance in *E. faecalis* is due to acquisition of penicillinase, the second common species *E. faecium* has developed resistance to all availabele β-lactam agents due to alterations of the penicillin binding (target) proteins.

Multiresistant *E. faecium* isolates with altered PBPs are often untreatable pathogens and have caused widespread concern, particularly in the USA.

Betalactam (but not multiply) resistant *E. faecium* have become increasingly common in Swedish hospitals in recent years.

Materials and methods

Clinical isolates of β-lactam resistant *E. faecium* (ampicillin MIC ≥ 16 mg/l, n = 102) were obtained from three Swedish counties 1993-94 where such strains have caused problems. As reference, a random sample of fecal isolates from healthy individuals from 13 of 35 counties 1990 (n = 25) were used. All isolates were typed using the computerized pheneplate system. Its modification for fecal streptococci (PhP-FS) has shown high reproducibility and as good discriminatory power as pulsed field gel electropheresis of chromosomal DNA (Kühn, Tullus, Hæggman, Murray, Burman, in preparation). The PhP-FS data based on optical registration of the kinetics of 24 biochemical reactions per isolate were clustered using the UPGMA method.

Results

The fecal *E. faecium* isolates from healthy individuals were of many distinct PhP-FS types. Two isolates were ampicillin resistant but had different PhP-FS type and place of isolation. In contrast (80%) of the ampicillin resistant clinicla isolates of *E. faecium* belonged to identical or closely related PhP-FS types (cluster A). One of the ampicillin resistant isolates from healthy individuals had nearly identical PhP-FS type as the cluster A isolates.

Conclusions

1. Fecal *E. faecium* isolates from healthy individuals in Sweden are biochemically diverse and usually do not express ampicillin/β-lactam resistance.
2. Recent Swedish clinical *E. faecium* isolates with acquired ampicillin resistance mostly belong to identical or closely related phenotypes (cluster A) suggesting a clonal origin.
3. A cluster A-like ampicillin resistant fecal isolate was found in a healthy carrier in 1990.

Swedish Institute for Infectious Disease Control, S-105 21 Stockholm, Sweden

Phase Variation of Class 1 outer Membrane Protein in *Neisseria meningitidis*

Arie van der Ende

The class 1 outer membrane protein code by the *porA* gene of *Neisseria meningitidis*, is a vaccine candidate against this pathogen. The expression of class 1 outer membrane protein displays phase variation between three expression levels.

Analysis by PCR showed two classes of class 1 protein phase variants; one with an intact *porA* gene and the other with the *porA* gene completely absent. Analysis of the *porA* specific transcripts of the first class of phase variants by Northern hybridization showed that these phase variants are modulated at the transcriptional level. The start site for transcription is located 59 base pairs upstream of the translational initiation codon. Sequence analysis the DNA region upstream of the coding region of the *porA* gene, revealed a poly G tract in the spacer between the -10 and -35 sequence of its promoter. Comparison of promoter sequences of different phase variants showed that the length of the poly G tract can be correlated with the expression level of the class 1 outer membrane protein. These results show that the transcription of *porA* gene is modulated by slipped strand mispairing of a poly G stretch within the intervening sequence of the -35 and -10 regions of its promoter. Sequence analysis of the DNA region upstream and downstream the *porA* gene also revealed regions with extensive homology at either side of the gene. The deletion of the *porA* gene of the second class of phase variants comprised the region between these sequences of extensive homology. From these data we suggest that the *porA* gene can be deleted by homologous recombination. The phase variation of class 1 outer membrane protein may provide a molecular mechanism to evade the host immune defence.

Department of Medical Microbiology, University of Amsterdam, AMC, and the Reference Laboratory for Bacterial Meningitis UVA/RIVM, Meibergdreef 15, 1105 AZ Amsterdam

The Structural Organization of Fimbrial Ashesins; Variation on a Common Theme: Aspects of Chaperones and Ushers

B. Oudega

The interaction of the *E. coli* K88 molecular chaperone FaeE with the K88 major fimbrial subunit FaeG was studied by isoelectric focusing, anion exchange FPLC, SDS-PAGE, native gel electrophoresis, immunoblotting and determination of N-terminal amino acid sequencing. FaeE and FaeG form a heterotrimer consisting of one molecule of FaeG and two molecules of the chaperone FaeE. Gel filtration, protein crosslinking analysis and a biophysical approach in which the rotation diffusion coefficient of the purified FaeE was determined showed that the native chaperone FaeE is a homodimer. As for FaeG also FaeH and FaeI were shown to form a heterotrimer with FaeE.

An outer membrane folding model for the fimbrial ushers FaeD was developed based on insertion mutagenesis, protease accessibility studies, subcellular localization experiments and computer analysis. Evolutionary aspects of both the molecular chaperone and the outer membrane ushers will be studied.

Faculteit Biologie, Vrije Universiteit, Dept. of Microbial Microbiology, De Boelelaan 1087, 1081 HV Amsterdam

Epidemiological Typing of Pathogenic Bacteria

J. Van der Plas[1], L. Schouls[2], H. Goossens[3] and H. Hofstra[1]

Bacterial species can be differentiated by rRNA gene restriction patterns generated after cleavage of total DNA with restriction enzymes and hybridization of the fragments with labelled 16S + 23S rRNA probes (ribotyping). We extended this methodology by development of RFLP probes based on other highly conserved sequences from common (eu)bacterial genes, ATPase, ribosomal protein S12, and elongation factor Ef-Tu, while preserving the generic approach.

RFLP probes were produced by PCR ampification using primers from highly conserved regions found in sequence alignment. A probe for the Campylobacter flagellin was also produced and applied in the same manner. RFLP analyses with these probes supplement the ribotyping data and add extra levels of discrimination, because the resolution level varies with the number and kind of restriction enzyme/probe combinations used. This DNA typing method successfully discriminated Campylobacter isolates on the strain level. The RFLP patterns obtained were reproducible and appeared to be stable.

RFLP-typing was applied to compare isolates from a *C. upsaliensis* outbreak in four day-care centres in Brussels and to investigate the possible route(s) of transmission of *C. coli* in pigs. In order to compare the RFLP-typing with the traditional serotyping according to Penner and Lior, and with the rapid PCR typing method called Random Amplified Polymorphic DNA (RAPD), 180 *Campylobacter* strains from various origins (humans, cattle, pigs, poultry) were collected, identified with our multiplex PCR assay for *C. jejuni/coli*, and subjected to the three typing methods in parallel. The resulting data were subsequently analyzed by nonlinear multivariate analysis.

Department of Bioprocessing & Biomonitoring[1], TNO Nutrition and Food Research, Zeist. The Netherlands.
Lab. of Molecular Microbiology[2], RIVM, Bilthoven, the Netherlands.
Department of Microbiology[3], University Hospital Antwerp, Belgium.

The Roles of IS630 Sequence in the Expression of the Form I Antigen of *Shigella sonnei*: Molecular and Evolutionary Aspects

Huo-Shu H. Houng*, Michael J. Zapor, Antoinette B. Hartman, Thomas L. Hale and Malabi M. Venkatesan

Infections by *Shigella* spp. are frequent causes of human diarrheal diseases. These organisms invade the colonic epithelium via the distinct processes of penetration, multiplication and intercellular dissemination. One of the four species in this genus, *S. sonnei* comprises a single serotype expressing an O-chain lipopolysaccharide (LPS) termed form I (smooth) antigen. Unlike the other enteric organisms, the form I antigen of *S. sonnei* is encoded by a 180 kilobase (kb) virulence plasmid which is also essential for *Shigella* to invade epithelial cells. The expression of the form I antigen in *S. sonnei* is not stably maintained, frequently giving rise to a form II (rough) phenotype when cultivated on artifical medium. The form II colonies are cured of the invasive plasmid and are uniformly avirulent.

We have genetically characterized the form I coding region of *S. sonnei* and have found that an 11.0 kb *Hin*dIII-*Xba*I fragment is sufficient to encode for the form I antigen as detected by slide agglutination using form I-specific antisera. Precise boundaries for the form I coding region were defined by *Exo*III exonuclease mapping. A total of 10 essential ORF's organized as an operon were predicted from the DNA sequence analysis of the form I coding region. These polypeptides share significant homology with the products encoded by the Vi antigen genes of *S. typhi* and the *rfb* loci of *S. typhimurium* and *V. cholerae*. We also identified an insertional element sequence, IS630, which encodes for the 5th ORF of the form I operon in *S. sonnei*. Southern hybridization experiments have shown that *Plesiomonas shigelloides* and *S. sonnei* share homologous form I coding sequences. Using polymerase chain reactions (PCR) and available oligonucleotide primers flanking the IS630 sequence, we demonstrated that the form I coding region of *P. shigelloides* shares extensive homologous DNA sequence with *S. sonnei* form I antigen, but lacks the IS630 sequence. This may account for the comparative stability of the form I antigen expression in *P. shigelloides* over *S. sonnei*. Clinical isolates of *S. sonnei* from south America, southeast Asia, U.S.S.R., and United States were obtained and examined for the existence of IS630 in the form I coding region, and it was found that all the strains examined contain an IS630 sequence locating at the same insertion site within the from I coding region. We further constructed a recombinant plasmid encoding for the functional form I region which is free of IS630 sequence. The resultant plasmid, pHH2062, is capable of expressing the form I antigen in *E. coli* K12, but fails to express the same form I antigen in its parental *S. sonnei* form II strain.

The form I coding regions of *S. sonnei* and *P. shigelloides* produce seriologically-identical O-antigen and have extensive homologous identities at DNA level. It is likely that the O-antigen operons for these two organisms evolved from the same origin. Results of this study indicated that the IS630 does not play any synthetic role in the form I antigen expression, but it plays an important role in terms of maintaining the form I expression and subsequent survival for the pathogenic *S. sonnei* in the human reservoir.

Department of Enteric Infections, Walter Reed Army Institute of Research, Washington, DC 20307-5100

Evolution of Capsule Synthesis Genes of *Streptococcus pneumoniae*

Piet Nuijten[2], Marc Kolkman[1] and Bernard van der Zeijst[1]

Most bacterial polysaccharides are synthesized via a similar route; the repeating oligosaccharide subunit is made on a lipid-carrier molecule at the cytoplasmic surface of the membrane and after polymerization of these subunits the polysaccharide is transported and exposed on the surface of the bacterium. The structure of an oligosaccharide subunit is determined by 1) transferases that link a specific monosaccharide to a growing structure and ii) synthetases that make the specific monosaccharides. The enormous diversity in polysaccharide structures is due to variation in i) the monosaccharide composition; ii) the specific linkage between the sugars within a subunit; iii) the linkage between the subunits; iv) modifications. The molecular basis of polysaccharide synthesis and of its structural diversity is investigated using *Streptococcus pneumoniae* capsule polysaccharides as a model. This species is divided into 85 different capsular serotypes each one having its own specific polysaccharide structure. We have cloned and sequenced a large part of the capsule locus of *S. pneumoniae* serotype 14 and identified 9 ORF's (*cps14A-I*). *Cps14A-D* are probably involved in regulation and transport, while *cps14E* and *cps14G* were identified as glycosyl transferase genes Cps14E links glucose-1-phosphate to the lipid carrier. The amino acid sequence at the carboxy-terminus shows homologies to other bacterial glycosyl transferases that all catalyze the transfer of the first sugar to the lipid carrier, but they differ in the type of the monosaccharide which is transferred. Glucosyl transferase activity (like Cps14E) is found in many *S. pneumoniae* serotypes that contain glucose in their polysaccharide structure, but they not all carry a *cps14E*-like gene. Thus, *S. pneumoniae* glucosyl transferase genes are not all homologous and probably originate from different sources.

[1] Dept. of Bacteriology, Institute of Infectious Diseases and Immunology, School of Veterinary Medicine, University of Utrecht, P.O.Box 80.165, 3508 TD Utrecht.
[2] Dept. of Bacteriology, Institute of Animal Science and Health (ID-DLO), P.O.Box 65, 8200 AB, Lelystad, the Netherlands.

The Effect of the Introduction of the Salmonella Plasmid Virulence (*spv*)genes of *Salmonella typhimurium* into other *Salmonella* serotypes

J.E. Olsen[1], D.J. Brown[1] and D.J. Platt[2]

The Salmonella Plasmid Virulence (*spv*) genes from *Salmonella typhimurium* have been introduced into 32 different serotypes of *Salmonella enterica* by means of a conjugative cointegrate plasmid, pOG669, derived from the serotype associated virulence plasmid (SAP) of *S. typhimurium* and a 54 kb IncX resistance plasmid (pOG670). The cointegrate was found to be incompatible with the serotype associated virulence plasmids (SAP) in *S. typhimurium*, *S. enteritidis*, *S. dublin*, *S. choleraesuis*, *S. gallinarum* biovar *gallinarum*. The SAP of *S. dublin* was also incompatible with pOG670.

Salmonella strains and their pOG669 and pOG670 containing derivatives were tested for mouse virulence following intraperitoneal (i.p.) inoculation in Balb/c mice. Replacement of the SAPs present in *S. typhimurium*, *S. enteritidis*, *S. dublin* or *S. choleraesuis* with pOG669 did not alter mouse virulence after intraperitoneal inoculation. Similarly, replacement of the SAP in a strain of *S. gallinarum* biovar *gallinarum* by pOG669 did not affect the virulence for chicks as ascertained by viable counts obtained at different times from organs after oral inoculation of day old chicks. No effect on mouse virulence was observed when pOG670 was introduced into any of the serotypes tested except that *S. dublin* became avirulent following displacement of the resident virulence plasmid by pOG670. The mouse virulence of 27 other *Salmonella* serotypes not associated with SAPs was not increased by the presence of pOG669.

These observations strongly suggest that whereas the *spv* locus is necessary for salmonella virulence in mice there appear to be host strain factors required for the expression of virulence.

[1] Department of Veterinary Microbiology, The Royal Veterinary and Agricultural University, Bülowsvej 13, DK 1870 Frederiksberg C., Denmark.
[2] University Department of Bacteriology, Royal Infirmary, Castle Street, Glasgow, G4 0SF, Scotland.

Molecular Determinants of Pathogenicity in *Leptospira*

Tom Olyhoek and Aart Lammers

The first step in bacterial infection is colonisation of host tissues, in some cases followed by invasion of host cells. Because culturing of *Leptospira* leads to loss of virulence, it might be that culturing leads to loss of expression of adhesion/invasion molecules. Our work shows, that long time cultured *Leptospira* do indeed adhere less to kidney cells. The possible role of leptospiral LPS in this process was studied by incubation of kidney cells with various extracts of leptospiral LPS. These experiments showed, that LPS does not function as an adhesion factor.

Another likely candidate virulence factor of *Leptospira* is haemolysin. Haemolysins have been shown to be important for pathogenesis in many bacteria. We have cloned and sequenced the gene for a leptospiral haemolysin. Our experiments showed, that the gene is present in many pathogenic strains of *Leptospira*. The gene bears no ressemblance to previously cloned haemolysins from *Leptospira*, nor to any of the DNA sequences published to date. Further characterisation of the gene product is needed to clarify a role in leptospiral pathogenesis.

Institute of Animal Science and Health (ID-DLO), Dept. of Bacteriology, Lelystad, the Netherlands

Identification and Characterization of Virulence Markers of *Streptococcus suis* type 2

Hilde Smith*, Uri Vecht, Henk Wisselink, Arno Gielkens and Mari Smits

Streptococcus suis infections are a common cause of meningitis, arthritis and polyserositis in young pigs and also cause meningitis in humans. Strains can differ in virulence. We have identified two proteins which are associated with pathogenic strains. Strains that express a 136-kDa muramidase-released protein (MRP) and a 110-kDa extracellular protein (EF) are pathogenic and cause specific signs of disease in piglets after intranasal inoculations. Strains that do not express MRP and EF and strains that express MRP and an enlarged form of EF (EF*) cause no or nonspecific signs of disease in piglets. The genes encoding MRP, EF and EF* have been cloned and characterized. Using those genes, we have constructed mutants of *S. suis* type 1 and 2 by inactivating the *mrp* and *epf* genes. For this purpose we developed an efficient DNA transfer system for *S. suis* by the use of electroporation. The pathogenicity of the mutant strains was tested in pigs. Mutant strains of serotype 2 were as virulent as the wild type. However, preliminary data indicate that a mutant MRP-EF-strain of serotype 1 is less virulent than the wild type strain of serotype 1.

Institute of Animal Science and Health (ID-DLO), Lelystad, the Netherlands

RTX Toxins of *Actinobacillus pleuropneumoniae*

Mari A. Smits, Elbarte M. Kamp and Ruud Jansen

Actinobacillus pleuropneumoniae, the causative agent of porcine pleuropneumonia, secretes three different toxins; ApxI, ApxII, and ApxIII. Each serotype reference strain secretes only one or two of these toxins. The toxins play a key role in the pathogenesis.

In the poster data are presented on the molecular structure of the Apx toxins, the organization of their genetic determinants, the dissemination of these determinants among field strains and other *Actinobacillus* species, and on the role of the Apx toxins in pathogenesis. We conclude that the Apx toxins are members of the pore forming RTX toxin family. They are encoded by (truncated) operons that consist of four genes: the posttranslational activator gene *apxC*; the toxin structural gene *apxA*; and the secretion genes *apxB* and *apxD*. The organization of the Apx operons in the various serotypes correlates well with their Apx secretion profiles. The presence of *apxI*, *apxII*, and *apxIII* genes is specific to a given serotype of *A. pleuropneumoniae*, but not specific for the species. Horizontal transfer of *apx* determinants seems to occur among different *Actinobacillus* species. The Apx toxins are the major virulence factors that prevent clearance of the pathogen from the lung by the inactivation of phagocytic cells.

Institute for Animal Science and Health (ID-DLO). P.O. Box 65, 8200 AB Lelystad, the Netherlands

Host Specificity in Pathogenic Leptospires

W.J. Terpstra, H. Korver and R.A. Hartskeerl

On the basis of antigenic similarities pathogenic leptospires are divided in 24 serogroups.

Leptospires from the serogroup Grippotyphosa occur worldwide in various reservoir host species. They belong to *Leptospira interrogans*, *L. santarosai* and *L. kirschneri*. On the basis of antigenic profiles as revealed by monoclonal antibodies a pattern can be observed that is characteristic for isolates from western Europe and another pattern that is characteristic for eastern European isolates. The European isolates belonged to *L. kirschneri*, at least those isolates in which the species was determined on the basis of DNA amplification with specific primers. An isolate from China displaying the eastern European antigenic profile was non-*L. kirschneri*.

Royal Tropical Institute, Amsterdam, the Netherlands

Putative Sphingomyelinase Genes among Pathogenic *Leptospira* Species

Ruud P.A.M. Segers[1], Jaap Wagenaar[2], Ivan Polgrossi[1], Bernard A.M. van der Zeijst[2] and Wim Gaastra[2]

Hemolytic activity of Leptospira is caused by sphingomyelinase, which is present in pathogenic leptospira only. A sphingomyelinase gene (designated *sphA*) was cloned from a bovine Dutch *Leptospira borgpetersenii* field isolate (1, 2) and shown to confer hemolytic and sphingomyelinase activities on *E. coli*. The *sphA* gene was shown to be homologous to Gram-positive sphingomyelinase genes. Low-stringency hybridization with the *sphA* gene revealed that multiple similar genetic elements are present in pathogenic *Leptospira* species (3, 4). Several of these hybridizing elements were cloned and were shown to contain ORF's, homologous to *sphA*. Judging from the cloning and hybridization experiments there are at least 8 different genes present among pathogenic *Leptospira* species. So far, the *sphA* and *sphB* genes from *L. borgpetersenii*, and the *sphD*, *sphE*, *sphG* and *sphX* genes from *L. interrogans* have been sequenced. Translated amino acid sequence identity among these sphingomyelinases varies between 46 and 68%. Hybridization experiments identify two clusters of pathogenic species: one cluster of *L. borgpetersenii*, *L. santarosai* and *L. weilii* hybridizing with *sphA* and *sphB*, the other cluster of *L. interrogans*, *L. noguchii* and *L. kirschneri* hybridizing with *sphD*, *sphE*, *sphF* and *sphG*.

The presence of 4 to 5 different *sph*-genes in the same pathogenic strain warrants further investigation. Are *sph*'s real genes? We are inclined to believe so, since at least *sphA* is actively expressed in *E. coli* and at least *sphB* and *sphG* seem to have transcription and translation control elements. Both strains with and without sphingomyelinase activity have very simular *sph*-gene patterns. Possibly, some genes are only expressed in vivo.

Do *sph*'s have different activities/functions? There are several functions, sphingomyelinase might have. The first and most obvious one, is the hemolysis of red blood cells for the subsequent acquisition of iron from hemoglobin. This however, would only be advantageous during infections in ruminants which have red blood cells with a high sphingomyelin content in the membrane. Human or canine red blood cells do not lyse upon incubation with sphingomyelinase. A second function could be de acquisition of long chain fatty acids (the sole source of carbon and energy for leptospira) by the degradation of sphingomyelin. A third possible function might be the modulation of the host cellular response. Minute degradation of sphingomyelin can have profound effects on a cell, since ceramide (a degradation product of sphingomyelin) acts as a second messenger and modulates cholesterol transport, inhibits cellular growth and induces cellular differentiation (5). This could be an explanation for the absence of hemolytic activity in some strains.

References

1. Del Real et al., 1989 - Infect. Immun. **57**, 2588–2590.
2. Segers et al., 1990 - Infect. Immun. **58**, 2177–2185.
3. Segers, 1991 - PhD Thesis, University of Utrecht, the Netherlands.
4. Segers et al., 1992 - Infect. Immun. **60**, 1707–1710.
5. Merril, 1992 - Nutrition Reviews **50**, 78–80.

[1] Dept. of Bacteriological Research. Intervet International B.V. P.O. Box 31, 5830 AA Boxmeer. The Netherlands.
[2] Dept. of Bacteriology, Inst. of Infectuous Diseases and Immunology, Faculty of Veterinary Medicine, University of Utrecht, 3508 TD Utrecht, the Netherlands.

Discrimination of Epidemic and Sporadic Methicillin-resistant *Staphylococcus aureus* Strains Based on Protein A Gene Polymorphism

H.M.E. Frenay, J.P.G. Theelen, L.M. Schouls, C.M.J.E. Vandenbroucke-Grauls, J. Verhoef, W.J. van Leeuwen and F.R. Mooi

The aim of the present study was to identify a genetic marker to discriminate epidemic from sporadic Methicillin-Resistant *Staphylococcus Aureus* (MRSA). We focussed on the X region of the protein A gene of *S. aureus* (*spa*) because it contains a highly polymorphic sequence, composed of repeats of 24 bp. The X region was amplified by PCR and cleaved with *Rsa*I in three fragments. One fragment contained the repetitive DNA, and from its size the number of repeats could be estimated. Twenty-four out of 33 epidemic MRSA strains contained more than seven repeats, 10 out of 24 sporadic strains contained seven or fewer repeats. This correlation was significant. Possibly, a longer X region results in better exposition of the Fc-binding region of protein A, which facilitates colonization of the host and dissemination of the epidemic phenotype.

Molecular Microbiology Unit and Laboratory of Bacteriology, Rijksinstituut voor Volksgezondheid en Milieuhygiene, Bilthoven, and Eykman-Winkler Institute of Medical Microbiology, Utrecht University, Utrecht, The Netherlands.

Genetic and Structural Studies on the Mu Gin Protein

E.H.A. Spaeny-Dekking, N. Goosen and P. van de Putte

Site-specific recombination involves the formation of ordered nucleoprotein complexes. For the recombination process that leads to the inversion of the G-region in Mu, a synaptic complex is formed between two Gin dimers bound to the inverted repeats that flank the G-region, and Fis molecules bound to the enhancer. Until now it is not clear what kind of interactions between the different molecules of Gin take place during the subsequent steps of the recombination reaction, and whether Fis is only needed for the formation of the complex or whether it has some additional role in the strand exchange.

To get more information about the protein interactions between the different molecules of Gin we did *in vitro* cross-link experiments on the purified protein in solution. We found that in the Gin molecule the N-terminal region of 61 amino acids is in close contact with a second Gin molecule upon dimer formation. Surprisingly we found that under oxidizing conditions, a dimer of Gin molecules is also formed without the presence of a chemical crosslinker. We can show that this dimerisation under oxidizing conditions is caused by disulfide bond formation between one or two of the cysteines which are present in the wildtype protein at the positions 24 and 27.

We have also tried to isolate mutants in Gin which are disturbed in the putative interaction with Fis. For this we have isolated 25 independent Gin mutants that still normally bind to the recombination site but are affected in one or more of the subsequent steps in the reaction. In these mutants we introduced a mutation which in the wildtype Gin protein causes a Fis-independent phenotype (A. Klippel et al., EMBO J. 7 (1988) 3983-3989). This was done because we expected that mutants that were only disturbed in the interaction with Fis will function again when they are Fis-independent. Among the Gin mutants we have isolated, we found several mutants with the expected phenotype. The location of these mutations in the protein structure and their properties will be discussed.

Department of Molecular Genetics, Leiden Institute of Chemistry, Leiden University, 2300 RA Leiden, the Netherlands.